Androgens and Reproductive Aging

Togas Tulandi MD MHCM FRCSC FACOG
Professor of Obstetrics and Gynecology
Milton Leong Chair in Reproductive Medicine
McGill University Department of Obstetrics and Gynecology
Montreal
Quebec
Canada

Morrie M Gelfand CM MD FRCSC FACS FACOG
Professor of Obstetrics and Gynecology
McGill University Department of Obstetrics and Gynecology
Montreal
Quebec
Canada

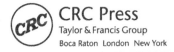

CRC Press
Taylor & Francis Group
Boca Raton London New York

CRC Press is an imprint of the
Taylor & Francis Group, an **informa** business

CRC Press
Taylor & Francis Group
6000 Broken Sound Parkway NW, Suite 300
Boca Raton, FL 33487-2742

Visit the Taylor & Francis Web site at
http://www.taylorandfrancis.com

and the CRC Press Web site at
http://www.crcpress.com

Contents

Contributors

Gloria A Bachmann, MD
Director
Women's Health Institute
The Robert Wood Johnson Medical School
University of Medicine and Dentistry
  of New Jersey
New Brunswick, NJ
USA

Hermann M Behre, MD
Professor
Andrology Unit, Department of Urology
University of Halle
Halle
Germany

Alain Bélanger, PhD
Molecular Endocrinology and Oncology
  Research Center
Le Centre Hospitalier de l'Université Laval
Québec City, Québec
Canada

Jennifer R Berman, MD
Director
Female Urology and Female Sexual Medicine
Rodeo Drive Women's Health Center
Beverly Hills, CA
USA

William M Buckett, MD, MRCOG
Assistant Professor
McGill Reproductive Center
McGill University Department of Obstetrics
  and Gynecology
Montreal, Québec
Canada

Orhan Bukulmez, MD
Fellow and Assistant Instructor
Division of Reproductive Endocrinology
Department of Obstetrics and Gynecology
University of Texas Southwestern
  Medical Center at Dallas
Dallas, TX
USA

Natalie Z Burger, MD
Fellow Reproductive Endocrinology
  and Infertility
Department of Obstetrics and Gynecology
University of Vermont College
  of Medicine
Burlington, VT
USA

Bruce R Carr, MD
Professor and Director
Division of Reproductive Endocrinology
Department of Obstetrics and Gynecology
University of Texas Southwestern
  Medical Center at Dallas
Dallas, TX
USA

Maurita H Carrejo, MS
AMRED Consulting LLC
Houston, TX
USA

Claus Christiansen, MD, DMSc
Center for Clinical and Basic Research
Ballerup
Denmark

Karine Chung, MD, MSCE
*Assistant Professor of Reproductive
    Endocrinology and Infertility*
*University of Southern California Keck School
    of Medicine*
Los Angeles, CA
USA

John W Culberson, MD
AMRED Consulting LLC
Houston, TX
USA

Susan R Davis, FRACP
Director
Women's Health Program
Monash University Department of Medicine
Melbourne, Victoria
Australia

Morrie M Gelfand, MD
Professor of Obstetrics and Gynecology
McGill University
Montreal, Québec
Canada

Crista E Johnson, MD
Clinical Lecturer
*Robert Wood Johnson Clinical Scholars Program
    Research Fellow*
University of Michigan Medical School
Ann Arbor, MI
USA

Julia V Johnson, MD
Professor and Vice Chair
Department of Obstetrics and Gynecology
University of Vermont College of Medicine
Burlington, VT
USA

Margaret Kilibwa, PhD
Clinical Assistant Professor
Women's Health Institute
The Robert Wood Johnson Medical School
University of Medicine and Dentistry of New Jersey
New Brunswick, NJ
USA

Claude Labrie, MD, PhD
*Molecular Endocrinology and Oncology
    Research Center*
Le Centre Hospitalier de l'Université Laval
Québec City, Québec
Canada

Fernand Labrie, MD, PhD
*Molecular Endocrinology and Oncology
    Research Center*
Le Centre Hospitalier de l'Université Laval
Québec City, Québec
Canada

Van Luu-The, PhD
*Molecular Endocrinology and Oncology
    Research Center*
Le Centre Hospitalier de l'Université Laval
Québec City, Québec
Canada

Luigi Mastroianni Jr, MD
*William Goodall Professor of Obstetrics and
    Gynecology*
*University of Pennsylvania School of
    Medicine*
Philadelphia, PA
USA

Richard Poulin, PhD
*Molecular Endocrinology and Oncology
    Research Center*
Le Centre Hospitalier de l'Université Laval
Québec City, Québec
Canada

Livia Rivera-Woll, MBBS
Endocrine Research Fellow
Women's Health Program
*Monash University Department of
    Medicine*
Melbourne, Victoria
Australia

Joseph S Sanfilippo, MD, MBA
*Professor of Obstetrics, Gynecology and
    Reproductive Sciences*
Division of Reproductive Endocrinology
*University of Pittsburgh School of
    Medicine*
Pittsburgh, PA
USA

Hermann PG Schneider, MD, PhD
Professor
Department of Obstetrics and Gynecology
University of Muenster
Muenster
Germany

Barbara B Sherwin, PhD
James McGill Professor
Department of Psychology and Department
  of Obstetrics and Gynecology
McGill University
Montreal, Québec
Canada

Jacques Simard, PhD
Molecular Endocrinology and Oncology
  Research Center
Le Centre Hospitalier de l'Université Laval
Québec City, Québec
Canada

Camille Sylvestre, MD, FRCSC
Assistant Professor
McGill Reproductive Center
McGill University Department of Obstetrics
  and Gynecology
Montreal, Québec
Canada

Robert S Tan, MD
AMRED Consulting LLC
Houston, TX
USA

László B Tankó, MD, PhD
Center for Clinical and Basic Research
Ballerup
Denmark

Ryan Zlupko, MD
Clinical Instructor
Division of Reproductive Endocrinology
Magee Womens Hospital
Pittsburgh, PA
USA

Foreword

The role of androgens in men and women is receiving increasing attention, not only among scientists and clinicians, but also by our patients. Controversial issues are inevitable when and where clear-cut evidence is either lacking or insufficient. Thus, many questions arise. For example, can the measurement of endogenous testosterone levels delineate a population of women with sexual dysfunction that would respond to testosterone treatment? Can testosterone treatment produce a desired response without achieving pharmacologic levels? What are the long-term consequences of testosterone treatment? Are there other androgens or agents that would provide treatment more easily and are potentially safer than testosterone? Questions like these can only be answered with a full understanding of the normal role of androgens in normal development and function and by assessing the quality of the available evidence.

The contents of *Androgens and Reproductive Aging* are comprehensive. Respected experts describe normal physiology and consider the consequences of androgen deficiency. Androgen treatment of both men and women receives the evidence-based consideration that is required. The controversial issues of long-term consequences, acute risks, and the effect on the risk of breast cancer are given appropriate attention. This is a major effort coming at a crucial time.

The publication of a book of this nature is worthwhile only if it fulfills a need. I am impressed by how often clinicians and patients are asking questions about the role of androgens in women, and therein lies the justification for this book. *Androgens and Reproductive Aging* provides clinicians and scientists with the current state-of-the-art information available. This required foundation of knowledge allows the clinician to address patient questions regarding testosterone deficiency and treatment and to provide appropriate counseling. Future research must evolve from a consideration of this knowledge by the scientist, leading to the formulation of study questions. For these reasons, the editors of *Androgens and Reproductive Aging* can feel confident that they have produced a meaningful and useful book for clinicians and scientists.

Leon Speroff, MD
Professor of Obstetrics and Gynecology
Oregon Health and Science University
USA

Preface

The role of androgens in reproductive aging remains controversial. The advantages and disadvantages of androgen treatment in menopausal women – and to a lesser extent, in aging men – are being asked not only by clinicians and scientists but also by patients. The most frequently asked questions include the possible masculinization effects of androgens, how to minimize this side effect, what preparation of androgens should be used, and whether concomitant estrogen should be given. Many studies have evaluated the benefits of androgens on psychosexual function; however studies on the effects of androgens on bone mass and breast tissue have just begun. It appears that there is a role of androgens in some menopausal women, although methods of administration and suitable doses still need to be perfected. In males, however, the role of androgens has not been fully investigated. *Androgens and Reproductive Aging* reflects the latest advances in the field. It addresses the pathophysiology of androgen deficiency, new concepts and novel treatment modalities, effects of androgens on osteoporosis and breast cancer, and effects of androgen deficiency in males.

The contributors are physicians and researchers who are acknowledged leaders in this field with many years of experience. Chapters 1–3 discuss physiology of androgens in women, and pathophysiology and endocrinology of androgen deficiency. Chapters 4–6 are dedicated to psychosexual aspects of menopause, including studies of androgen receptors and the effects of estrogen and androgen on sexual function. Clinical use including the new transdermal administration of androgens and antiandrogens, the role of androgens in premenopausal women, and the practical aspects of androgen treatment are discussed in Chapters 7–11. The last three chapters deal with the possible effects of androgen on breast cancer, the side effects, and androgen deficiency in aging males.

As this is a multiauthored book, different authors might discuss a same subject, each with their own opinions or approaches. Different opinions stimulate research and we intentionally leave them to the readers' critical judgment.

This is a book for clinical and basic researchers as well as for practicing physicians, students, residents, and fellows. Readers will gain an understanding of the role of androgens in women and men, and androgen treatment including the route of administration, dose, and other practical aspects of treatment. They will also learn about new developments in androgen treatment. We hope that this book will be helpful in directing new investigations and in managing patients.

Togas Tulandi, MD, MHCM, FRCSC, FACOG
Morrie M Gelfand, CM, MD, FRCSC, FACS, FACOG

Chapter 1
Androgen production in women

Natalie Z Burger and Julia V Johnson

Summary

The production and effects of testosterone in men have been widely studied, and a testosterone deficiency state has been clearly identified. However, investigation of the physiologic and pathologic roles of testosterone in women has been limited.

Androgen dynamics in women

In women the circulating androgens have simply been considered as byproducts of adrenal cortical or ovarian estrogen production, with little independent clinical relevance. As a result androgen dynamics in women, both in the reproductive and postreproductive years, are poorly understood. If one considers the contribution of the adrenal cortex and ovary, androgens levels would exceed those of other steroid hormones (Table 1.1). Testosterone level is usually higher than serum estradiol (E_2) level. This suggests the possibility that androgens serve a fundamental and independent physiologic purpose in women, and a deficiency of these hormones may result in adverse consequences.

Source of androgens in women

The three sources of androgens in women are: the adrenal cortex, the ovarian theca cells (and to a lesser degree, ovarian stromal cells), and peripheral bioconversion of circulating androgenic prohormones. The adrenal gland produces about 95% of circulating serum dehydroepiandrosterone sulfate (DHEAS, production rate 19 mg/day in young women) and 50% of

Table 1.1 Androgens in women: levels, potencies, and bioconversion

Androgen	Serum level	Potency (relative to testosterone)
DHEAS	200 µg/dL	0.001
DHEA	500 ng/dL	0.01
Δ⁴A	100 ng/dL	0.1
Testosterone	50 ng/dL	1.0
DHT	5 ng/dL	5

DHEAS, dihydroepiandrosterone sulfate; DHT, dihydrotestosterone.

dehydroepiandrosterone (DHEA, production rate 16 mg/day). Thirty percent of the circulating DHEA is produced by peripheral conversion of DHEAS, and the remaining 20% is produced by the ovary.[1] DHEAS circulates unbound to protein and with a half-life of 10 hours. It has limited androgenic action and primarily acts as a circulating prohormone for production of DHEA and the more potent downstream androgens both in the circulation and in the peripheral tissues. There is also ongoing turnover of DHEA and about 31% is sulfated to DHEAS.[2,3] The production of both DHEAS and DHEA is stimulated by adrenocorticotropin (ACTH) through its effect on the zona reticularis see Figure 1.1. Negative feedback is controlled by circulating cortisol.

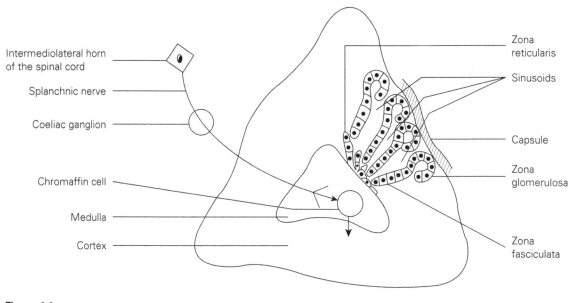

Figure 1.1

The adrenal gland showing zonation of adrenal cortex and the relationship between adrenal cortex and medulla.

Androstenedione (Δ^4A) is produced in about equal portions by the adrenocortical cells and by the theca cells of the ovary. In addition, about 40% of Δ^4A is produced by peripheral bioconversion of DHEA.[1] The ovary produces both Δ^4A and testosterone under the stimulation of luteinizing hormone (LH). The circulating level of Δ^4A is subject to significant short-term variation secondary to the diurnal nature of its adrenal contribution and the variation in ovarian contribution over the menstrual cycle.

Testosterone, the most clinically relevant circulating androgen, has both an adrenal contribution (25%) and an ovarian contribution (25%). The remaining 50% comes from peripheral bioconversion of circulating Δ^4A.[1] By virtue of its relatively large ovarian contribution, serum testosterone is probably the best measure of ovarian androgen production. Dihydrotestosterone (DHT) is produced almost exclusively in target tissues by 5α-reductase action on circulating testosterone. The circulating levels are negligible and believed to be a result of spillover from the primarily local action of this hormone.

Androgen levels in women are subject to three temporal phenomena: ovarian cyclicity, decline of the adrenal androgens with age, and ovarian

follicular depletion at climacterium. Throughout the course of the normal ovulatory cycle changing patterns of LH secretion, including a mid-cycle LH surge, result in varying ovarian follicular thecal cell stimulation of testosterone and Δ^4A production. In turn, the thecal Δ^4A acts as a substrate for granulosa cell estrogen production. These changes result in a mid-cycle peak in circulating Δ^4A and testosterone production.

With age, the adrenal androgen levels decrease in both men and women. The circulating DHEA and DHEAS levels undergo a steady decline after 25 years of age and have been used as a hormonal marker for normal aging. There is a reduction in the size of zona reticularis as men and women age, and this decrease in adrenal androgens has been termed as andropause.

Apart from the normal adrenal changes with aging, women undergo a loss of ovarian hormone production during the climacterium. A modest decrease in testosterone and androstenedione levels following menopause, but the decrease is less pronounced than that of estradiol. Additionally, the decrease in sex hormone binding globulin increases the level of free testosterone.[4] The decrease in circulating androgen levels following menopause does not offer a clear explanation

Table 1.2 Distribution of androgen receptors

Reproductive tissue	Expression level	Nonreproductive tissue	Expression level
Prostate	1.0	Endometrial carcinoma	0.8
Testis	0.9	Prostate carcinoma	0.5
Seminal vesicles	0.7	Kidney	0.4
Ejaculatory duct	0.4	Thyroid carcinoma	0.4
Endometrium	1.8	Breast	0.3
Ovary	1.5	Colon	0.1
Uterus	1.4	Lung	0.07
Fallopian tube	1.0	Adrenal	0.03
Myometrium	0.6		

for the physical and behavioral changes associated with this transition.

Physiologic effects of androgens in women

The primary function of androgens during fetal development and during the reproductive years, is on the reproductive tract. In the fetus, androgens have multiple reproductive effects including directing the development of sexual dimorphism and mainteinance of secondary sexual characteristics. During pubarche, adrenal androgens stimulate pubic and axillary hair growth and contribute to linear growth. Following the onset of menarche, androgens produced during the follicular phase, stimulated by LH, act as the prohormone for estradiol production by the granulosa cells.

Androgens are not simply reproductive hormones. Both in women as well as in men, they act on multiple organ systems including the skin and its appendages. They also enhance bone, potentiate certain cognitive behaviors, and enhance erythropoiesis. They modify hepatic protein secretion, stimulate kidney and muscle hypertrophy and modify patterns of adipose tissue deposition. They may have certain immune-enhancing effects. Evidence of the potential multisystem role of androgens is demonstrated by a wide distribution of androgen receptor expression in human tissues.[5] As shown in Table 1.2, there is significant androgen receptor expression in male and female nonreproductive tissues, including kidney, thyroid, breast, colon, lung, and adrenal glands. There is also androgen receptor expression in female reproductive tissues including endometrium, ovary, uterus, fallopian tube, and myometrium.

It has been speculated that androgens are physiologically important hormones in women, and there may be parallels between female and male androgen deficiency. Testosterone deficiency in men, from either surgical or natural hypogonadism, is a well defined state. These men are obese, insulin resistant, at risk for heart disease, have decreased muscle mass and strength, at risk for osteoporosis, and have diminished sexual function. Data on the role of androgen in women are still limited. The vast majority of testosterone deficiency in females is secondary to iatrogenic causes such are ovarian suppression or prophylactic oophorectomy.[6]

Androgen changes with age

With follicular depletion and the onset of menopausal transition, ovarian E_2 production declines precipitously, leading to loss of negative feedback at the pituitary and the hypothalamus. In response, circulating serum LH and follicle stimulating hormone levels increase dramatically, and the circulating LH drives the ovarian theca/stroma to produce increasing amounts of testosterone.[7] The increased LH production following menopause allows the ovary to continue production of androgens. This effect appears to continue well into the postmenopausal years, with limited attenuation.[8]

The adrenocortical androgen production diminishes with age. With a diminution of cells in the zona reticularis, there is a decline in circulating steroids as well as their responses to ACTH stimulation. Andropause is the term used for this senescent, cortisol-independent decline of adrenocortical secretion of androgens. It occurs in a linear fashion from about the age of 20 or 25 onward to the point where a woman in her eighties would have about 10% of the circulating DHEAS in a woman of early reproductive age.[9] Because the adrenal androgens circulate in such high quantities and provide a substantial proportion of circulating Δ^4A and testosterone by peripheral conversion, andropause represents a significant loss of substrate for circulating testosterone and thus creates an age-related gradual decline in testosterone levels, independent of menopause.

The cumulative effect of andropause and the continued production of ovarian testosterone lead to variability in serum testosterone levels in aging women. Several large cross-sectional studies have demonstrated that circulating testosterone levels do not reproducibly change in relation to the menopausal transition. This is best illustrated by the Melbourne Women's Midlife Health Project.[4] Because of diminution of E_2 and a subsequent decline in hepatic production of sex hormone binding globulin, the free androgen index, a marker of free testosterone, increases over the menopausal transition. Subsequent testosterone effects may increase over the menopausal transition, an explanation for the widely observed clinical phenomenon of menopausal hirsutism. However, there appears to be a small but significant decline in serum testosterone levels in older women of reproductive age presumed to be due to decreased availability of adrenal androgen precursors.

Conclusion

The role of androgens in women remains unclear. However, recent studies have demonstrated their importance in fetal development, reproductive health, and in the menopausal years. By determining the role of androgen in normal female physiology, researchers can develop diagnostic parameters for androgen deficiency in women. This will allow clinicians to understand the symptoms associated with this disorder and develop effective treatment options for women.

References

1. Burger HG. Androgen production in women. Fertil Steril 2002; 77(Suppl 4):S3–S5.
2. Haning RV Jr, Chabot M, Flood CA et al. Metabolic clearance rate (MCR) of DHEAS, its metabolism to DHEA, androstenedione, T, and DHT, and the effect of increased plasma DS on DS MCR in normal women. J Clin Endocrinol Metab 1989; 69:1047.
3. Bird CE, Murphy J, Boroomand K et al. Dehydroepiandrosterone: kinetics of metabolism in normal men and women. J Clin Endocrinol Metab 1978; 47:818.
4. Burger HG. A prospective longitudinal study of serum testosterone, dehydroepiandrosterone sulfate, and sex hormone-binding globulin levels through the menopause transition. J Clin Endocrinol Metab 2000; 85:2832–2838.
5. Wilson CM, McPhaul MS. A and B forms of the androgen receptor are expressed in a variety of human tissues. Mol Cell Endocrinol 1996; 120:51–7.
6. Davis SR. When to expect androgen deficiency other than at menopause. Fertil Steril 2001; 77:S68–S71.
7. Adashi EY. The climacteric ovary as a functional gonadotropin-driven androgen-producing gland. Fertil Steril 1994; 62:20–27.
8. Meldrum DR, Davidson BJ, Tataryn IV, Judd HL. Changes in circulating steroids in postmenopausal women. Obstet Gynecol 1981; 57:624–628.
9. Orentreich N, Brind JL, Rizer RL, Vogelman JH. Age changes and sex differences in serum dihydroepiandrosterone sulfate concentration throughout adulthood. J clin Endocrinol Metab 1984; 59:551–5

Chapter 2
Pathophysiology of androgen deficiency

Gloria Bachmann and Margaret Kilibwa

Summary

Women with hypopituitarism, adrenal insufficiency following adrenalectomy or oophorectomy, and men with either primary or secondary hypogonadism may become deficient in androgens. Also, premenopausal and naturally menopausal women may have symptoms of androgen decline due to age-related effects on the adrenals and the ovaries. In men, it is generally accepted that the principal cause of age-related decrease in testosterone production is testicular atrophy although diminished gonadotropin production may play a role.

Introduction

The importance of androgens in female health is often apparent when a woman's androgen concentrations are in excess. Androgen hypersecretion, either from an ovarian or from an adrenal source causes androgen excess disorders such as polycystic ovary syndrome and congenital adrenal hyperplasia, universally recognized clinical entities that often require intervention. Androgen deficiency (used interchangeably with insufficiency) in women is also recognized by many researchers and clinicians as an endocrinopathy with significant pathophysiologic consequences similar to those observed in men. Typical signs and symptoms of diminished androgen levels in men are given in Table 2.1. Inadequate androgen levels equally affect women's health and the signs and symptoms of androgen deficiency can be just as dramatic (Table 2.2).

It is not generally recognized that androgens are prohormones to estrogen synthesis across the adult female life cycle. The major androgens found in women in descending order of their serum concentration include dehydroepiandrosterone sulfate (DHEAS), dehydroepiandrosterone (DHEA), androstenedione, testosterone,

Table 2.1 Symptoms of androgen deficiency in men

- Decreased sexual desire (libido) and erectile quality
- Changes in mood (depression, fatigue)
- Decreased lean body mass, and muscle strength
- Increased visceral fat
- Alterations in skin and body hair
- Decreased bone mineral density

Source: Morales & Tenover.[1]

and dihydrotestosterone (DHT). Relative to testosterone potency (which has a relative androgenic potency of 1), DHEA has a potency of 0.01 and DHEAS has a potency of 0.001. In the unbound state, testosterone may act directly on specific cell receptors or be aromatized to estrogen to exert its effect. With advancing age and increasing weight, aromatization of androgens to estrogens increases; androstenedione aromatizes to estrone and testosterone to estradiol. In premenopausal women, a large portion of circulating testosterone is produced by the ovaries, with the remainder coming from peripheral conversion of DHEA and androstenedione from the adrenals and ovaries. Most production of DHEAS occurs in the adrenal glands. Although DHEA and androstenedione levels decrease dramatically with age,

Table 2.2 Symptoms of androgen deficiency in women

- Reduced
  - Sex motivation
  - Sex fantasy
  - Sex arousal
  - Bone and muscle mass
- Changes in quality of life
  - Changes in mood (depression, fatigue)
- More frequent
  - Vasomotor symptoms
  - Insomnia
  - Headache

Source: Bachmann.[2]

circulating testosterone decrease less dramatically. Most of the circulating testosterone is bound tightly to sex hormone binding globulin (SHBG) and loosely to albumin.

Circulating androgen levels also decline with advancing age in men, so that 20% of men over age 60 and 40% of men over age 80 have serum testosterone levels that are markedly decreased compared with levels in young adult men. In men the physiologic decline in circulating androgen levels is compounded by testicular disorders, acute stressful illnesses, such as surgery, and wasting diseases such as cancer and acquired immunodeficiency syndrome. The decrease of androgen levels in the female can be attributed to the gradual reduction in adrenal androgen production with age and to the loss of cyclical ovarian androgen production in the late reproductive years. Reduced ovarian function, either natural or due to induced menopause (from excision of the ovaries or other destructive processes to the ovaries, such as chemotherapy or radiation therapy to the pelvis), further contributes to this overall androgen decline. In addition to this, adrenal function reduces not only due to age but also due to extrinsic glucocorticoid administration and other adrenal pathologies associated with androgen decline in women. Further, women with pituitary disease characterized by hypogonadism and/or hypoadrenalism have a significant reduction in androgen production.

When androgen insufficiency is suspected from clinical signs and symptoms, measurements of serum androgen levels may not always confirm the diagnosis as clearly as an elevated fasting glucose level is diagnostic of diabetes mellitus.

A significant obstacle to an accurate evaluation is the difficulty of measuring low levels of androgen. Unlike other hormonal measurements, the measurement of testosterone is limited by the lack of routinely available sensitive assays for low circulating levels of both total and free testosterone. Most testosterone assays show poor reliability at the lower end of the circulating serum female concentration range. Added to this, is the controversy regarding the normal androgen values for women. The lack of a large normative database of androgen levels for women makes it difficult to definitely state the absolute level at which female androgen deficiency or, as more commonly referred to, insufficiency exists. Furthermore, there is a lack of evidence from clinical trials on testosterone levels in menstruating women; geriatric women, and women with chronic illnesses making it difficult to define androgen deficiency in different cohorts of women in precise quantitative terms. This is further confounded by psychosocial and relationship issues as well as the changing hormonal status in women during times of rapid hormonal change such as during the perimenopausal transition and later with aging changes superimposed on endocrinologic changes. Testosterone insufficiency also shares symptoms with various medical and psychologic conditions such as depression and chronic illness. As a result, health problems resulting from androgen insufficiency such as low sexual desire may be attributed to psychosocial and interpersonal relationship issues rather than to diminished testosterone levels.

Androgen therapy may benefit men and women presenting with androgen deficiency not only from the point of view of quality of life but also from correction of a specific pathophysiologic deviation from the endocrinologic norm. Currently, many women can expect to live about 30 years after midlife and emerging data from clinical trials increasingly support androgen therapy for symptomatic, older women. Thus, addressing the laboratory inadequacies of measuring low levels of androgens, the lack of clear guidelines regarding normal testosterone levels for women, the consensus on optimum therapeutic doses, and the type and delivery system of androgens remain research priorities.

Even in lighty of the growing pool of data on androgen loss with aging and with menopause, there continue to be researchers who request more data to confirm the diagnosis of androgen insufficiency in women. Since the most common symptom of androgen insufficiency is decreased libido – which is a common and nonspecific complaint associated with stress, marital discord, and depression – reasons other than hormonal ones are often inferred. Similarly, sexual dysfunction and lack of wellbeing in women, both highly complex with multifactorial causes, may erroneously be wholly ascribed to androgen insufficiency.

Therapy with androgens, especially testosterone, has played a role in women's health since the 1930s and data on its efficacy and safety are available since that time. Early investigators observed that testosterone treatment in women with signs of androgen insufficiency positively affects sexual desire, energy level, bone mass, muscle mass and strength, and a sense of wellbeing. In the 1940s a prospective study by Geist and Salomon demonstrated that 422 postmenopausal women treated with testosterone and estrogen for the relief of menopausal symptoms had greater relief of symptoms than estrogen alone could provide.[3] In another prospective, double blind, placebo controlled study performed in the 1950s, 31 subjects (65%) who were treated with methyltestosterone reported increased libido as compared with women (12%) who received estrogen alone.[4] In 1959, Waxenberg and coworkers reported an association between decreased sexual desire and decreased testosterone levels in women.[5] Other investigators have since noted a similar effect on wellbeing with androgen therapy usually in an environment with adequate circulating estrogen.[6] The literature continues to expand in this century as several well controlled clinical trials have evaluated the therapeutic effects and tolerance of testosterone therapy in women with low levels of androgens and the effect of a diminution or elimination of symptoms with this pharmacologic intervention.[7–9] For the improvement of sexual function and general wellbeing in women, especially women who have undergone surgical menopause, a combination of estrogen for the vasomotor and urogenital symptoms and androgen for the sexual and quality of life symptoms appears to be effective.

Production of androgens

In the female, androgen production occurs in both adrenals and ovaries. The adrenocorticotropic hormone (ACTH) stimulates adrenal secretion of androgens, and ovarian secretion is stimulated by the luteinizing hormone (LH). Unlike in the male, a physiologic negative feedback system that regulates androgen production has not been demonstrated in the female. Approximately 25–35% of circulating testosterone is produced by the ovaries and 50–75% from circulating precursors.[10] Testosterone levels fluctuate during the menstrual cycle, being lowest in the early follicular phase, peaking at midcycle, and then dropping off again in the luteal phase.

In the male, a large proportion of circulating testosterone is produced in the testes at a rate of about 0.24 μmol/day, in contrast with the adrenal cortex which produces 0.002 μmol/day of androgens, mostly as androstenedione. The production of testosterone by the male testes is stimulated by LH which is secreted in a pulsatile manner in response to the stimulation by gonadotropin hormone releasing hormone from the hypothalamus.[11] LH is then inhibited through a negative feedback loop by increased concentrations of serum testosterone and its metabolites. There also is a fluctuation in testosterone levels in males. For example, in young men the highest serum testosterone levels are measured in the morning as compared with the evening. This circadian rhythm either declines or is lost in older men.[12]

In addition to the female gonads, the adrenal gland produces androgens (testosterone, DHEAS, DHEA, and androstenedione) that contribute significantly to circulating levels in women. DHEAS is mainly produced by the adrenal glands in premenopausal women, with approximately 90% of circulating DHEAS coming from adrenal sources. The remaining 10% is formed from the conversion of DHEA in peripheral tissues.[13] DHEA is produced by both organs, but the adrenal gland produces more (50%) than the ovaries (20%). Approximately 30% of the circulating DHEA comes from peripheral conversion of DHEAS.

Androstenedione levels are similar in young women and men.[14] In ovulating women, the serum androstenedione levels rise in the follicular phase and peak in the late luteal phase, with an approximate 15% increase.[15] This increase has been attributed to an increase in ovarian secretion of the hormone rather than from adrenal sources. Androstenedione accounts for about 50% of the testosterone produced in the peripheral tissues of premenopausal women. But at menopause, although androstenedione continues to be aromatized to estradiol, its serum level begin to decrease in most women regardless of the type of menopause, and therefore estradiol levels decrease as well.[16]

Measurement of androgen levels

The measurement of androgen levels may be useful for the investigation of androgen insufficiency in women. In healthy women, about 50–66% of testosterone is bound to SHBG, 30–40% to albumin, and only 0.5–2% is unbound.[17] The SHBG-bound portion is not considered bioavailable. In men, compared with women, at least 2% of the serum testosterone is free and available to target tissues for androgen action. The rest of the testosterone is bound to SHBG and albumin. Therefore, the amount of testosterone in women that is bound to protein is higher than the proportion that is bound in men. In contrast, androstenedione, DHEAS, and DHEA are not strongly bound to SHBG. Almost 95% of circulating androstenedione is available for androgen action.[17] Characterization of androgen levels is more comprehensive in male cohorts compared with females and prepubetal males, since most testosterone assays are not sensitive enough to measure low circulating levels.[18]

In most large clinical and reference laboratories, testosterone assays are performed on automated platforms using nonradioactive methods. For men, the testosterone immunoassay with enhanced efficiency, reduced cost, and improved sensitivity is used effectively to measure total testosterone and is considered the gold standard for diagnosing hypogonadism.[19] Some investigators argue that free testosterone levels are the most helpful to clinicians who are evaluating androgen status in both men and women. This is because free testosterone is the most biologically active and is representative of the actual concentration of testosterone to which tissues are exposed. This may be true but accurate free testosterone assays are not available to most clinicians and true normal ranges have not been established for women. In addition, total levels of testosterone (both free and protein-bound), may be affected by changes in SHBG concentrations. For example, total testosterone levels are decreased

in conditions associated with reduced SHBG levels (e.g. moderate obesity, hypothyroidism, androgen therapy, glucocorticoid or progestin use) and increased in situations associated with increased SHBG levels (e.g. aging, androgen deficiency, estrogen therapy, hepatic cirrhosis). Therefore, in these conditions the total testosterone levels will give false information about the actual level of testosterone that is present and that which is biologically active.[20] The rise in SHBG concentrations in men as they age indicates that assays measuring total testosterone levels may produce unreliable results. In women, use of estrogens and oral contraceptive pill increases SHBG concentrations, binding testosterone to SHBG with high affinity, and affecting measurements of free testosterone. If total testosterone levels in women are to be used for clinical decision making, it has been suggested that total testosterone levels in or below the lower quartile of normal or accompanied by elevated SHBG levels should be considered when contemplating the diagnosis of androgen insufficiency.[21]

To date, a relation between specific levels of free testosterone and symptoms of androgen insufficiency has not been established.[22] It has been demonstrated, however, that serum levels of total testosterone do not always correlate with androgen insufficiency symptoms in women if SHBG levels are also not evaluated. Serum levels of free testosterone levels correlate more closely with symptoms of androgen insufficiency in women. In the absence of a reliable free or total testosterone assay, a calculated value for free testosterone, using the mass action equation, may be an acceptable substitute for measurement of free testosterone by equilibrium dialysis.

Androgen deficiency and aging

Female androgen insufficiency symptoms in women may be part of the natural aging process or can be exacerbated by underlying etiologies that also effect testosterone production or metabolism. Circulating androgen levels, total and free testosterone, DHEA, and DHEAS fall continuously with age, starting in the sixth decade preceding the average age of natural menopause.[23] A recent cross-sectional study of 60 healthy premenopausal women, aged 20–49 years with cyclic menses and no complaints of sexual dysfunction, reported a progressive decline of androgen levels with advancing age. Androgen values in the 20–29-year-old cohort compared with those in the 40–49-year-old cohort were 195 µg/dL versus 140 µg/dL for DHEAS, 51.5 ng/dL versus 33.7 ng/dL for serum total testosterone, and 1.51 pg/mL versus 1.03 pg/mL for free testosterone, respectively.[24] The investigators noted that testosterone levels declined irrespective of whether measurements were made by total testosterone immunoassay, free testosterone by the analog method, or calculated by the Free Androgen Index.

In the male, aging is associated with a decrease in total, free, and bioavailable concentrations of testosterone in serum. SHBG levels also increase, that leads to increased serum SHBG–testosterone binding and a decrease in metabolic clearance rate of testosterone.[25] The lowest levels of testosterone are seen in men older than 70 years. The New Mexico Aging Process Study, a longitudinal, 15-year study of 77 healthy older men ages 61–87, demonstrated a progressive decline in testosterone and progressive increases in the LH and follicle stimulating hormone (FSH). Levels SHBG, in particular, increased significantly with age ($P < 0.0001$).[26]

Although many research studies have noted the dramatic decline of DHEA, testosterone, and androstenedione in the elderly compared with young adults, there has been no clear explanation for the cause of this decline in adrenal output with age. Parker et al. reported that the total adrenal output of DHEA was reduced after ACTH stimulation in postmenopausal women when compared to premenopausal women.[27] Also, the reduction in androstenedione in older women may be due to the reduction in circulating levels of DHEA that can be converted to androstenedione in peripheral tissues. Histologically, adrenal androgen dysfunction with aging is confirmed by the decreased number of cells of the zona reticularis, as compared to the cells of the cortex. Additionally, the DHEA sulfotransferase enzyme in the adrenals of aging men and women is reduced compared with that in young adults. Other studies have confirmed that aging is associated with a decrease in adrenal DHEAS secretion[28] in association with a change in 17-α-hydroxylase enzyme activity such that there is a decrease in 17,20 desmolase.[29] These alterations parallel the decrease in lean body mass associated with and increased body fat seen in advancing age. It appears that decreased testosterone production with age could be a result of decreased DHEA and DHEAS formation due to a defect in the enzyme system. However, what causes the ages-related changes in the functional and morphologic integrity of the zona reticularis that affects adrenal androgen production is still a pressing research question.

Table 2.3 Mean steroid levels in women (pg/mL)

	Reproductive age	Natural menopause	Surgical menopause
E$_2$	150	10–15	10
T	400	290	110
Δ⁴A	1900	1000	700
DHEA	5000	2000	1800
DHEAS	3 000 000	1 000 000	1 000 000

See text for abbreviations.

Ovarian androgen deficiency with menopause

Serum testosterone levels are lower in older women than in young, regularly menstruating women. The decline in testosterone may begin in the decade prior to menopause and this decline continues across the life cycle with testosterone levels for women in their sixties at approximately 50% as compared to women in their twenties.[8] Unlike the tenfold drop in estrogen levels that occurs with natural or surgical menopause, the reduction in androgens is not that abrupt, unless menopause has been surgically induced (Table 2.3). Androgen decline at menopause does not appear to be related to follicular depletion, but rather to gradual atrophy of ovarian stroma, which is also consistent with decreasing ovarian size with aging. A large cross-sectional study in Australia reported no abrupt changes in serum testosterone concentrations in women progressing from their reproductive years to their postreproductive years, suggesting that the ovarian androgen secretion is not significantly attenuated in most women at the point of menopause but is a gradual phenomenon.[30]

Because androgens produced by the ovaries significantly contribute to the serum concentration it follows that pathologic disorders that affect the ovaries will result in decreased androgen levels. Ovarian disorders include premature ovarian failure, ovarian tumors, Turner syndrome, oophorectomy, and ovarian damage from either chemotherapy or radiotherapy. For example, women with Turner syndrome, which is characterized by strick ovaries in which there are no functional follicles, have low circulating levels of androstenedione, and total and free testosterone, and increased levels of SHBG.[31] Because young women with loss of ovarian function are often prescribed oral contraceptive pills, a further decrease in free androgen levels may occur as a result of increased SHBG levels.

Androgens and oophorectomy

Ovarian androgen production continues well into the postmenopausal years as confirmed by the cross-sectional, Rancho Bernado community-based study of 684 women between the ages of 50 and 89 years. The most dramatic decline in ovarian androgen production occurred in the oophorectomized cohort whose total and bio-available testosterone levels were 40% lower and androstenedione levels 10% lower than a matched cohort with intact ovaries.[32] Further, studies of women before and after bilateral oophorectomy provide evidence of the relative contribution of the ovaries to androgen production as compared to adrenal glands in women. In the classic study by Judd et al. the mean testosterone level, which was within normal range before surgery in post-reproductive aged women, decreased by about 50% after oophorectomy.[16] In younger, pre-menopausal women, oophorectomy resulted in an even greater reduction in testosterone levels than those reported in postmenopausal women. These data support findings that ovaries may account for about half of the circulating testosterone in postmenopausal women and an even larger proportion in reproductive-aged women.

Women who have either undergone oophorectomy or experienced chemical/radiation-induced ovariectomy are more likely to report symptoms of fatigue, low energy, and decreased sexual motivation and desire with estrogen-only therapy. Shifren et al. evaluated 75 surgically menopausal women who complained of sexual dysfunction despite estrogen therapy use. In this clinical trial, each woman received three different treatments that were administered temporally but in a random order: placebo, 150 μg/day of testosterone, and 300 μg/day of testosterone every day for 12 weeks. Treatment with higher dose of transdermal testosterone resulted in a significant improvement in sexual function and quality of life compared to placebo and estrogen alone.[33]

Impact of estrogen therapy in postmenopausal women

Postmenopausal women with intact ovaries who complain of distressing vasomotor symptoms are offered estrogen (without uterus present) or estrogen/progestin (with uterus present) therapy, when there are no contraindications to this intervention. Exogenous oral estrogen therapy improves vasomotor symptoms but increases SHBG levels and suppresses the pituitary LH production. LH suppression may further decrease the stimulus for ovarian androgen production.[34] Raisz and coworkers, who studied a group of women presenting with natural menopause, reported an effect of estrogen therapy on LH and SHBG. The women were treated with 1.25 mg of conjugated equine estrogens for 9 weeks. Their SHBG increased by 184% and LH levels decreased by 47%.[35] Using the mathematical calculations of testosterone levels developed by Vermuelen and coworkers, the calculated free testosterone levels decreased by 57%, from a baseline value of 3 pg/mL to 1.3 pg/mL with the use of oral estrogens.

Androgens in women with pituitary disease

Central nervous system causes of androgen deficiency include disorders affecting the pituitary or the hypothalamus. Panhypopituitarism is related to a decreased secretion of both ovarian and adrenal androgens. Patients with panhypopituitarism have lower circulating concentrations of total and free testosterone and androstenedione than the concentrations found in patients with either adrenal or ovarian failure.[36] Miller et al.

demonstrated a 73% reduction in androgen levels in a cohort of women with hypopituitarism relative to an age-matched group of normal women. Serum concentrations of testosterone, free testosterone, androstenedione, and DHEAS in 55 women who had either central hypogonadism or hypoandrenalism from pituitary disease were markedly lower than in 92 control women. It did not matter whether the women who had pituitary disease were perimenopausal or postmenopausal, or if they were estrogen depleted or repleted. The long-term effects of low androgen levels on body composition and libido in women with hypopituitarism have not been established.

Androgen deficiency and medications

The use of glucorcoticoids is associated not only with reduced levels of circulating androgens, but with corticosteroids as well. In a study of nine young healthy females on dexamethasone suppression, Arlt et al. reported a decrease of 8% in serum cortisol, 16% in DHEAS, 18% in DHEA, 26% in androstenedione, and 28% in testosterone from baseline.[37] The net effect of glucocorticoid therapy is suppression of corticotropin releasing hormone (CRH) and ACTH. In a similar study, Abraham evaluated testosterone production in regularly cycling, reproductive-age females before and after dexamethasone therapy.[15] In this study, testosterone levels were reduced by 50% following dexamethasone therapy. It follows that women on dexamethasone for autoimmune diseases and reproductive disorders may experience androgen insufficiency symptoms, including sexual dysfunction and impaired wellbeing.

In a small, randomized, double blind, controlled study of 24 women with adrenal insufficiency, the administration of DHEA (50 mg/day) restored DHEAS and androstenedione to normal range values and testosterone levels to low normal range values.[37] Subjects reported a significant reduction in depression and anxiety, and a marked improvement in mood and overall wellbeing. Davis and coworkers[38] added to these observations by conducting a prospective, single blind randomized trial and administered either a combination of 50 mg of testosterone implants plus 50 mg of estradiol implants or 50 mg of estradiol implant alone to post menopausal women. The treatments were administered every 3 months for 2 years. Sexual fantasies, orgasm, and several other aspects of sexual function in women treated with combined therapy were greater than with estradiol alone.

Androgen deficiency states in men

In the male, the majority of testosterone production occurs in the testes, an integral part of the hypothalamic–pituitary–gonadal axis. In the testes, LH stimulates Leydig cells to secrete testosterone, and, along with the testes, which produce about 0.24 μmol/day of testosterone, the adrenal cortex produces 0.002 μmol/day of androgens, mostly as androstenedione.[39] Data available on androgen deficiency in the male link its development to either testicular failure or hypogonadotropic hypogonadism. The gonadal failure results from a decrease in the number and volume of the Leydig cells and impaired blood supply to the gonads.[40] Secondary hypogonadism is caused by tumors of the pituitary gland or testicles, meningitis, head trauma affecting the hypothalamus, surgery, and effects of chemotherapy and radiation.[41] Other conditions that have been associated with systemic causes of androgen deficiency include rheumatoid arthritis and human immunodeficiency virus infection. The resulting loss of androgen production leads to physical alterations and behavioral symptoms.

There is a progressive reduction in the hypothalamic–pituitary–gonadal axis activity in aging men and not only do testosterone levels decline but there is a subsequent loss of the circadian rhythm of testosterone secretion. This decline is thought to be responsible for fatigue, decreased muscle and bone mass, abdominal obesity, decreased sexual dysfunction and increased rates of depression often reported by elderly men.[42–44]

In older men, the most common presenting symptoms associated with androgen deficiency are loss of libido along with diminished sexual thoughts and enjoyment.[45] Bioavailable testosterone levels have been shown to correlate strongly with nocturnal penile tumescence, particularly in men 55–64 years of age.[46] Men with primary hypogonadism who have high SHBG levels because of enhanced production of estradiol from a rise in intratesticular aromatization have been shown to develop weakness of the limb girdle muscles. In young hypogonadal men, administration of supraphysiologic levels of testosterone increases muscle mass and strength.[44] These clinical consequences of androgen deficiency, including the increased risk of osteoporosis are well documented in men.[47] In one study, the risk of hip fractures was twice as great in older men with hypogonadism compared with in those without this condition.[48] Young men with testosterone deficiency are also reported to have lower bone density compared with age-matched controls.[49]

Like menopause in women, cross-sectional studies support a hormonal shift in men with aging such that older men have reduced concentrations of circulating testosterone.[50-53] One study using longitudinal data from the Massachusetts Male Aging Study which included men aged 39–70 years, reported a decrease of 1.6% per year for total testosterone and about 3% per year for bioavailable testosterone.[54] It is clear that there is a gradual and progressive decline in serum testosterone after the age of 30 years, Vermeulen et al. found that 7% of men at age 40–60 years have testosterone levels below the normal value established in young men, 22% at age 60–80 years and, 37% at over age 80.[50]

In addition to testosterone therapy, other androgens may be of benefit. In one study, DHEAS enhanced mitogenesis in bone cells by inducing transforming growth factor beta mRNA and by enhancing the binding of insulin-like growth factor II to osteoblasts.[55] In a 6-month study in which DHEA (50 mg/day) was administered to eight elderly men, there was noted improvement in bone mineral density and a favorable effect on body composition.[56]

Androgen insufficiency states in women

The deleterious clinical consequences of androgen insufficiency have also been reported in women. Loss of libido, which affects more than 15 million women in the USA, is often the presenting complaint of women with inadequate testosterone.[57] It follows that therapy with testosterone ameliorates this complaint and restores sexual frequency, sexual fantasy, and pleasure with orgasm as well as improving overall wellbeing and depressed mood.[31,58] No Food and Drug Administration (FDA)-approved androgen preparations formulated for women are currently available. The adverse effects resulting from diminished androgens in some women suggest that an androgen formulation for women, especially for those who have had a surgical menopause, is a pressing need.

Androgen products currently available are approved for the treatment of male hypogonadism. The only commercially available, prescription testosterone preparation for women is a combination of oral esterified estrogen (EE) and methyltestosterone (MT). This formulation is recommended for the treatment of vasomotor menopausal symptoms not responsive to estrogen alone and not for female sexual dysfunction or other indications. Some studies comparing EE alone with EE plus MT have demonstrated that daily oral administration of the combined hormones when the MT portion was 1.25 mg or 2.5 mg significantly improves sexual function.[59,60] Bone mineral density also increased with the therapy of EE plus MT daily compared to EE alone.[35] Testosterone preparations formulated for men, which result in serum testosterone levels that are 10–20 times higher than necessary for women, are not recommended for use in women.

DHEA also has been used for androgen therapy in women and men.[61] In studies using pharmaceutical grade DHEA, doses above 30 mg/day may improve sexual function, although results from many DHEA trials are conflicting. Because the FDA considers DHEA a dietary supplement, it is available without a prescription. Unfortunately, over-the-counter preparations demonstrate a wide range of efficacy and many lack consistent delivery of the stated amount of DHEA. One study found that some of the DHEA supplements contain from 0% to approximately 150% the potency of the stated amount of DHEA.[62]

Conclusions

It is clear that women with hypopituitarism, adrenal insufficiency, or history of adrenalectomy or oophorectomy, and men with either primary or secondary hypogonadism, may become deficient in androgens. Also, premenopausal and naturally menopausal women may develop symptoms of androgen decline due to age-related effects on the adrenals and the ovaries. In men, it is generally accepted that the principal cause of age-related decrease in testosterone production is testicular atrophy although diminished gonadotropin production may play a role. Data also support that women may develop androgen insufficiency with aging or with other conditions that compromise ovarian or adrenal function. Androgen deficiency may severely impair the quality of men and women's lives but the physiologic mechanisms especially of female androgen insufficiency and the subsequent symptoms have not been characterized as clearly.

Many clinicians prescribe testosterone therapy for men with marked symptoms of androgen deficiency. A level below 300 ng/dL is proposed as a cut-off point for considering therapy in symptomatic men. Women with low levels of bioavailable testosterone relative to reference intervals shown in women in their twenties and thirties have been found to suffer similar symptoms to those observed in hypogonadal men. Therefore, testosterone supplementation has also been suggested for women with symptoms of androgen insufficiency, especially after surgical menopause. Although testosterone supplementation has been shown to improve sexual function and psychologic wellbeing in women with decreased testosterone caused by surgical removal of their ovaries, there are no FDA-approved testosterone products for women with androgen insufficiency. Basic science research to better characterize adrenal and ovarian changes with aging and clinical trials to expand the database that characterizes androgen insufficiency in the female and the results of androgen therapy are research imperatives.

References

1. Morales A, Tenover JL. Androgen deficiency in the aging male: when, who, and how to investigate and treat. Urol Clin North Am 2002; 29:975–982.
2. Bachmann GA. The hypoadrogenic woman: pathophysiologic overview. Fertil Steril 2002; 77:S72–S76.
3. Geist SH, Salmon UJ. Androgen therapy in gynecology. JAMA 1941; 117:2207–2213.
4. Greenblatt RB, Barfield WE, Garner JF et al. Evaluation of an estrogen, androgen and estrogen-androgen combination and a placebo in the treatment of the menopause. J Clin Endocrinol Metab 1950; 10:1547–1558.
5. Waxenberg SE, Drelich MG, Sutherland AM. The role of hormones in human behavior: changes in female sexuality after adrenalectomy. J Clin Endocrinol Metab 1959; 19:193–202.
6. Sherwin BB, Gelfand MM. Differential symptoms response to parenteral estrogen and/or androgen administration in the surgical menopause. Am J Obstet Gynecol 1985; 151:153–160.
7. Burger H, Hailes J, Neslon J. Effect of combined implants of oestradiol and testosterone on libido in post-menopausal women. Br Med J 1987; 294:936–7.
8. Watts NB, Notelovitz M, Timmons MC et al. Comparison of oral estrogens and estrogens plus androgen on bone mineral density, menopausal symptoms, and lipid-lipoprotein profiles in surgical menopause. Obstet Gynecol 1995; 85:529–537.
9. Casson PR, Carson SA, Buster JE. Testosterone delivery systems for women: present status and future promise. Semin Reprod Endocrinol 1998; 16:153–159.
10. Zumoff B, Strain GW, Miller LK, Rosner W. Twenty-four hour mean plasma testosterone concentration declines with age in normal premenopausal women. J Clin Endocrinol Metab 1995; 80:1429–30.
11. Ismail AAA, Astley P, Burr WA et al. The role of testosterone measurement in the investigation of androgen disorders. Ann Clin Biochem 1986; 23:113–134.
12. Bremner WJ, Vitielo V, Prinz PN. Loss of circadian rhythmicity in blood testosterone levels with aging in normal men. J Clin Endocrinol Metab 1983; 56:1278–1281.
13. Longcope C. Adrenal and gonadal androgen secretion in normal females. Clin Endocrinol Metab 1986; 15:213–228.
14. Baird D, Horton R, Longcope C, Toit JF. Steroid prehormones. Perspect Biol Med 1968; 11:384–421.
15. Abraham GE. Ovarian and adrenal contribution to peripheral androgens during the menstrual cycle. J Clin Endocrinol Metab 1974; 39:340–346.
16. Judd HL, Lucas WE, Yen SS. Effect of oophorectomy on circulating testosterone and androstenedione levels in patients with endometrial cancer. Am J Obstet Gynecol 1974; 118:793–798.
17. Dunn JF, Nisula BC, Rodbard D. Transport of steroid hormones: binding of 21 endogenous steroids to both testosterone-binding globulin and corticosteroid-binding globulin in human plasma. J Clin Endocrinol Metab 1981; 53:58–68.
18. Guay AT. Screening for androgen deficiency in women: methodological and interpretive issues. Fertil Steril 2002; 77:S6–S10.
19. Dechaud H, Lejuene H, Garoscio-Cholet M et al. Radioimmunoassay of testosterone not bound to sex-steroid binding protein in plasma. Clin Chem 1989; 35:1609–1614.

20. Vermuelen A, Verdonck L, Kaufman JM. A critical evaluation of simple methods for the estimation of free testosterone in serum. J Clin Endocrinol Metab 1999; 84:3666–3672.
21. Davis S, Schneider H, Donarti-Sarti C et al. Androgen levels in normal and oophorectomized women. Proceedings of the 10th International Congress on the Menopause, Berlin 10–14 June 2002. Climacteric 2002; 5:219–228.
22. Dennerstein L, Randolph J, Taffe J et al. Hormones, mood, sexuality, and the menopausal transition. Fertil Steril 2002; 77:S42–S48.
23. Mushayandebvu T, Castracane VD, Gimpel T et al. Evidence for diminished midcycle ovarian androgen production in older reproductive aged women. Fertil Steril 1996; 65:721–723.
24. Guay A, Munarriz R, Jacobson J et al. Serum androgen levels in healthy premenopausal women with and without sexual dysfunction: Part A. Serum androgen levels in women aged 20–49 years with no complaints of sexual dysfunction. Int J Impot Res 2004; 16(2):112–120.
25. Kandeel FR, Koussa VK, Swerdloff RS. Male sexual function and its disorders: Physiology, pathophysiology, clinical investigation, and treatment. Endocr Rev 2001; 22:342–388.
26. Morley JE, Kaiser FE, Perry HM et al. Longitudinal changes in testosterone, luteinizing hormone, and follicle-stimulating hormone in healthy older men. Metabolism 1997; 46:410–413.
27. Parker RC, Scott M, Slayden RZ et al. Effects of aging on adrenal function in the human: Responsiveness and sensitivity of adrenal androgens and cortisol to adrenocorticotropin in premenopausal and post-menopausal women. J Clin Endocrinol Metab 2000; 85:48–54.
28. Orentreich N, Brind JL, Rizer RL, Vogelman JH. Age changes and sex differences in serum dehydroepiandrosterone sulfate concentrations throughout adulthood. J Clin Endocrinol Metab 1984; 59:551–555.
29. Liu CH, Laughlin GA, Fischer UG, Yen SS. Marked attenuation of ultradian and circadian rhythms of dehydroepiandrosterone in postmenopausal women: evidence for a reduced 17,20 desmolase enzymatic activity. J Clin Endocrinol Metab 1990; 71:900–906.
30. Burger HG, Dudley EC, Cui J, et al. A prospective longitudinal study of serum testosterone, dehydroepiandrosterone sulfate, and sex hormone-binding globulin levels through the menopause transition. J Clin Endocrinol Metab 2000; 85:2832–2838.
31. Hojbjerg GC, Svenstrup B, Bennett P, Sandahl CJ. Reduced androgen levels in adult turner syndrome: influence of female sex steroids and growth hormone status. Clin Endocrinol (Oxford) 1999; 50:791–800.
32. Laughlin GA, Barrett-Conner E, Kritz-Silverstein D, von Muhlen D. Hysterectomy, oophorectomy, and endogenous sex hormone levels in older women: the Rancho Bernado Study. J Clin Endocrinol Metab 2000; 85:645–651.
33. Shifren JL, Braunstein GD, Simon JA et al. Transdermal testosterone treatment in women with impaired sexual function after oophorectomy. N Engl J Med 2000; 343:682–688.
34. Mathur RS, Landgrebe SC, Moody LO et al. The effect of estrogen treatment on plasma concentrations of steroid hormones, gonadotropins, prolactin and sex hormone-binding globulin in post-menopausal women. Maturitas 1985; 7:129–133.
35. Raisz LG, Wiita B, Artis A et al. Comparison of the effects of estrogen alone and estrogen plus androgen on biochemical markers of bone formation and resorption in postmenopausal women. J Clin Endocrinol Metab 1996; 81:37–43.
36. Miller KK, Sesmilo G, Schiller A et al. Androgen deficiency in women with hypopituitarism. J Clin Endocrinol Metab 2001; 86:51–57.
37. Arlt W, Callies F, van Vlijmen JC et al. Dehydroepiandrosterone replacement in women with adrenal insufficiency. N Engl J Med 1999; 341:1013–1020.
38. Davis SR, McCloud P, Strauss BJ et al. Testosterone enhances estradiol's effects on postmenopausal bone density and sexuality. Maturitas 1995; 21:227–236.
39. Neaves WB, Johnson L, Porter JC et al. Leydig cell numbers, daily sperm production and serum gonadotrophin levels in aging men. J Clin Endocrinol Metab 1984; 59:756–763.
40. Suoranta H. Changes in small blood vessels of the adult human testes in relation to age and some pathological conditions. Virchows Arch (Pathol Anat) 1971; 352:765–781.
41. AACE medical guidelines for clinical practice for the evaluation and treatment of hypogonadism in adult male patients. Endocr Pract 2002; 8:439–456.
42. Forbes GB & Reina JC. Adult lean body mass declines with age: some longitudinal observations. Metabolism 1970; 19:653–663.
43. Kallman DA, Plato CC, Tobin JD. The role of muscle loss in the age-related decline of grip strength: cross-sectional and longitudinal perspectives. J Gerontol 1990; 45:M82–M88.
44. Bhasin S, Storer TW, Berman N, et al. Testosterone replacement increases fat free mass and muscle size in hypogonadal men. J Clin Endocrinol Metab 1997; 82:407–413.
45. Seidman NS. The aging male: androgens, erectile dysfunction, and depression. J Clin Psychiatry. J Clin Psychiatry 2003; 64:31–37.

46. Schiavi CR, White D, Mandeli J. Pituitary-gonadal function during sleep in healthy aging men. Psychoneuroendocrinology 1993; 17:599–609.

47. Drinka PJ, Bauwens, SF. Male osteopenia: a brief review. J Am Geriatr Soc 1987; 35:258–261.

48. Jackson JA, Riggs MW, Spiekerman AM. Testosterone deficiency as a risk factor for hip fractures in men: a case–control study. Am J Med Sci 1992; 304:4–8.

49. Finkelstein JS, Klibanski A, Neer RM et al. Increase in bone density during treatment of men with idiopathic hypogonadotropic hypogonadism. J Clin Endocrinol Metab 1989; 69:776–783.

50. Vermuelen A, Kaufman JM, Giagulli VA. Influence of some biological indexes on sex-hormone-binding globulin and androgen levels in aging and obese males. J Clin Endocrinol Metab 1996; 81:1821–1826.

51. Plymate SR, Bremner WJ. The effects of aging in normal men on bioavailable testosterone and luteinizing hormone secretion: response to clomiphene citrate. J Clin Endocrinol Metab 1987; 65:1118–1126.

52. Vermuelen A, Rubens R, Verdonck L. Testosterone secretion and metabolism in male senescence. J Clin Endocrinol Metab 1972; 34:730–735.

53. Gray A, Berlin JA, McKinlay JB, Langcope C. An examination of research design effects on the association of testosterone and male aging: results of meta-analysis. J Clin Epidemiol 1991; 44:671–684.

54. Feldman HA, Longcope C, Derby CA et al. Age trends in the level of serum testosterone and other hormones in middle-aged men: longitudinal results from the Massachusetts Male Aging Study. J Clin Endocrinol Metab 2002; 87:589–598.

55. Kasperk CH, Wergedal JE, Farley JR et al. Androgens directly stimulate proliferation of bone cells in vitro. Endocrinology 1989; 124:1576–1578.

56. Villareal DT, Holloszy JO, Kohrt WM. Effects of DHEA replacement on bone mineral density and body composition in elderly women and men. Clin Endocrinol (Oxford) 2000; 53:561–568.

57. Laumann EO, Paik A, Rosem RC. Sex dysfunction in the United States: prevalence and predictors. JAMA 1999; 281:537–544.

58. Goldstat R, Biganti E, Tran J et al. Transdermal testosterone therapy improves well-being, mood, and sexual function in premenopausal women. Menopause 2003; 10:390–398.

59. Lobo RA, Rosen RC, Yang HM et al. Comparative effects of oral esterified estrogens with and without methyltestosterone on endocrine profiles and dimensions of sexual function in postmenopausal women with hypoactive sexual desire. Fertil Steril 2003; 79:1341–1352.

60. Sarrel P, Dobay, B, Wiita B. Estrogen and estrogen-androgen replacement in postmenopausal women dissatisfied with estrogen-only therapy. Sexual behavior and neuroendocrine responses. J Reprod Med 1998; 43:847–856.

61. Morales AJ, Haubrich RH, Hwang JY et al. The effect of six months treatment with a 100 mg daily dose of dehydroepiandrosterone (DHEA) on circulating sex steroids, body composition and muscle strength in age-advanced men and women. Clin Endocrinol (Oxford) 1998; 49: 421–432.

62. Parasrampuria J, Schwartz K, Petesch R. Quality control of dehydroepiandrosterone dietary supplement products. JAMA 1998; 280:1565.

Chapter 3

Endocrine aspects of reproductive aging in men and women

Ryan Zlupko and Joseph Sanfilippo

Summary

The population of the world is aging, and the increase in lifespan has been in years with compromised functioning. The prospect of male hormone replacement and the role of androgens in female hormone replacement has been the subject of increasing study. This chapter reviews the normal male and female sex hormone physiology. Attention to the regulatory mechanisms and pathways in the reproductive age is followed by endocrine states through the natural aging process. Emphasis is placed on current evidence for these physiologic changes. As will be clear from this chapter, there are still substantial gaps in our knowledge base that will continue to be fertile areas of research in the future.

Epidemiology of aging

The aging of the human body has received increasing attention over the past several decades. The average lifespan for humans is 75–78 years with an anticipated increase to 85 years over the next two decades. As lifespan increases, the proportion of various age groups is changing. In 2003, the United Nations issued a report on world trends in aging.[1] The report revealed that by 2050, the world proportion of persons older than 60 years is expected to exceed the younger population. The proportion of older persons was 8% in 1950, 10% in 2000, and is estimated to reach 21% by 2050 (Figure 3.1). The most rapid growth is occurring in the oldest age group. Persons aged 80 years and older have shown a growth rate of 3.8% per year. At such a rate, this segment of the population will increase to represent one fifth of the world population.

Besides the major economic and societal implications for this shift in age distribution, there are significant medical consequences as well. The major gain in lifespan thus far has been in years spent with compromised social, mental, or physical functions. According to the 2004 report of vital

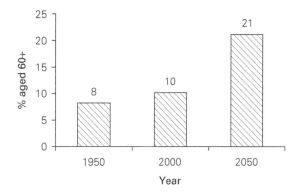

Figure 3.1

Proportion of population 60 years or older: world, 1950–2050.[1]

statistics from the US Department of Health, the percentage of US citizens having limitations of both activities of daily living and/or instrumental activities of daily living increases from 9% in the 65–74 age group to almost 30% in the over 75 age group.[2]

Multiple physiologic systems show signs of decline with age.[3] These include decreased cellular protein synthesis, decreased immune function, increased fat mass, decreased muscle mass and strength, and a decrease in bone mineral density. The five leading causes of mortality in the USA are heart disease, malignant neoplasms, accidents, cerebrovascular diseases, and chronic obstructive pulmonary disease.[4] However, for the healthy 'oldest old', loss of muscle strength is the limiting factor for independent living. Physical frailty is the outcome of this altered body composition and decreased function.[5,6]

Many endocrine functions also decline as we age. Two common examples include the pancreas and thyroid.[7] Active screening for changes in insulin sensitivity and age-related thyroid diseases are standard. Treatment is given accordingly. Age-related changes also occur in the hypothalamic–pituitary–gonadal axis, adrenal axis and growth hormone–insulin-like growth factor (IGF) axis. These changes, conversely, have been treated as physiologic although they are associated with significant physical, mental, and social impairment.

Much debate has surrounded the role of sex hormones in successful aging. The concept of endocrine factors playing a central role in human aging is not new.[8] Although there is no known 'fountain of youth', increasing interest in hormonal replacement strategies and controversy as to the appropriateness and safety of these treatments reveal a need for understanding of these systems in the overall functioning of humans with age.

For the purposes of this chapter, a brief review of this hormonal axis is warranted to highlight the changes observed as well as sex differences during aging. End-organ effects of androgens and estrogens are beyond the scope of this chapter and are covered elsewhere.

Review of basic male reproductive physiology

The male reproductive hormonal axis is geared for the production of sperm and testosterone. Most of the hormonal signals and pathways are homologous to the female system. The main difference between the male and female axes is the former's lack of a significant cyclic nature and its relative longevity throughout the male lifetime.

Pulsatile gonadotrophic releasing hormone (GnRH) secretion by the hypothalamus induces follicle stimulating hormone (FSH) and luteinizing hormone (LH) secretion by basophilic pituitary cells. Regulation by the preoptic area and the medial basal region of the hypothalamus (particularly the arcuate nucleus) maintains normal GnRH pulse frequency and amplitude.

The Leydig cells are the main targets for LH action in the testis. LH binds to Leydig cell receptors to increase cAMP thus increasing conversion of cholesterol to testosterone. FSH binds to Sertoli cell receptors at the basal membrane. This binding leads to an increase in cAMP. Elevated cAMP levels act to increase production of androgen binding protein, aromatase, transferrin, inhibin, and plasminogen activators. The binding of FSH thus increases the aromatization of testosterone to estradiol within the Sertoli cells. The exact mechanisms under FSH regulation in the Sertoli cells that lead to spermatogenesis are poorly understood. These mechanisms also depend on high local levels of testosterone thus illustrating that both LH and FSH effects are essential for normal development of spermatogenesis in the male.

Testicular hormones feed back to the pituitary and hypothalamus complete the endocrine circuit. Estradiol and inhibin B play the main role in regulating FSH release.[9] These hormones negatively feedback to the pituitary and diminish FSH. Activin and follistatin also play a role in local regulation of FSH secretion, modifying inhibin B effects at the pituitary level. Autocrine and paracrine functions of activin and follistatin may also play a role in the male gonads. Inhibin A does not appear to play a major regulatory role in male reproductive physiology.

The testosterone produced in the testes is converted peripherally to dihydrotestosterone (DHT) by 5α-reductase. Both testosterone and DHT provide feedback to the pituitary, directly decreasing LH release. Local conversion of testosterone to estradiol may play a role in this mechanism.[10] Feedback to the hypothalamus by these hormones will also slow the GnRH pulse frequency thus decreasing LH pulse frequency.

Although the male axis lacks the monthly cyclic variance of the female system, there is a daily variation in testosterone levels. This circadian rhythmicity leads to higher testosterone levels in the early morning and declining levels in the late afternoon. This may have few implications in the young healthy male but may lead to confounding factors in the laboratory assessment of androgens in the later phases of life.[11]

Review of basic female reproductive physiology

The hypothalamic–pituitary–ovarian axis in women utilizes many of the same signals and pathways outlined in male section above. However, if the male axis produces a relatively constant and long-lived hormonal milieu, the female axis produces a tightly coordinated waxing and waning monthly cycle. This string of hormonal events facilitates the production of ovarian sex steroid precursors, the selection of a dominant follicle, and proper preparation of the uterine lining for conception. This cycle in women is also finite, demonstrated by the complete cessation of menses in later life.

GnRH pulses from hypothalamic peptidergic neurons located in the arcuate nucleus of the medial basal hypothalamus and the preoptic area of the anterior hypothalamus stimulate pulsatile secretion of LH and FSH from gonadotrophs in the anterior pituitary. The number of GnRH receptors on the cell surface of gonadotrophs is influenced by the chronicity of GnRH pulses with increasing numbers of receptors seen with shorter pulse intervals but a decrease in receptors with continuous stimulation.

Gonadotropin

FSH and LH are heterodimer structures consisting of alpha and beta subunits. The alpha unit is shared between FSH, LH, thyroid stimulating hormone (TSH), and human chorionic gonadotropin (hCG). The beta unit is unique to each alpha-beta heterodimer and confers the specific activity. FSH, as opposed to LH, does have some GnRH independent secretion influenced most likely by intrapituitary activin stimulation.[12]

The ovarian follicle within the ovarian cortex is the functional unit of the ovary, comprised of the oocyte and the surrounding granulosa and theca cells. Of the original 6–7 million oogonia present by 16–20 weeks in fetal life, roughly 300 000 primordial follicles are present at the time of menarche. Hormonal recruitment transforms primordial follicles to primary follicles. Primary follicles that fail to become the selected-dominant follicle undergo follicular atresia.

Hormonal recruitment and follicular development depends on both the specific hormonal signal and timing to create a functional oocyte. LH acts on theca cells of the ovary to produce testosterone. FSH targets the granulosa cells, and drives the production of aromatase to convert testosterone to estrogen in the granulosa cells via a G-protein family receptor. The granulosa cells surrounding a large, preovulatory follicle will also demonstrate LH receptors. Development of LH receptors in these cells is believed to be under FSH control. The stromal cells of the ovary may also respond to LH and hCG stimulation with production of androstenedione. Progesterone is produced by the granulosa-lutein cells of the corpus luteum following ovulation.

Inhibin

Inhibin and activin are glycoprotein hormones and members of the transforming growth factor β (TGF-β) family of peptides. Inhibin is a heterodimer composed of a common alpha subunit and a unique beta subunit producing either inhibin A or B. Both originate from the granulosa cells although there may be a small component from the theca cells. Inhibins have a negative feedback effect on FSH from the anterior pituitary. The mechanism is still poorly understood but likely involves a signal pathway involving betaglycan and p120.[13,14]

Inhibin A is primarily a product of the dominant follicle. The pattern of release shows a late follicular peak then a luteal rise parallel to progesterone from the corpus luteum. The levels of estradiol, progesterone, and inhibin A decrease in the late luteal phase.[15,16]

Inhibin B is produced from the pool of growing follicles in the early follicular phase. Under the influence of increasing FSH in the early follicular phase, the level of inhibin B rises. Inhibin B peaks with inhibin A in the late follicular phase but then falls and stays at a constant low until the next round of follicular recruitment.[15]

Additional regulators of pituitary–ovarian function have been a subject of interest for researchers expanding the molecular pathways involved in sex hormone regulation.[17] Activin is a homodimer of any combination of beta subunits and seems to play multiple roles in development and aging. In the pituitary, it stimulates the release of FSH via a pathway that interacts with the inhibin/betaglycan moiety at the activin type II receptor.[18] Binding of follistatin also modifies activin activity. Follistatin is a single chain polypeptide that binds and inactivates the activin homodimer. Thus follistatin is an indirect regulator of FSH. Direct binding of follistatin to inhibin is known but its impact on inhibin activity is limited secondary to weak binding kinetics. The overall impact this system has on FSH release is still unclear as almost all activin is follistatin bound.

Estradiol

Estradiol exerts a negative feedback on FSH and LH secretion, mostly by acting at the level of hypothalamus. The relative weight of estradiol and inhibin in the regulation of central signaling to the gonads is roughly 50:50.[19] The net effect of this network of hormone products is an early, rising FSH level that drives the recruitment of ovarian follicles. Estradiol and inhibin increase as a result of FSH stimulation. A dominant follicle is selected and inhibin A levels spike in concordance with the LH peak, signaling ovulation, and FSH levels fall. Estradiol production remains high and progesterone from the corpus luteum is elevated until the end of this phase of the menstrual cycle. In the absence of an ongoing pregnancy, the prepared endometrial lining sheds with the beginning of the subsequent cycle.

Androgen

Androgen production in women involves both the ovaries and the adrenal glands. The principal androgens include dehydroepiandrosterone (DHEA), DHEA sulfate (DHEAS), androstenedione, and testosterone. The ovary and adrenals evenly split the production of androstenedione.[20] In contrast, 90% of DHEAS is of adrenal origin.[21] Men and premenopausal women have similar levels of circulating androstenedione.[22] Total testosterone levels in premenopausal women are approximately 10% of that of male levels.[20] The ovaries directly secrete 25% of the total testosterone with the remainder being split equally from peripheral conversion of androstenedione and from the adrenals.

Sex hormone binding globulin

Normative data for the levels of various androgens in women from early reproductive age to postmenopausal is lacking. Additionally, at least for testosterone, the measurement itself is under debate. Sex hormone binding globulin (SHBG) binds approximately 66% of the total serum testosterone with another significant minority being bound by other plasma proteins. It is estimated that only 1–2% of the total testosterone is bioavailable at any one time. Factors such as oral estrogen and thyroxine can increase SHBG while obesity, growth hormone, hyperinsulinemia, and glucocorticoids all decrease SHBG concentration. Measurement of a free T index would likely reflect the bioavailable concentrations of testosterone but the accuracy of the current analog assays is questionable.

Sinha-Hikim et al.[23] reported total testosterone levels of 1.2 nmol/L and free testosterone levels of 12.8 pmol/L in 34 healthy women with normal menstrual cycles. The levels of total and free T and androstenedione show a cyclic variation with the menstrual cycle with the peak occurring in the middle third of the cycle and the nadir during menstruation.[22–24] This cycle variation is not seen with DHEAS because of its primary adrenal origin. Circulating testosterone levels also demonstrate a diurnal variation with higher serum levels in the morning hours. Thus between the natural variations in secretion and the inherent error noted with measurement assays an accurate representation of androgen physiology is a challenging task.

Hormonal changes in aging men

In contrast with the abrupt changes seen during the menopausal transition in women, aging men experience longer, less dramatic changes to their levels of sex hormones. The magnitude and clinical relevance of these changes continues to be the source of debate and research but the general concept of decreasing sex hormone availability was demonstrated in multiple cross-sectional studies of aging men.

Testosterone

The Baltimore Longitudinal Aging Study[25] reported the levels of various sex hormones and gonadotropins, and testosterone response to hCG, in 69 healthy men aged 25–89 years. This study failed to show any effect of age on levels of serum testosterone, 5α-DHT, estrone, and estradiol. There was an increase in serum binding of testosterone in response to an elevated SHBG but no change in the free T index. The authors noted a slightly elevated basal LH and a blunted testosterone response to hCG with aging that suggested a small peripheral resistance to LH at the level of the Leydig cell. They concluded that the effect of age-related illnesses were more responsible for the decreases in sex hormones reported by previous studies considering the excellent health of the study subjects. One criticism of this study is that blood was collected in the afternoon when the natural circadian rhythm would be at its nadir.

Decreases in total and free testosterone have been documented in aging men in subsequent longitudinal studies. Morley et al. reported results from the New Mexico Aging Process Study.[26] Samples from 77 men aged 61–87 years old were obtained from multiple time points and evaluated for change over time. Samples were drawn in the morning between 8 am and 11 am. This study demonstrated a steady decline in testosterone levels of 110 ng/dL every 10 years. Levels of LH, FSH, and SHBG were shown to rise over this same time period. Similar results were also reported by Zmuda et al.[27] A larger longitudinal study from the Baltimore Longitudinal Aging Study reported the results for 890 men. In contrast to the earlier cross-sectional report, this reported data showed a linear decline in both total and free testosterone levels. SHBG levels appeared to increase in a curvilinear fashion over time. The estimated rate of decline was reported as 3.2 ng/dL per year. Gonadotropin levels were not reported.[28]

The Massachusetts Male Aging Study reported data for 1709 men.[29] Results showed that both testosterone and DHEA declined after the age of 40. Testosterone declined 1.6% per year and DHEA fell 2–3% per year. When coupled with a rise in SHBG of 1.6% per year, the free T Index declined faster at 2–3% per year. FSH rose 3% per year and LH rose 1% per year. Estrone remained steady in the cross-sectional analysis but fell 0.8% per year in the longitudinal data (Figure 3.2).

In looking at the above levels of sex hormones and gonadotropins, one must question the physiology of these changes. Obviously these data suggest a change in the hypothalamic–pituitary–gonadal axis but the exact nature of the regulatory changes occurring is an ongoing subject of research.

Inhibin

Inhibins arising from the testis serve as a main feedback mechanism in sex hormone regulation. Inhibin B is produced by the Sertoli cells in response to FSH stimulation. Circulating inhibin B has been correlated with sperm counts, spermatogenesis, and testicular volume in fertile and infertile men.[30–32] Basal levels decrease over time with the steepest drop in the fourth decade then modestly afterward. Inhibin B production is not provoked by LH or hCG in the male testis thus it serves as a measure of testicular reserve, similar to ovarian reserve in women. However, unlike women, this is less tightly linked to fertility potential. Studies suggest that there is only moderate change of semen parameters up to age 50, however, this is a poor surrogate for reproductive potential.[33] Testicular volume can act as a surrogate for tubular volume, and thus spermatogenesis. Studies of testicular volume suggest that there is no significant drop in volume until the eighth decade of life.[34] Thus the drop in testosterone observed seems less a function of Sertoli/Leydig cell number but more of a function or responsiveness to LH and FSH.

Luteinizing hormone

Central defects in the hypothalamic–pituitary axis have been proposed as the cause of hormonal profiles in men. LH secretion has been shown to rise over time but does not always directly correlate to the level of testosterone in older men. Mulligan et al. demonstrated both a central and peripheral effect of aging on the reproductive axis by stimulating LH secretion using pulsatile GnRH infusions in both younger and older men.[35] LH pulse amplitude and frequency could be normalized with

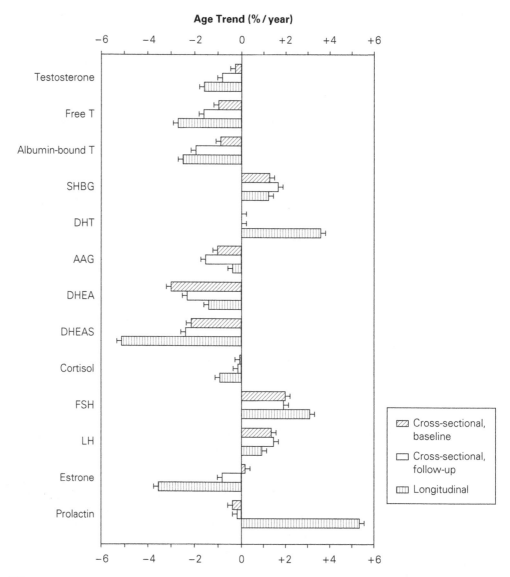

Figure 3.2

Hormonal changes in aging men. Data from the Massachusetts Male Aging Study.[29] SHBG, sex hormone binding globulin; DHT, dihydro testosterone; DHEA(s), dehydro-epiandrosterone (sulfate); FSH, follicle stimulating hormone; LH, luteinizine hormone; AAG, androstanediol glucoronide.

this method but testosterone response was not normalized in the older cohort. This suggests not only a peripheral but also a central defect of the reproductive axis associated with aging. Similar findings using direct LH stimulation in healthy men under GnRH blockade has also been reported.[36]

Dehydroepiandrosterone

Androgen is also produced in the adrenal gland. DHEA is a universal androgen and estrogen precursor transformed by a host of enzymatic systems in peripheral tissues. DHEA levels are

10× higher than plasma cortisol levels in healthy adults. DHEA and its sulfated form are dramatically reduced as men age such that levels are 5× lower than in 20–30-year-olds by age 85.[37] Plasma cortisol is, however, maintained. This drop in DHEA production seems to be a function of decreased numbers of zona reticularis cells rather than a central change in signaling from the hypothalamus.[38] This change also occurs in women.

The clinical impact of this overall drop in sex hormones is felt to be significant. Hypogonadal mid-adult men experience muscle weakness, anemia, decreased bone mass, and mood changes. There is rapid normalization with replacement of testosterone. Similar hormonal changes are seen in elderly men, i.e. decreased muscle strength, muscle mass, decreased bone density, and increased total body fat. There also appears to be an increased rate of depression.[39] Replacement strategies in older men, though, have not been shown to overwhelmingly improve functional status. Androgen treatment either with testosterone or DHEA has been shown to decrease fat mass (6–14%) and increase lean muscle mass (3.2–5%) in most studies. Most studies also document a subjective increase in general sense of well-being in men.[39] Despite these gains, there are few data showing that these replacement regimens improve overall functioning. Safety data for long-term hormone replacement are also lacking.

Ultimately one is left with some general conclusions: serum sex hormone levels decrease with age; the decline is likely due to age-related changes in both the gonads and the hypothalamus; the exact physiology of this interaction remains an area of great research interest both for its implications of male infertility and for decreasing age-related morbidity.

Hormone changes in women

Women, as opposed to men, have a defining marker of reproductive aging in the spontaneous, complete cessation of menstrual flow. This inevitable occurrence is the result of morphologic changes to the ovary and accompanying alterations to the hormonal pathways. The menopausal transition has been further characterized as a progressive series of changes rather than a solitary event. The Stages of Reproductive Aging Workshop (STRAW) proposed a classification system of the menopausal transition. The current classification proposed by STRAW is based on both menstrual cycle pattern and FSH levels (Figure 3.3).[40]

Follicle stimulating hormone

The most striking, albeit silent, change for women still having normal menstrual periods is the progressive rise in early follicular and mid-cycle FSH levels without significant change in LH, estradiol, or progesterone.[41] Although there is a decrease in fertility prior to the onset of increased FSH levels, the monotropic rise in FSH is felt to be the most readily available marker of reproductive aging. Other markers that also have been studied include inhibin B, anti-mullerian hormone and ultrasound antral follicle counts.[42–46] Elevated FHS levels occur late in the reproductive phase of the STRAW staging system and precedes the onset of variable menstrual cycles that are seen early in the perimenopausal stage.

The rise in FSH has been explained by falling levels of inhibin B from the ovary. Inhibin levels fall secondary to the declining number and quality of ovarian follicles and may be thought of as measures of 'ovarian reserve'. Follicular atresia begins before birth and long before puberty. This early, accelerated loss translates into a reduction from a peak of 6–7 million follicles at around 20 weeks' gestation to 1–2 million follicles at birth. This rate of follicular atresia is independent of gonadotropic stimulation. Follicle loss continues throughout the reproductive phase of a woman's life but accelerates again in the thirties and forties.[47] Follicular number in women in this age group with cycle irregularity is approximately one-tenth that of similar aged women with regular cycles. The menstrual irregularity has been linked to the rising FSH recruiting a larger cohort of remaining follicles with a stable or even slightly increased estradiol (E_2) level in older reproductive age women.[41,48,49] An increased E_2 level has been thought to be associated with the breast tenderness experienced at this time. The continued loss of follicular number and decreased function leads to the eventual decline in E_2 levels despite continued rises in FSH.[50–52] By the time menses cease, fewer than 1000 follicles are left.[53] FSH is approximately 50% of its peak level and estradiol will be about 50% of its early follicular phase level.[19] Nadirs in hormone

Final menstrual period
(FMP)

Stages	−5	−4	−3	−2	−1	0	+1	+2
Terminology	Reproductive			Menopausal transition			Postmenopause	
	Early	Peak	Late	Early	Late*		Early*	Late
				Perimenopause				
Duration of stage	Variable			Variable		ⓐ 1 yr	ⓑ 4 years	Until demise
Menstrual cycles	Variable to regular	Regular		Variable cycle length (>7 days different from normal)	≥2 skipped cycles and an interval of amenorrhea (≥60 days)	Amen × 12mos	None	
Endocrine	Normal FSH		↑FSH	↑FSH			↑FSH	

Figure 3.3

Classification of menopausal transition (Stages of Reproductive Aging Workshop[40]).
*Stages most likely to be characterized by vasomotor symptoms; ↑=elevated; FSH, follicle stimulating hormone.

production are reached 2–3 years after the last menstrual period along with peak FSH. Inhibin B and A are also very low or undetectable.

Longitudinal data from the Melbourne Women's Midlife Health Project imply that hot flushes, night sweats, and vaginal dryness are the only symptoms that have been clearly related to the profound drop in E_2 levels seen in the transition between early and late menopause,[54] breast tenderness also decreases around this time. The fall in E_2 levels has most definitively been associated with an accelerated loss of bone mineral density. This accelerated rate of loss may continue for a period of 5–8 years after the last menstrual period.[55]

Androgen

The effects of aging on androgen production in women have much more conflicting data at the present time. Zumoff et al.[56] showed a 50% decline in total testosterone levels in 33 normally cycling women stratified by age. Cross-sectional data from Burger et al. in 1995[57] showed a 1.7% decline in total testosterone for women 45–55

years old. However, when these women were stratified according to menstrual status, women without menstrual flow for at least 3 months had a 16% higher total testosterone level than women with no cycle disturbances. In 1999, a Norwegian longitudinal study of 59 women showed that in the years leading up to the final menstrual period, FSH and LH rose along with declining E_2 levels but also falling rates of DHEAS, androstenedione, testosterone, and SHBG of roughly 15%. Androgen levels then began to rise in the 1–2 years after the final menstrual period. Similar documentation of this postmenopausal rise in androgen levels has both been supported[57–59] and refuted[60,61] in various studies. Burger et al. reported a larger, longitudinal cohort in 2000 that correlated hormonal values in relation to the final menstrual period. Yearly collections in 172 women showed a fall in SHBG and no change in total testosterone or calculated free androgen index over the 6 year follow-up. DHEAS declined 1.5% per year and was not related to menopausal status.

Intracycle variation of androgen production may also be seen as a result of aging. Mushayandebvu et al. reported a loss of the mid-cycle surge of testosterone in women in the decade preceding menopause.[24]

Adrenal and ovarian androgen

The differential role that the adrenals and the ovaries play in this androgen transition may also be less than clear (Figure 3.4). Classically, the postmenopausal ovary is felt to be a gonadotropin-responsive, androgen-secreting organ: thus preservation, if possible, may be beneficial to women in the long run.[63] Couzinet et al. refuted this view in 2001 with a small study of adrenally compromised women either naturally postmenopausal or after oophorectomy and compared them with normal, postmenopausal, or oophorectomized controls. In their analysis, very low to undetectable levels of total testosterone, free testosterone, androstenedione, and DHEA were seen in the adrenal insufficiency cohort regardless of the presence or absence of ovaries. Those women with normal adrenal function had similar androgen levels regardless of ovarian status. No response was measured after hCG administration, and immunohistologic evaluation revealed low to absent levels of both steroidogenic enzymes and LH/FSH receptors.

Taken together, the literature supports a more gradual decline in androgen levels in women in the years leading up to the menopause starting from as early as the third decade of life.[56] This decline slows, stops, and may reverse in the years following the last menstrual period perhaps influenced by elevated levels of LH during this time.[64] Falling DHEA levels appear to be age related and not necessarily associated with menstrual status of the women. Lack of clear data regarding normal androgen physiology and the role of the ovary in androgen production will continue to be a driving force for research in this field. Obviously, absolute levels of hormone may be of less clinical utility than some measure of androgen activity given our current difficulties both with accurate androgen assays and lack of standardized values to base the diagnosis of androgen insufficiency.[65]

Conclusion

Both men and women show age related derangements of sex hormone production and regulation. The health implications for society as a whole given the relationship that these hormones have

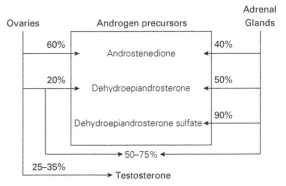

Figure 3.4

Androgen production in women during reproductive years. Most of the testosterone is produced from androgenic precursors created in the adrenal glands and the ovaries. The ovary makes a moderate amount of testosterone directly, but the contribution from the adrenal glands is negligible. Adapted from Davis (1999).[66]

to physical frailty are massive. Whether hormone replacement therapies may play a role in treating age-related decline in hormonal function remains to be fully elucidated.

References

1. World Population Ageing 1950–2050. 2002:xxvii–xxxi. Population Division of the Department of Economic and Social Affairs, United Nations.
2. Schiller JS, Bernadel L, Summary Health Statistics for the U.S. Population: National Health Interview Survey, 2002, in Vital Health Stat 10 (220), 2004.
3. Fried LP, Ferrucci L, Darer J, Williamson JD & Anderson G. Untangling the Concepts of Disability, Frailty, and Comorbidity: Implications for Improved Targeting and Care. J Gerontol Med Sci 2004; 59:255–263.
4. Anderson RN, Smith BL. Deaths: Leading Cases for 2002. Natl Vital Stat Rep 2005; 53:1–89.
5. Buchner DM, Wagner EH, Preventing frail health. Clin Geriatr Med 1992; 8:1–17.
6. Stuck AE, Walthert JM, Nikolaus T et al. Risk factors for functional status decline in community-living elderly people: a systematic literature review. Soc Sci Med 1999; 48:445–469.
7. Lamberts SWJ, Endocrinology and Aging. In: Williams Textbook of Endocrinology, Larsen (Ed.). WB Saunders. 2003:1287–1301.
8. Horani MH, Morley JE, Hormonal fountains of youth. Clin Geriatr Med 2004; 20:275–292.

9. Meachem SJ, Nieschlag E., Simoni M. Inhibin B in male reproduction: pathophysiology and clinical relevance. Eur J Endocrinol 2001; 145:561–71.

10. Hayes FJ, Seminara SB, Decruz S et al. Aromatase inhibition in the human male reveals a hypothalamic site of estrogen feedback. J Clin Endocrinol Metab 2000; 85:3027–3035.

11. Bremner WJ, Vitiello MV, & Prinz PN. Loss of circadian rhythmicity in blood testosterone levels with aging in normal men. J Clin Endocrinol Metabol 1983; 56:1278–1281.

12. Corrigan AZ, Bilezikjian LM, Carroll RS et al. Evidence for an autocrine role of activin B within rat anterior pituitary cultures. Endocrinology 1991; 128:1682–1684.

13. Chong H, Pangas SA, Bernard DJ et al. Structure and expression of a membrane component of the inhibin receptor system. Endocrinology 2000; 141:2600–2607.

14. Lewis KA, Gray PC, Blount AL et al. Betaglycan binds inhibin and can mediate functional antagonism of activin signaling. Nature 2000; 404:411–414.

15. Groome NP, Illingworth PJ, O'Brien M et al. Measurement of dimeric inhibin B throughout the human menstrual cycle. J Clin Endocrinol Metab 1996; 81:1401–1405.

16. Roberts VJ, Barth S, el-Roeiy A, Yen SS. Expression of inhibin/activin subunits and follistatin messenger ribonucleic acids and proteins in ovarian follicles and the corpus luteum during the human menstrual cycle. J Clin Endocrinol Metab 1993; 77:1402–1410.

17. Hurwitz JM, Santoro N, Inhibins, activins, and follistatin in the aging female and male. Semin Reprod Med 2004; 22:209–217.

18. Bilezikjian LM, Blount AL, Corrigan AZ, et al. Actions of activins, inhibins and follistatins: implications in anterior pituitary function. Clin Exp Pharmacol Physiol 2001; 28:244–248.

19. Burger HG, Dudley E, Mamers P et al. The ageing female reproductive axis I. Novartis Found Symp 2002; 242:161–171.

20. Judd HL, Judd GE, Lucas WE, Yen SSC. Endocrine function of the post-menopausal ovary. Concentrations of androgens and estrogens in ovarian and peripheral venous blood. J Clin Endocrinol Metab 1974; 39:1020–1024.

21. Abraham GE. Ovarian and adrenal contribution to peripheral androgens during the menstrual cycle. J Clin Endocrinol Metab 1974; 39:340–346.

22. Judd HL, Yen SS, Serum androstenedione and testosterone levels during the menstrual cycle. J Clin Endocrinol Metab 1973; 36:475–481.

23. Sinha-Hikim I, Arver S, Beall G et al. The use of a sensitive equilibrium dialysis method for the measurement of free testosterone levels in healthy, cycling women and in human immunodeficiency virus-infected women. J Clin Endocrinol Metab 1998; 83:1312–1318.

24. Mushayandebvu T, Castracane VD, Gimpel T et al. Evidence for diminished midcycle ovarian androgen production in older reproductive aged women. Fertil Steril 1996; 65:721–723.

25. Harman SM, Tsitouras PD, Reproductive hormones in aging men. Measurement of sex steroids, basal luteinizing hormone, and Leydig cell response to human chorionic gonadotropin. J Clin Endocrinol Metab 1980; 51:35–41.

26. Morley JE, Kaiser FE, Perry III HM et al. Longitudinal changes in testosterone, luteinizing hormone, and follicle–stimulating hormone in healthy older men. Metabolism 1997; 46:410–413.

27. Zmuda JM, Cavely JA, Kriska A, et al. Kriska A. Longitudinal relation between endogenous testosterone and cardiovascular disease risk factors in middle aged men. A 13-year follow-up of former multiple risk factor intervention trial participants. Am J Epidemiol 1997; 146:609–617.

28. Harman SM, Melter EJ, Tobin JD et al. Longitudinal effects of aging on serum total and free testosterone levels in healthy men. J Clin Endocrinol Metab 2001; 86:724–731.

29. Feldman HA, Longcope C, Derby CA et al. Age trends in the level of serum testosterone and other hormones in middle-aged men: longitudinal results from the Massachusetts Male Aging Study. J Clin Endocrinol Metab 2002; 87:589–598.

30. Anawalt BD, Bebb RA, Matsumoto AM, et al. Serum inhibin B levels reflect Sertoli cell function in normal men and men with testicular dysfunction. J Clin Endocrinol Metab 1996; 81:3341–3345.

31. Hayes FJ, Pitteloud N, DeCruz S et al. Importance of inhibin B in the regulation of FSH secretion in the human male. J Clin Endocrinol Metab 2001; 86:5541–5546.

32. Illingworth PJ, Groome NP, Byrd W, et al. Inhibin B: a likely candidate for the physiologically important form of inhibin in men. J Clin Endocrinol Metab 1996; 81:11321–1325.

33. Handelsman DJ. Male reproductive ageing: Human fertility, androgens, and hormone dependent disease. Novartis Foundation Symposium 242 2002; 66–81.

34. Handelsman DJ, Staraj S, Testicular Size: the effects of aging, malnutrition, and Illness. J Androl 1985; 6:144–151.

35. Mulligan T, Iranmanesh A, Kerzner R, et al. Two-week pulsatile gonadotropin releasing hormone infusion unmasks dual (hypothalamic and Leydig cell) defects in the healthy aging male gonadotropic axis. Eur J Endocrinol 1999; 141:257–266.

36. Veldhuis JD, Veldhuis NJ, Keenan DM, Iranmanesh A. Age diminishes the testicular steroidogenic response to repeated intravenous pulses of recombinant human LH during acute GnRH-receptor blockade in healthy men. Am J Physiol Endocrinol Metab 2005; 288:E775–E781.

37. Ravaglia G, Forti P, Maioli F et al. The relationship of dehydroepiandrosterone sulfate (DHEAS) to endocrine-metabolic parameters and functional status in the oldest-old. Results from an Italian study on healthy free-living over-ninety-year-olds. J Clin Endocrinol Metab 1996; 81:1173–1178.

38. Hornsby PJ. Biosynthesis of DHEAS by the human adrenal cortex and its age-related decline. Ann NY Acad Sci 1995; 774:29–46.

39. van den Beld AW, Lamberts SW, Endocrine aspects of healthy ageing in men. Novartis Foundation Symposium 2002; 242:3–25.

40. Soules MR, Sherman S, Parrott E et al. Executive summary: Stages of Reproductive Aging Workshop (STRAW). Fertil Steril 2001; 76:874–878.

41. Lee SJ, Lenton EA, Sexton L, et al. The effect of age on the cyclical patterns of plasma LH, FSH, oestradiol and progesterone in women with regular menstrual cycles. Hum Reprod 1988; 3:851–855.

42. van Rooij IA, Tonkelaar I, Broekmans FJ, et al. Anti-mullerian hormone is a promising predictor for the occurrence of the menopausal transition. Menopause 2004; 11:601–606.

43. van Rooij IA, Broekmans FJ, te Velde ER et al. Serum anti-Mullerian hormone levels: a novel measure of ovarian reserve. Hum Reprod 2002; 17:3065–3071.

44. Welt CK, McNicholl DJ, Taylor AE, et al. Female reproductive aging is marked by decreased secretion of dimeric inhibin. J Clin Endocrinol Metab 1999; 84:105–111.

45. de Vet A, Laven JS, de Jong FH et al. Anti-mullerian hormone serum levels: a putative marker for ovarian aging. Fertil Steril 2002; 77:357–362.

46. Scheffer GJ, Broekmans FJ, Dorland M et al. Antral follicle counts by transvaginal ultrasonography is related to age in women with proven natural fertility. Fertil Steril 1999; 72:845–851.

47. Richardson SJ, Senikas V, Nelson JF. Follicular depletion during the menopausal transition: evidence for accelerated loss and ultimate exhaustion. J Clin Endocrinol Metab 1987; 65:1231–1237.

48. Klein NA, Illingworth PJ, Groome NP et al. Decreased inhibin B secretion is associated with the monotropic FSH rise in older, ovulatory women: a study of serum and follicular fluid levels of dimeric inhibin A and B in spontaneous menstrual cycles. J Clin Endocrinol Metab 1996; 81:2742–2745.

49. Lenton EA, de Kretser DM, Woodward AJ, et al. Robertson DM. Inhibin concentrations throughout the menstrual cycles of normal, infertile, and older women compared with those during spontaneous conception cycles. J Clin Endocrinol Metab 1991; 73:1180–1190.

50. Burger HG, Dudley EC, Hopper JL et al. Prospectively measured levels of serum follicle-stimulating hormone, estradiol, and the dimeric inhibins during the menopausal transition in a population-based cohort of women. J Clin Endocrinol Metab 1999; 84: 4025–4030.

51. MacNaughton J, Banah M, McCloud P, et al. Age related changes in follicle stimulating hormone, luteinizing hormone, oestradiol and immunoreactive inhibin in women of reproductive age. Clin Endocrinol 1992; 36:339–345.

52. Sherman BM, West JH, Korenman SG. The menopausal transition: analysis of LH, FSH, estradiol, and progesterone concentrations during menstrual cycles of older women. J Clin Endocrinol Metab 1976; 42:629–636.

53. Faddy MJ, Gosden RG, Gougeon A et al. Accelerated disappearance of ovarian follicles in mid-life: implications for forecasting menopause. Hum Reprod 1992; 7:1342–1346.

54. Dennerstein L, Dudley EC, Hopper JL et al. A prospective population-based study of menopausal symptoms. Obstet Gynecol 2000; 96:351–358.

55. Guthrie JR, Ebeling PR, Hopper JL et al. A prospective study of bone loss in menopausal Australian-born women. Osteoporosis Int 1998; 8:282–290.

56. Zumoff B, Strain GW, Miller LK, et al. Twenty-four-hour mean plasma testosterone concentration declines with age in normal premenopausal women. J Clin Endocrinol Metab 1995; 80:1429–1430.

57. Burger HG, Dudley EC, Hopper JL et al. The endocrinology of the menopausal transition: a cross-sectional study of a population-based sample. J Clin Endocrinol Metab1995; 80:3537–3545.

58. Jiroutek MR, Chen MH, Johnston CC, et al. Changes in reproductive hormones and sex hormone-binding globulin in a group of postmenopausal women measured over 10 years. Menopause 1998; 5:90–94.

59. Laughlin GA, Barrett-Connor E, Silverstein D, et al. Hysterectomy, oophorectomy, and endogenous sex hormone levels in older women: the Rancho Bernardo Study. J Clin Endocrinol Metab 2000; 85:645–651.

60. Longcope C, Franz C, Morello C et al. Steroid and gonadotropin levels in women during the peri-menopausal years. Maturitas 1986; 8:189–196.

61. Bancroft J, Cawood EH, Androgens and the menopause; a study of 40–60-year-old women. Clin Endocrinol 1996; 45:577–587.

62. Guay A, Davis SR, Testosterone insufficiency in women: fact or fiction? World J Urol 2002; 20:106–110.

63. Adashi EY. The climacteric ovary as a functional gonadotropin-driven androgen-producing gland. Fertil Steril 1994; 62:20–27.

64. Davison SL, Davis SR, Androgens in women. J Steroid Biochem Mol Biol 2003; 85:363–366.

65. Bachmann G, Bancroft J, Braunstein G et al. Female androgen insufficiency: the Princeton consensus statement on definition, classification, and assessment. Fertil Steril 2002; 77:660–665.

66. Danis SR. Androgen treatment in women. Med J Aust 1999; 170:545–549.

Chapter 4

Androgen receptor expression in women and its relationship to sexual function

Crista E Johnson and Jennifer R Berman

Summary

Androgens play a vital role in maintaining women's sexual health and overall wellbeing. Basic science research and clinical trials have begun to delineate the role of androgens in women throughout the reproductive cycle. The pathophysiologic mechanism of androgen receptor expression has been documented in numerous tissue sites including the central nervous system, vagina, pelvic floor, lower urinary and reproductive tracts, as well as in breast tissue, bone, muscle, and the cardiovascular system. The impact of advancing age and estrogens on androgen bioavailability, as well as the psychophysiologic role of androgen receptor expression on sexual function demands further research to better define treatment paradigms for improving the quality of life for women across the reproductive life cycle.

Introduction

In recent years, increased attention to women's sexual health has propelled basic science research and clinical trials exploring paradigms for improving quality of life amidst a growing population of menopausal women. As the prevalence of female sexual dysfunction has become manifest, the knowledge of the intricate pathophysiologic role of androgens has fostered a clearer understanding of the biosynthesis pathways and mechanism of action of the androgen receptor and its impact on numerous tissue and cellular sites throughout the body. Understanding androgen physiology and the pathways by which advancing age and medical conditions can alter androgen production will aid in the comprehension of the impact of androgens on female sexual health.

Androgen biosynthesis pathways in women

Androgens are important for the development of reproductive function and hormonal homeostasis, and are the precursors for the biosynthesis of estrogens. The physiologic role of androgens in women is confounded by the fact that synthesis and metabolism of androgens take place in three compartments: the ovary, adrenal glands, and peripheral tissues; this suggests a complex regulation of androgen synthesis by various organs, tissues, and enzymes involved in biotransformation. The major androgens in women, in descending order of serum concentration, include: dehydroepiandrosterone sulfate (DHEAS), dehydroepiandrosterone (DHEA), androstenedione, testosterone, and 5α-dihydrotestosterone (DHT). Androgen secretion is regulated by stimulation from the adrenocorti-cotropic hormone (ACTH) to the adrenal glands, and by the luteinizing hormone (LH) to the ovary, along with other intraglandular autocrine and paracrine mechanisms.[1] Testosterone and DHT have the most potent biologic activity of the androgenic steroids. In women, approximately 25% of androgen biosynthesis occurs in the ovaries, 25% is produced by the adrenal gland, and the remainder is produced in the peripheral tissue. Circulating testosterone functions as a prohormone, converting to DHT or estradiol in target tissues. Furthermore, testosterone can be synthesized in target tissue on demand; consequently resulting in levels of plasma testosterone which may not provide the critical information on the availability of other metabolites. DHEAS, DHEA, and androstenedione are the major sources of peripheral androgen production in women.

Serum androgens may be either unbound or bound, and it is the unbound androgens that are biologically active to exert their effects on target tissue. Following secretion from the adrenal glands and ovaries, testosterone is strongly bound by sex hormone binding globulin (SHBG) in the peripheral blood such that only ~1% of testosterone and DHT circulates freely. SHBG has a low capacity, but high affinity, for testosterone, and has a low affinity for androstenedione, DHEA and DHEAS.[2]

Androgens have been shown to regulate the development, growth, and maintenance of secondary sex characteristics as well as modulate the physiologic function of multiple receptors and tissue sites including the central nervous system, bone, breast, pilosebaceous unit, skeletal muscle, adipose tissues, and genital organs and tissues. Androgens not only have direct effects on target sites, but also their effects on these tissues may be mediated by its conversion to estrogens. Hence an imbalance in androgen biosynthesis or metabolism may have ill-effects on female general health, wellbeing, and sexual function.

Biochemical mechanism of androgen action

Androgens enter target and nontarget cells by passive diffusion, and once inside the cell, the biologically active androgens (testosterone, DHT) bind to a specific, soluble intracellular receptor protein molecule localized in the cytoplasm or in the nucleus.[3-6] The binding energy of the hormone to its receptor results in physiochemical changes in the receptor complex, converting the receptor from a biologically inactive form to a biologically active state.[3-6] These reactions initiated by hormone binding lead to interaction of the hormone receptor complex with unique and specific DNA enhancer elements referred to as androgen response elements (AREs).[4,7] The interaction of the activated androgen receptor complex with the AREs results in recruitment and binding of transcriptional factors, coactivators, or corepressors into the transcriptional complex and regulation of androgen-dependent gene transcription.[4,8]

Structural and functional domains of the androgen receptor

Androgens exert their effects by first binding to androgen receptors (AR). The *AR* gene is located on the X chromosome with no corresponding allele on the Y, so it functions solely as a single-copy gene, as shown by the complete loss of androgen effect in XY individuals with an inactivating mutation of the AR.[9] The AR, which comprises 918 amino acids with an estimated molecular weight of 110 kDa,[4] is a ligand-dependent nuclear transactivating factor and a member of the steroid-thyroid hormone-retinoic acid nuclear receptor superfamily.[3,5-8] The members of this superfamily are characterized by distinct functional domains comprised within a unique protein structure which includes: the hormone-binding domain, DNA-binding domain, and amino terminal domain encompassing a transactivation function, the nuclear localization domain, and the dimerization domain.[4]

The hormone-binding domain is located near the carboxyl terminal region and comprises a hydrophobic region, which forms the hormone-binding site.[4] The two predominant and naturally occurring androgens that bind to the AR are testosterone and DHT. In vivo and in vitro studies have demonstrated that DHT binds with greater affinity to the AR than testosterone and is more potent in inducing biologic responses.[10,11] The higher potency of DHT is attributed to DHT binding to the AR with greater affinity and thereby dissociating more slowly, and the AR–DHT complex being more stable.[12]

The AR gene shares significant homology with both the estrogen receptor and progesterone receptor genes. Two isoforms of the AR have been identified in a variety of human tissues and are similar in structure to the isoforms of the progesterone receptor. Despite the differences in structure and abundance, the two AR isoforms do not appear to differ in their regulation or in their ability to bind with ligands and activate target genes.[13]

Recent studies have suggested that different genes may be activated by different ligands and that this may be reconciled by the presence of cell-specific and limiting transcription factors and coactivators. In addition, the local concentration of the androgen hormone depends on the expression and activity of steroid-converting enzymes such as dehydrogenases and reductases; the latter of which play important roles in the peripheral conversion of androgens to active or inactive metabolites. Furthermore, the tissue and cell-specific expression of different coactivators or corepressors in different target cells plays an important role in specific gene expression by androgens in various target tissues. The conformational changes in the hormone receptor complex are induced by ligand binding of testosterone versus DHT. The energy of binding and the conformational changes in the protein determine which transcriptional factors, coactivators, and corepressors are to be assembled in the transcription complex and determine which genes are regulated by androgens and therefore act as a discriminatory mechanism of gene activation.[4]

The DNA-binding domain, a region highly conserved among all members of this superfamily, consists of 68 amino acids. This region folds into a tertiary structure resulting in the formation of two distinct zinc fingers that bind to the DNA in the major groove. The first zinc finger confers specificity, while the second zinc finger contributes to an increased binding affinity for DNA.[2–6] The AR binds to the palindromic ARE in a dimer form and in a cooperative manner, which is suited to interaction with the ARE half-sites of the palindromic response elements.[4]

Several other regions of the AR protein contribute to stabilization of the dimer molecule, among which include the ligand-binding domain and the loop of the second zinc finger.[3–7] Considerable homology exists between the DNA-binding domain of AR and that of progesterone, glucocorticoid, and mineralocorticoid receptors. Hence, regulation of gene expression by these proteins involves a complex mechanism that requires interaction of the transactivation domains with other accessory factors such as transcriptional factors, coactivators, and corepressors.[3–8]

The transactivational functional domain (TAF1) of the AR is localized in the amino terminal region of which unique sequences within this region interact with transcription factors and other accessory coactivators and corepressors.[4] A second transactivation functional domain (TAF2) is localized to the hormone-binding region. Consequently, regulation of gene expression by the AR and the physiologic response to androgens which is observed in various target tissues may be modulated by one or all of the following factors: binding of a specific ligand (testosterone versus DHT) to the AR, tissue-specific expression of the AR, differential binding of AR to AREs, or tissue and cell-specific expression of accessory transcriptional factors (coactivators and corepressors) necessary for interactions with the transactivation domain of the AR.[4]

Effect of age on androgen status

Advancing age has a much larger impact on androgen status than menopause. Several studies have examined androgen changes across the menopausal transition. Total testosterone does not change appreciably until women are much older (71–95 years of age), while androstenedione levels decrease much earlier.[14] Mean 24-h levels of testosterone decrease in women from age 20 to age 50, however this decline reflects aging, in that the ratio of DHEAS/T is constant over this time span.[15] DHEA and DHEAS concentrations begin to decline in the second decade of life, and by the age of 80, serum levels are approximately 20–30% of peak levels.[15] Data from a large longitudinal study demonstrate a 13% decline in mean DHEAS and a 46% decline in mean testosterone levels between the ages of 42 and 50.[16] These data confirm that although aging affects levels of testosterone, these levels are not much different before and after the menopause transition, and the small reduction in ovarian production is thought to result from declines in androstenedione.[14]

Androgen function in the postmenopausal ovary

Androgens are produced by ovarian theca lutein cells, are present in ovarian follicular fluid, and are the principal sex steroid of growing follicles. AR are found in the normal surface epithelium of the ovaries, suggesting that androgens are active in the organ. It is currently believed that after menopause, the ovaries are a major site of androgen production.[18–23] In the postmenopausal ovary, the loss of ovarian follicles and granulosa cells eliminates its estrogen-producing ability.[24] However, secondary interstitial cells and hilar cells may persist in the postmenopausal ovary;[25] which for many years were thought to remain continuously activated by the high levels of circulating LH, and thus remained steroidogenically active.[19] Furthermore, some of the most convincing data which suggested an important contribution of the postmenopausal ovary to steroidogenesis came from the analysis of ovarian and peripheral vein hormone levels.[26] However, postmenopausal ovaries are atrophic with limited blood flow. Hence ovarian vein sampling may be difficult and cross-contamination of adrenal venous blood can occur at the sampling site. Thus, herein lies the difficulty in assessing true hormonal activity in the postmenopausal population.[27]

The reduction in postmenopausal ovarian androgen production is not precipitous. Instead, ovarian testosterone production decreases slowly over the 5–10 years following the last menstrual period, whereas ovarian androstenedione production decreases substantially more at the time of menopause than does testosterone production.[28] Couzinet et al.[24] has recently concluded that the commonly held belief of a consistent and significant androgenic capability of the postmenopausal ovary is false. He demonstrated that in the absence of adrenal function, postmenopausal women averaging 12 years after menopause had no detectable circulating androgens and that their postmenopausal ovaries were devoid of gonadotropin receptors and steroidogenic enzymes.[24] These observations suggest that the postmenopausal ovary as early as 5 years after menopause is not a source of androgens. Instead, postmenopausal androgens are derived primarily from an adrenal rather than ovarian source.[15]

Furthermore, it is important to also consider that most of the androgens in women, particularly after menopause are synthesized in peripheral tissues from DHEAS and DHEA.[29] In this fashion, DHEA and DHEAS are converted into more potent androgens or estrogens in peripheral target tissues, and they exert their action in the same cells in which their synthesis took place without significant diffusion into the circulation – a process defined as intracrine production.[27] Consequently, this process may limit the interpretation of serum levels of active sex steroids as the sex steroids made in peripheral tissues may never enter the circulation, but are instead inactivated locally into more water-soluble compounds which then diffuse into the general circulation where they can be measured.[27]

On the other hand, realization of the precursor role of circulating androgenic steroids leads to the prediction that lower than average levels of these steroids could lead to inadequate synthesis of estradiol in peripheral tissues such as bone and brain. Changes that have been traditionally considered ensuing sequelae of estrogen insufficiency, such as loss of bone mineralization and possibly changes in brain-derived functions, may paradoxically turn out to be a consequence of insufficiency of circulating androgenic steroids.[30]

In addition, genetic and ethnic variation has been demonstrated in postmenopausal ovarian androgenic activity. Recent studies have shown that DHEAS levels are related to ovarian function in older women which varies with ethnicity.[17,31] In defining the relationship of adrenal steroid production during declining ovarian function, Lasley et al. demonstrated that log circulating DHEAS concentrations were highest among Chinese and Japanese women, and lowest among African–American and Hispanic women in a prospective cohort of 3029 women between the ages of 42 and 54 across five ethnic groups;[17] and this pattern persisted after adjustment for age, smoking, and log body mass index (BMI).

Impact of estrogen on androgen bioavailability

Estrogens play an important role in maintaining genital sensation, blood flow and function; as vaginal wall thickness, rugae and lubrication have been shown to be estrogen dependent.[4,32–35] Low estrogen levels are associated with sexual complaints during menopause, particularly vaginal dryness and dyspareunia,[36] due to thinning of the vaginal walls, diminished vaginal acidity with resultant vulnerability to infection, trauma, and decreased ability to heal.[37] Estrogen may affect smooth muscle cell growth in the vagina and the clitoris, regulate connective tissue metabolism and nitric oxide synthesis, and may be important in maintaining the functional integrity of vaginal and clitoral smooth muscle function.[4]

In premenopausal women, the ovaries are the principal source of estrogen, which functions as a circulating hormone to act on distal target tissues.[30] However in postmenopausal women, the primary source of estrogen is from the aromatization of DHEA, androstenedione, and testosterone to estrone and estradiol in the peripheral tissues, which include adipose tissues, osteoblasts and chondrocytes of bone, the vascular epithelium and aortic smooth muscle cells, and numerous sites in the brain. This circulating estrogen originates in extragonadal sites where it acts locally and enters the circulation if it escapes local metabolism;[30] consequently reflecting, instead of directing, estrogen action in postmenopausal women. Consequently, circulating levels of testosterone, androstenedione, DHEA, and DHEAS become extremely important in terms of providing adequate substrate for estrogen biosynthesis in these sites. The increased aromatase activity following menopause results in the peripheral tissues taking on a greater role in the production of estrogen compared with this process in younger women.[28] This increased aromatase activity is due to the progressive increase in body fat with aging, and an increase in aromatase activity per unit of fat with decreased endogenous estrogen.[38] Increased total body fat has an inverse effect on SHBG, in that the greater the BMI, the lower the SHBG concentration,[39] which has significant implications for the bioavailability of androgens.[28]

Estrogen therapy has been shown to provide significant relief of menopausal somatic symptoms, such as hot flashes, night sweats, and vaginal dryness.[28] However, it often does not provide adequate restoration of sexual desire, potentially because of its effect on SHBG and androgens. Estrogen replacement therapy, particularly at higher doses, and when administered orally (as oral contraceptives or hormone replacement therapy), increases SHBG thereby increasing the binding of testosterone; and decreases the endogenous production, metabolism, and bioavailability, of both ovarian and adrenal androgens.[28,40–42]

Effect of androgens on the central nervous system, mood, and psychosexual function

Androgens appear to play a key role in the psychophysiology of women before and after menopause. The effects of androgens on the brain are mediated through androgen receptors as well as by the aromatization of testosterone to estrogen. The cortical and pituitary actions of androgens are mediated through the AR. ARs have been identified in the cortex, pituitary, hypothalamus, preoptic region, thalamus, amygdala, and brain stem. Hypothalamic and limbic system aromatization leads to estrogen receptor-mediated actions. Androgen effects in the brain influence sexual behavior, libido, temperature control, sleep control, assertiveness, cognitive function, and learning capacities, including visuospatial skills and language fluency.[43]

The relation between mood and symptoms of menopause including depression, mood swings, irritability, lethargy, difficulty concentration, insomnia, anxiety and loss of sexual function has been studied extensively. The biologic factors influencing mood disorders and menopause are based on the premise that alterations in reproductive hormone activity cause changes in mood and behavior as a result of their impact on central neurotransmitter release.[44] In addition, psychosocial factors also have an impact on mood in postmenopausal women as there may be variation in sensitivity to sudden (oophorectomy) versus gradual (natural menopause) decline in ovarian function as symptoms of depression may significantly increase after surgical menopause.[45] Furthermore, women who have undergone surgical menopause have been shown to demonstrate lower levels of androgens than age-matched, naturally menopausal women.[46]

Androgens play an important role in women's sexual functioning, particularly sexual desire, as the psychologic significance of loss of sexual function can have profound impact on a woman's psychosexual health. Many studies have sought to delineate the role of androgens in maintaining sexual function. Increasing evidence suggests that women with androgen insufficiency not only experience alleviation of their psychologic symptoms but also note improvement in concentration, energy, fatigue, libido, sexual response, and wellbeing with androgen replacement therapy.[47]

Androgen receptor expression in vaginal tissue

Although androgens influence clitoral, labial, and vaginal physiology, its role in female sexual function is controversial and poorly understood. There is limited biochemical and physiologic data on the role of androgens in regulating female genital tissue structure and in modulating female genital sexual response. However, improved libido and orgasmic response as well as increased sexual satisfaction have been reported in women undergoing androgen therapy to alleviate menopausal symptoms.

Hemodynamic events during genital sexual arousal are regulated by estrogens and enhanced by androgen supplementation.[33,34], Furthermore, genital sexual arousal in women, which is characterized by an increase in genital blood flow, leads to vasocongestion of the vagina, vulva, and clitoris, and increased genital sensation, vaginal lengthening, and lubrication.[4] Changes in the hormonal milieu can alter these physiologic processes. Vaginal lubrication is a combination of basal mucin production and vaginal vascular transudate, which constitutes the major estrogen-dependent lubrication component during genital arousal: while mucin production and proliferation of vaginal epithelial cells are regulated by androgens.[48,49]

Immunohistochemical detection of androgen and estrogen receptors in vaginal tissues has been reported.[50] In animal models, the labia majora, labia minora, and vagina stain positive for the androgen receptor and vaginal epithelium responds to testosterone replacement in a similar manner to estrogen replacement, even in the absence of estrogen.[51] Although ARs are present in the human vagina, it is unclear whether testosterone acts directly on the receptor or by conversion to DHT or aromatization to estrogen. The enzymes necessary for metabolism of testosterone, aromatase and 5α-reductase, have been found to be expressed in the human vagina, which suggests that they play a role in the conversion of testosterone to DHT and estrogen in the vagina. The presence of aromatase mRNA indicates that some of the effects of testosterone in the vagina are also mediated through conversion to estrogen. In estrogen-depleted women, this residual source of estrogen could be beneficial. Varying levels of aromatase in the vagina may help to explain why postmenopausal women receiving hormone therapy present with different degrees of vaginal maturation and atrophy, sometimes requiring the addition of topical estrogen therapy.[51]

Berman et al.[51] confirmed the presence of ARs, mediating both testosterone and DHT actions, in

the human vagina, with their density affected by age, menopausal status, and estrogen replacement. Postmenopausal women receiving oral or transdermal estrogen replacement had lower vaginal androgen receptor densities than those who were not. This suggests that estrogen replacement may downregulate vaginal ARs. Fewer ARs in vaginal subepithelium of women on hormone therapy may result from estrogenic stimulation of SHBG, leading to less free testosterone and therefore, less production of ARs.[52] Furthermore, the current study revealed that androgen density is lower in the mucosa of postmenopausal women, irrespective of type or route of hormone therapy. Hence a reduction of androgen receptors in postmenopausal women combined with a gradual age-related decline in serum androgen levels in women may further decrease the androgen responsiveness of vaginal tissue.

Nitric oxide, vasoactive intestinal peptide (VIP), and serotonin are among several biochemical factors implicated in the signaling pathway of genital smooth muscle relaxation. Nitric oxide, which is a product of the conversion of arginine by nitric oxide synthase, has been recognized as an important molecule with a broad range of functions in the lower urinary tract and vagina. Estrogens may affect smooth muscle cell growth in the vagina and the clitoris as well as regulate connective tissue metabolism and nitric oxide synthesis, which may be important in maintaining the functional integrity of vaginal and clitoral smooth muscle function.[4] Thickness, rugae of the vaginal wall, and vaginal lubrication have been shown to be estrogen dependent as estrogen deficiency results in thin vaginal walls which are more susceptible to trauma, impaired healing, and a less acidic environment predisposed to infection. Vaginal epithelium of ovariectomized mice treated with testosterone or aromatase inhibitors demonstrate an increased number of layers, thickness, and mitotic rates compared with controls.[51] In addition, estrogen replacement therapy has been shown to increase pelvic blood flow in menopausal women and in women with surgical or medical oophorectomy.[37]

The physiologic response in vaginal tissues to androgens is also mediated by specific ARs. These effects may be related to maintenance of nonvascular smooth muscle function in the vagina and of vascular smooth muscle in the clitoris. Traish et al.[4] characterized androgen expression in proximal and distal vaginal tissues from control and ovariectomized animals treated with or without estrogen and/or androgen replacement therapy. It was demonstrated that androgens enhance nitric oxide synthase expression and activity and downregulated arginase (a substrate for nitric oxide synthase) activity in the proximal vagina, which may be manifested in facilitation of vaginal smooth muscle relaxation to electric field stimulation and VIP in androgen-treated animals. Estrogens, on the other hand, downregulate nitric oxide synthase activity and increase arginase activity which may result in attenuation of vaginal tissue relaxation to electric field stimulation and to VIP.[4] These observations suggest that androgens play an important role in modulating the physiology of vaginal tissue and may contribute to modulation of the genital sexual response in women.

Androgen receptor expression in the female pelvic floor and lower urinary tract

Disorders of the pelvic floor, including urinary and fecal incontinence as well as pelvic organ prolapse are major health problems for women, as the incidence of these disorders increase with age, particularly in postmenopausal women. Muscles of the pelvic floor and lower urinary tract are involved in the support of the pelvic organs and micturition, and damage to these muscles or lack of hormonal stimulation may cause pelvic organ prolapse and/or urinary incontinence in women.

The presence of ARs in levator ani muscle in animal rat models is well documented and have been used widely as a bioassay of androgenic activity.[52,54] In fact, higher levels of AR expression have been found in the levator ani muscle than in other skeletal muscles of the rat. Furthermore, androgen responsiveness depends not only on the AR expression within the particular muscle, but also on the particular cell type within that muscle.[55] ARs have also been found in the urethral and trigonal epithelium, detrusor muscle, and smooth muscle of the urethra in rabbits.[56] In addition, studies on male rats have demonstrated that ARs and β-estrogen receptors were coexpressed in the urothelium, neurons, bladder smooth muscle cells, and proximal urethra striated muscle

cells, suggesting that androgens may play an important role in the regulation of voiding function either by direct effects and/or indirect effects through interaction with estrogen in the lower urinary tract.[52,57]

Nnodim demonstrated the marked changes in muscle mass of the levator ani that occurs after castration and testosterone supplementation in rats.[53,54] In the group of denervated levator ani muscle but gonad-intact rats, myofiber cross-sectional area was markedly diminished and satellite cell nuclei increased significantly. In the group of castrated rats, pronounced myofiber atrophy was observed but satellite cells were not affected. The combination of castration and denervation of levator ani produced the same degree of myofiber atrophy as denervation alone but had no impact on the satellite cells. These results demonstrated that removal of androgen source caused an atrophic effect on levator ani in a similar fashion as denervation as well as diminished the muscle's ability to recruit and proliferate satellite cells. The administration of exogenous testosterone to the castrated adult rats restored the myofiber cross-sectional areas and increased satellite cell proliferation. Hence the anabolic effects of androgen play an important role in the levator ani of rats.

In human studies, the expression of AR in levator ani muscle and its fascia has been shown. Copas et al. demonstrated the expression of androgen and progesterone receptors in the striated muscle fibers, stromal cells and fascia of levator ani. Estrogen receptors were also present in the stromal cells and fascia of the levator ani, but not in the muscle fibers.[58] Ewies et al. compared the expression of androgen receptors in human cardinal ligaments of prolapsed uteri with nonprolapsed controls[59] and demonstrated that the cardinal ligaments of women with uterine prolapse expressed three to four times more androgen receptors than women without prolapse, implying that androgens may play a role in pelvic organ prolapse.

Androgens may also play a role in stress urinary incontinence as urinary levels of androgens have been demonstrated to be significantly higher in postmenopausal patients with stress urinary incontinence compared to postmenopausal women without incontinence. Concentrations of androgen metabolites in the urine of patients with incontinence were positively related to bladder neck descencus as measured by perineal ultrasound.[60]

Androgen receptor expression in endometrial cancer

Androgens are aromatized to estrogens in several tissues, including the endometrium. During menopause, extraglandular production of estrogens may play a role in the development of certain forms of endometrial carcinoma that depend on estrogenic stimulation for their growth. Therefore, local intratumor aromatization of androgens may play a critical role in stimulating the growth of estrogen-dependent endometrial carcinomas.

Maia et al. demonstrated immunohistochemical presence of ARs in the stroma of nonmalignant endometrium which is in accordance with previous studies indicating that the levels of mRNA transcripts for ARs are much higher in the endometrial stromal cells than in the glandular epithelium.[61] However in endometrioid endometrial adenocarcinoma, there is a shift of ARs towards the malignant epithelium with little staining of the intervening stroma, which may suggest a role for ARs in the mechanism of cellular growth in estrogen-dependent endometrial carcinomas. Previous studies have shown that the stimulatory effects of testosterone on the growth of certain cell lines of endometrial carcinoma in vitro were only observed in tumors that were capable of responding to estrogens.[62] This stimulatory effect was dependent on the presence of an aromatase enzymatic system capable of converting androgens into estrogens. Thus intratumor aromatization of androgen precursors may therefore generate a hyperestrogenic milieu in the carcinoma, stimulating tumor growth during menopause despite the presence of low plasma levels of estrogens. Consequently during menopause, as most estrogens originate from the extraglandular conversion of androgen precursors, patients with estrogen-dependent endometrial carcinoma will demonstrate strong immunohistochemical staining for testosterone receptors in the glandular epithelium.[61]

Androgen receptor expression in ovarian cancer

Epidemiological evidence supports the possibility of an androgen–ovarian cancer link as most ovarian cancers express ARs, and antiandrogens inhibit ovarian cancer growth.[13] Oral contraceptives, the most effective chemoprotective agents against ovarian cancer, suppress ovarian testosterone production by 35–70%.[13] In contrast, there is evidence that the AR gene may have an ovarian tumor suppressor function. Androgen receptor mRNA and protein are downregulated in ovarian cancer. Furthermore, loss of heterozygosity in the region containing the gene has been reported in approximately 40% of ovarian cancers. In addition, nonrandom X-inactivation has been reported in invasive ovarian cancer, with expression potentially favoring the allele producing the less active receptor protein.[13] While androgens, acting through ARs have been implicated in the disease, progestins, acting through progesterone receptors, may provide protection against the disease. Based on mounting evidence in support of the role of androgens and progestins in ovarian cancer, polymorphisms in the androgen and progesterone receptor genes may act as risk factors for ovarian cancer and/or as modifiers of risk associated with exposure to hormonal factors including oral contraceptive use, parity, and BRCA 1/2 mutation status.[13] Future studies across large, diverse populations are necessary to identify more precisely the contribution of genetic factors and/or environmental exposures to the etiology of ovarian cancer.

Androgen receptor expression in breast cancer

Numerous studies indicate that 70–80% of primary breast tumors express ARs, as well as 75% of breast cancer metastases, and AR is the sole sex steroid receptor expressed in approximately 25% of metastatic disease.[63] However it is unknown at this time whether there is any relation between exogenous androgen therapy and the incidence of breast cancer, as epidemiologic studies have shown both positive and negative associations between endogenous androgen levels and breast cancer risk.[9,64] For instance, experimental data suggest that conventional estrogen treatment regimens, as oral contraceptives or hormone replacement therapy, may upset the normal estrogen–androgen balance and promote unopposed estrogenic stimulation of mammary epithelial proliferation which may potentiate breast cancer risk.[9] In addition, endogenous androgen activity may be suppressed as oral estrogen therapy reduces free androgens by stimulating hepatic production of SHBG and suppressing LH, thereby inhibiting ovarian androgen production.[9] A recent study found that a low-dose oral contraceptive induced robust mammary epithelial proliferation in rats but addition of methyltestosterone to the therapy significantly suppressed the proliferation.[9] In addition, testosterone added to estrogen therapy significantly inhibits estrogen-induced mammary epithelial proliferation in ovariectomized rhesus monkeys.[8] There is also the theoretical risk of aromatization of androgens into estrogens in target tissue which may have potential deleterious impact on women with a history of breast cancer or any estrogen-dependent neoplasia.

Androgens have been shown in vitro to have either inhibitory or stimulatory effects on the growth of human breast cancer cells, and androgens either upregulate or downregulate AR mRNA expression in breast cancer cell lines.[65] ARs have also been associated with longer survival in women with operable breast cancer and a favorable response to hormone treatment in advanced disease.[66,67] Although androgens have not been used as a primary hormonal treatment for breast cancer since the 1960s due to their masculinizing side effects (i.e. hirsutism, acne), androgens such as fluoxymesterone have a therapeutic efficacy comparable to current hormonal therapies such as tamoxifen.[68] In fact, clinical observations and experimental data indicate that androgens inhibit mammary growth and have been used with success similar to that of tamoxifen to treat breast cancer.[9]

In vivo studies using the hormone-dependent dimethylbenz(a)anthracene (DMBA) rat mammary tumor model have shown that treatment with testosterone results in tumor regression and a concomitant reduction in estrogen receptor levels.[65] One possible mechanism for this decrease in estrogen receptor levels in the tumors is that androgen directly regulates their expression. An alternative explanation is that pharmacologic doses of testosterone may be aromatized to estrogen resulting in autologous downregulation of estrogen receptors. Furthermore, androgens bind with a low affinity to ER, which may result in an apparent reduction in ER levels following treatment with high doses of testosterone propionate due to interference with ligand binding in biochemical assays for estrogen receptors.[65]

Further studies are needed to evaluate the efficacy of supplementing hormone therapy with androgens and ensuing breast cancer risk. Furthermore, as current forms of estrogen in oral contraceptives and oral estrogen replacement therapy suppress endogenous androgen activity, there is a need for future studies on the efficacy of supplementing both oral contraceptive and estrogen replacement therapy with physiologic replacement androgen, in a nonaromatizable form, to maintain the natural estrogen–androgen ratios typical of normal women.

Androgen receptor expression in bone

Sex steroids are directly involved in bone remodeling. Androgens, acting either directly or via aromatization to estrogen, have profound impact on the physiology and preservation of bone mineral density in women. Androgens also increase muscle mass and strength and induce mechanical factors that alter the balance between bone resorption and formation in favor of formation, with the net result being an increase in bone mass and strength.[69]

ARs are found in all three bone cells: osteoblasts, osteoclasts, and osteocytes. However ARs are predominantly expressed in active osteoblasts and to a greater degree in cortical rather than cancellous bone at the site of bone formation. ARs are also found in bone marrow cells that regulate osteoclastogenesis. Osteoclast function is regulated by estrogen primarily, although indirect aromatization of testosterone to estrogen can also occur. ARs can also be found embedded in osteocytes within the bone matrix.[69]

Androgens have an important function in regulating bone matrix production and organization. ARs are upregulated by androgens in bone and also by exposure to glucocorticoids, estrogen and vitamin D. Androgen exposure enhances osteoblast differentiation and the synthesis of extracellular matrix proteins. Androgens also stimulate bone mineralization and influence bone cell function through the effect on local and systemic factors that control the bone cell microenvironment. The synthesis of transforming growth factor (TGF)-β, a potent osteoblast mitogen, as well as insulin-like growth factor (IGF) II and fibroblast growth factor are all influenced by DHT and testosterone. Androgens also decrease osteoclastogenesis by inhibiting the production of interleukin-6 (IL-6) in the stromal cells of the bone marrow, resulting in diminished maturation and development of osteoclast precursors and osteoclasts.[69] The reduction of IL-6 has been demonstrated for testosterone, DHT, androstenedione and DHEA. Furthermore, testosterone and DHT also regulate osteoclast activity, thereby reducing bone turnover by inhibiting both parathyroid hormone and IL–1-stimulated prostaglandin E_2 production.[69]

Anabolic effects of androgen

There are clear associations among muscle mass, muscle strength, and bone density in that muscle exerts a greater load on bone than does weight-dependent gravity. Mechanical loading when combined with estrogen, results in a greater osteogenic response than either separately. This is probably the result of estrogen's antiresorptive effect and of the stimulation of bone formation with exercise.[69] Approximately 4% of muscle mass is lost during the first 3 years after menopause, which is associated with a significant decline in muscle strength.[70] In men, muscle strength is preserved until age 60 and reaches levels found in menopausal women at about 75 years of age, which may explain the greater tendency for falls in older women.[71]

Androgens have direct anabolic effects on skeletal muscle as testosterone increases lean body mass and decreases fat mass in a dose and concentration-dependent fashion. In addition, the administration of androgens is associated with the upregulation of androgen receptors and resultant increased responsiveness of skeletal muscle.[72] The action of testosterone on muscle involves multiple mechanisms including its effects on inducing protein synthesis, recruiting satellite cells, and modulating the commitment of pluripotent mesenchymal cells to myogenic lineage.[52] Testosterone supplementation has been shown to increase muscle mass in older men and men with human immunodeficiency virus infection with low testosterone, chronic debilitative illnesses and healthy, but hypogonadal men, with the anabolic effects on muscle mass dependent on dose and plasma concentration.[52,73] The testosterone-induced muscle

fiber hypertrophy was also associated with a dose-dependent increase in myonuclear number inside the muscle fiber.[72] In addition to the stimulation of muscle protein synthesis, testosterone also affected satellite cells, which are quiescent precursors of skeletal muscle. In response to testosterone, satellite cells proliferated and then fused subsequently with the muscle fibers resulting in an increase in myonuclear number and muscle fiber hypertrophy. The observed increase in the number of satellite cells were seen in men who were treated with supraphysiologic doses of testosterone.[52,72]

Administration of testosterone and DHT has been shown to be associated with increasing muscle mass and decreasing fat mass. Bhasin et al.[74] demonstrated that testosterone supplementation in older men, young hypogonadal men, and middle-aged men with visceral obesity resulted in a decrease in fat mass which was proportional to the administered testosterone doses. Hence supraphysiologic doses of testosterone may produce a strong anabolic effect and testosterone may also influence additional steps in the myogenic and adipogenic pathways, muscle protein synthesis, and satellite cell replication.[52]

Androgen effects on the cardiovascular system

In recent years, there has been a dramatic increase in research into androgen effects on the cardiovascular system. Whereas previously androgens were considered harmful (and estrogens protective) for the cardiovascular system, current evidence suggests that androgens have beneficial or neutral cardiovascular effects and that they exert different effects at early (plaque formation) and late (rupture, thrombosis, vasospasm) stages of atherosclerosis.[75] An increasing number of studies demonstrate protective effects of androgens on cardiovascular function. However these findings derive almost entirely from male patients, and hold undetermined relevance for women's cardiovascular health. Nonetheless, limited human data do suggest that testosterone exposure does not shorten lifespan of either sex, and oral estrogen treatment increases the risk of cardiovascular death in men as it does in women. Patterns of age-specific cardiovascular death rates provide little support for the gender gap being due to estrogen protection. Rather, androgen exposure in early life (perinatal androgen imprinting) may predispose males to earlier onset of atherosclerosis, but the subsequent tempo of atherosclerotic progression is similar in men and women.[75] Future research on women's cardiovascular health will promote a better understanding of AR coregulators, nongenomic androgen effects, tissue-specific metabolic activation of androgens, and androgen sensitivity.

Conclusion

The importance of androgens in women is now being recognized as an essential component in maintaining sexual health and overall wellbeing. Extensive research has documented the physiologic role of androgen receptors throughout the body as well as its involvement in cancers of the reproductive tract. However, further basic science and clinical trials are needed to assess the role of androgens in premenopausal women as well as during the natural decline that occurs with aging and menopause, and the abrupt losses that occur with surgical menopause. In addition to quality of life and sexual outcomes, the impact of androgens on the pelvic floor and genital tract, muscle, bone, and cognitive and cardiovascular function requires improved characterization in future studies.

References

1. Burger HG. Androgen production in women. Fertil Steril 2002; 77(4 Suppl):S3–S5.
2. Vermuelen A. Plasma androgens in women. J Reprod Med 1998; 43 (Suppl 8): 725–733.
3. Maclean H, Warne G, Zajac J. Localization of functional domains in the androgen receptor. J Steroid Biochem Mol Biol 1997; 62:233–242.
4. Traish AM, Kim N, Min K et al. Role of androgens in female genital sexual arousal: receptor expression, structure and function. Fertil Steril 2002; 77: S11–S18.
5. Keller E, Ershler W, Chang C. The androgen receptor: a mediator of diverse responses. Front Biosci 1996; 1:d59–d71.
6. Lamb D, Weigel N, Marcelli M. Androgen receptors and their biology. Vitam Horm 2001; 62:199–230.
7. Lobacarro J, Poujol N, Chiche L et al. Molecular modeling and in vitro investigations of the human androgen receptor DNA-binding domain: application for the study of two mutations. Mol Cell Endocrinol 1996; 116:137–147.
8. Mckenna N, Lanz R, O'Malley B. Nuclear Receptor coregulators: cellular and molecular biology. Endocr Rev 1999; 20:321–344.
9. Dimitrakakis C, Zhou J, Bondy CA. Androgens and mammary growth and neoplasia. Fertil Steril 2002; 77(suppl 4):S26–S33.
10. Wilburt D, Griffin J, Wilson J. Characterization of the cytosol androgen receptor of the human prostate. J Clin Endocrinol Metab 1983; 56:113–120.
11. Wilson E, French F. Binding properties of androgen receptors. Evidence for identical receptors in rat testis, epididymis, and prostate. J Biol Chem 1976; 251:5620–5629.
12. Zhou Z, Lane M, Kemppainen J et al. Specificity of ligand-dependent androgen receptor stabilization: receptor domain interactions influence ligand dissociation and receptor stability. Mol Endocrinol 1995; 9:208–218.
13. Modugno F. Ovarian cancer and polymorphisms in the androgen and progesterone receptor genes: a HuGE review. Am J Epidemiol 2004; 159: 319–335.
14. Lobo RA. Androgens in postmenopausal women: production, possible role, and replacement options. Obstet Gynecol Surv 2001; 56:361–376.
15. Burger H, Dudley EC, Cui J et al. A prospective longitudinal study of serum testosterone dehydroepiandrosterone sulphate and sex hormone binding globulin levels through the menopause transition. J Clin Endocrinol Metab 2000; 85: 2832–2938.
16. Labrie F, Belanger A, Cusan L et al. Marked decline in serum concentrations of adrenal C19 sex steroid precursors and conjugated androgen metabolites during aging. J Clin Endocrinol Metab 1997; 82: 2396–2402.
17. Lasley BL, Santoro N, Randolf JF et al. The relationship of circulating dehydroepiandrosterone, testosterone, and estradiol to stages of the menopausal transition and ethnicity. J Clin Endocrinol Metab 2002; 87:3760–3767.
18. Longcope C. Metabolic and blood production rates of estrogen in postmenopausal women. Am J Obstet Gynecol 1971; 111:778–781.
19. Vermuelen A. The hormonal activity of the postmenopausal ovary. J Clin Endocrinol Metab 1976; 42:247–253.
20. Adashi EY. The climacteric ovary as a functional gonadotropin-driven androgen-producing gland. Fertil Steril 1994; 62:20–27.
21. Judd HL, Lucas WE, & Yen SCS. Endocrine function of the postmenopausal ovary: concentration of androgens and estrogens in ovarian and peripheral vein blood. J Clin Endocrinol Metab 1974; 39:1020.

22. Dowsett M, Cantwell B, Lal A et al. Suppression of postmenopausal ovarian steroidogenesis with the lutenizing hormone-releasing hormone agonist Goserelin. J Clin Endocrinol Metab 1988; 66:672–677.

23. Sluijmer AV, Heineman MJ, De Jong FH et al. Endocrine activity of the postmenopausal ovary: the effects of pituitary down-regulation and oophorectomy. J Clin Endocrinol Metab 1995; 80:2163–2167.

24. Couzinet B, Meduri G, Lecce MG et al. The postmenopausal ovary is not a major androgen-producing gland. J Clin Endocrinol Metab 2001; 86:5060–5066.

25. Erickson GF, Magoffin DA, Dyer C et al. The ovarian androgen producing cells: a review of structure/function relationships. Endocr Rev 1985; 6:371–398.

26. Heineman MJ, Sluijmer AV, Ever JLH. Utero-ovarian vein blood sampling in postmenopausal women. Fertil Steril 1993; 60:184–186.

27. Rinaudo P, Strauss JF. Endocrine function of the postmenopausal ovary. Endocr Metabol Clin 2004; 33:661–674.

28. Simon JA. Estrogen replacement therapy: effects on the endogenous androgen milieu. Fertil Steril 2002; 77:S77–S82.

29. Labrie F, Luu V, Labrie C et al. Endocrine and intracrine sources of androgens in women: inhibition of breast cancer and other roles of androgens and their precursor dehydroepiandrosterone. Endocr Rev 2003; 24:152–182.

30. Simpson ER. Aromatization of androgens in women: current concepts and findings. Fertil Steril 2002; 77(suppl 4):S6–S10.

31. Ukkola O, Rankinen T, Gagnon J et al. A genome-wide scan for steroids and SHBG levels in black and white females: the HERITAGE Family Study. J Clin Endocrinol Metab 2002; 87:3708–3720.

32. Laan E, Van Lunsen RH. Hormones and sexuality in postmenopausal women: a psychophysiological study. J Psychosom Obstet Gynaecol 1997; 18:126–133.

33. Sarrel PM. Sexuality and menopause. Obstet Gynecol 1990; 75(Suppl):S26–30.

34. Sarrel PM. Ovarian hormones and vaginal blood flow using laser doppler velocimetry to measure effects in a clinical trial in postmenopausal women. Int J Impot Res 1998; 10:S91–S93.

35. Simon JA, Klaiber E, Wiita B et al. Differential effects of estrogen-androgen and estrogen-only therapy on vasomotor symptoms, gonadotropin secretion, and endogenous androgen bioavailability in post-menopausal women. Menopause 1999; 6:138–146.

36. Sarrel PM. Effects of hormone replacement therapy on sexual psychophysiology and behavior in postmenopause. J Womens Health Gend Based Med 2000; 9(Suppl 1):S25–S32.

37. Stenberg A, Heimer G, & Ulmsten U. The prevalence of urogenital symptoms in postmenopausal women. Maturitas 1995; 22(Suppl):S17–S20.

38. Bulun SE, Simpson ER. Competitive reverse transcription-polymerase chain reaction analysis indicates that levels of aromatase cytochrome P450 transcripts in adipose tissue of buttocks, thighs and abdomen of women increase with advancing age. J Clin Endocrinol Metab 1994; 78:428–432.

39. Longcope C, Baler S. Androgen and estrogen dynamics: relationships with age, weight and menopause status. J Clin Endocrinol Metab 1993; 76:601–604.

40. Laughlin GA, Barrett-Connor E, Kritz-Silverstein D et al. Hysterectomy, oophorectomy, and endogenous sex hormone levels in older women: the Rancho Bernardo Study. J Clin Endocrinol Metab 2000; 85:645–651.

41. Tazuke S, Shaw KT. Exogenous estrogen and endogenous sex hormones. Medicine 1992; 71:44–51.

42. Judd HL. Hormonal dynamics associated with the menopause. Clin Obstet Gynecol 1976; 19:775–788.

43. Sarrel PM. Psychosexual effects of menopause: role of androgens. Am J Obstet Gynecol 1999; 180:S319–S324.

44. Sherwin BB. Hormones, mood, and cognitive functioning in postmenopausal women. Obstet Gynecol 1996; 87:S20–S26.

45. Avis N, Brambilla D, Mckinlay S et al. A longitudinal analysis of the association between menopause and depression: results from the Massachusetts Women's Health Study. Ann Epidemiol 1994; 4:15–21.

46. Sarrel P. Androgen deficiency: menopause and estrogen-related factors. Fertil Steril 2002; 77: S63–S67.

47. Sherwin BB, Gelfand MM. The role of androgen in the maintenance of sexual functioning in oophorectomized women. Psychosom Med 1987; 49:397–409.

48. Sourla A, Flamand M, Belanger A et al. Effect of dehydroepiandrosterone on vaginal and uterine histomorphology in the rat. J Steroid Biochem Mol Biol 1998; 66:137–149.

49. Kennedy T, Armstrong D. Induction of vaginal mucification in rats with testosterone and 17beta-hydroxy-5alpha-androstan-3–one. Steroids 1976; 27:423–430.

50. Hodgins M, Spike RC, Mackie R, Maclean A. An immunohistochemical study of androgen, oestrogen and progesterone receptors in the vulva and vagina. Br J Obstet Gynaecol 1998; 105:216–222.

51. Berman J, Almeida F, Jolin J et al. Correlation of androgen receptors, aromatase, and 5-alpha reductase in the human vagina with menopausal status. Fertil Steril 2003; 79:925–931.

52. Ho M, Bhatia N, & Bhasin S. Anabolic effects of androgens on muscles of female pelvic floor and lower urinary tract. Curr Opin Obstet Gynecol 2004; 16:405–409.

53. Nnodim J. Quantitative study of the effects of denervation and castration on the levator ani muscle of the rat. Anat Rec 1999; 255:324–333.

54. Nnodim J. Testosterone modifies satellite cell activation in denervated rat levator ani muscle. Anat Rec 2001; 263:19–24.

55. Monks D, O'Bryant E, Jordan C. Androgen receptor immunoreactivity in skeletal muscle: enrichment at the neuromuscular junction. J Comp Neurol 2004; 473:59–72.

56. Rosenweig B, Bolina P, Birch L et al. Location and concentration of estrogen, progesterone and androgen receptors in the bladder and urethra of the rabbit. Neurourol Urodyn 1995; 14:87–96.

57. Salmi S, Santti R, Gustafsson J et al. Co-localization of androgen receptor with estrogen receptor beta in the lower urinary tract of the male rat. J Urol 2001; 166:674–677.

58. Copas P, Bukovsky A, Asbury B et al. Estrogen, Progesterone, and androgen receptor expression in levator ani muscle and fascia. J Women Health Gend Based Med 2001; 10:785–795.

59. Ewies A, Thompson J, Al-Azzawi F. Changes in gonadal steroid receptors in the cardinal ligaments of prolapsed uteri; immunohistomorphometric data. Hum Reprod 2004; 19:1622–1628.

60. Bai S, Jung B, Chung B et al. Relationship between urinary profile of the endogenous steroids and postmenopausal women with stress urinary incontinence. Neurourol Urodyn 2003; 22:198–205.

61. Maia H, Maltez A, Fahel P et al. Detection of testosterone and estrogen receptors in the postmenopausal endometrium. Maturitas 2001; 38:179–188.

62. Tada A, Sasaki H, Nakamura J, et al. Aromatase activity and the effect of estradiol and testosterone on DNA synthesis in endometrial carcinoma cell lines. J Steroid Biochem Mol Biol 1993; 44:661–666.

63. Lea O, Kvinnsland S, Thorsen T. Improved measurement of androgen receptors in human breast cancer. Cancer Res 1989; 49:7162–7167.

64. Davis S. Androgen replacement in women: a commentary. J Clin Endocrinol Metab 1999; 84:1886–1891.

65. Birrell S, Hall R, Tilley W. Role of the androgen receptor in human breast Cancer. J Mamm Gland Biol Neoplasia 1998; 3:95–103.

66. Recchione C, Venturelli E, Manzari A et al. Testosterone, dihydrotestosterone, and oestradiol levels in postmenopausal breast cancer tissues. J Steroid Biochem Mol Biol 1995; 52:541–546.

67. Bryan RM, Mercer RJ, Rennie GC et al. Androgen receptors in breast cancer. Cancer 1984; 54: 2436–2440.

68. Tormey D, Lippman M, Edwards B et al. Evaluation of tamoxifen doses with and without fluoxymesterone in advanced breast cancer. Ann Intern Med 1983; 98:139–144.

69. Notelovitz M. Androgen effects on bone and muscle. Fertil Steril 2002; 77:S34–S41.

70. Aloia J, McGowan D, Vaswani A et al. The relationship of menopause to skeletal and muscle mass. Am J Clin Nutr 1991; 53:1378–1383.

71. Phillips S, Rook K, Siddle N et al. Muscle weakness in women occurs at an earlier age than men, but strength is preserved by hormone replacement therapy. Clin Sci 1993; 84:94–98.

72. Sinha-Hakim I, Artaza J, Woodhouse L et al. Testosterone-induced increase in muscle size in healthy young men is associated with muscle fiber hypertrophy. Am J Physiol Endocrinol Metab 2002; 283:E154–E164.

73. Sinha-Hakim I, Roth S, Lee M et al. Testosterone-induced muscle hypertrophy is associated with an increase in satellite cell number in healthy young men. Am J Physiol Endocrinol Metab 2003; 285:E197–E205.

74. Bhasin S, Taylor W, Singh R et al. The mechanism of androgen effects on body composition: mesenchymal pluripotent cell as the target of androgen action. J Gerontol 2003; 58A:1103–1110.

75. Liu P, Death A, Handelsman D. Androgens and cardiovascular disease. Endocr Rev 2003; 24:313–340.

Chapter 5
Psychosexual effects of menopause

Karine Chung and Luigi Mastroianni Jr

Summary

Female reproductive aging is associated with dramatic biologic, psychologic, and social changes. These can negatively impact sexuality. Four different models for normal female sexual function are presented and diagnostic categories of sexual dysfunction are described. The challenge is to define normal and abnormal sexual function, which has proven difficult due to the multidimensional nature of female sexuality. The menopausal transition is a period of hormonal flux and resulting anatomic changes, vasomotor symptoms, and mood disorders can further impair the sexual experience, and the loss of reproductive capacity can be a source of severe emotional distress. This period frequently coincides with major medical events such as hysterectomy or the development of concomitant medical illnesses. These may exacerbate disturbances in sexuality. This chapter summarizes current literature on the prevalence of sexual dysfunction, its relationship to aging and menopause, and the influences of hormonal, psychological and medical factors.

Introduction

Sexuality is an important component of health and overall wellbeing in women of all ages. It is a complex entity determined by multiple factors, including biologic, psychologic, social, and cultural influences. To understand the potential effects of menopause on sexuality and sexual dysfunction, it is important to be familiar with normal sexual functioning in the female patient. Masters and Johnson first described the female sexual response cycle as consisting of four phases: excitement, plateau, orgasm, and resolution.[1] During sexual excitement, the clitoris and labia minora become engorged, fluid is released along the vaginal lining, and the clitoris and vagina lengthen. Estrogen plays an essential role in this physiologic component of sexual response. The model of female response has since evolved to include the concepts of desire and satisfaction. Kaplan and colleagues proposed a three-phase model of sexual response in 1974,[2] which consisted of desire, followed by sexual arousal, and orgasm. It is this three-phase model that serves as the basis for the American Psychiatric Association's definition of sexual dysfunction in the *Diagnostic and Statistical Manual of Mental Disorders* (DSM-IV).[3] Other investigators have suggested that healthy sexual function in the female depends upon the interplay between four essential domains: libido, arousal, orgasm, and satisfaction.[4] More recently, a five-phase model of female sexual response has been introduced, depicting a cyclic progression from intimacy needs to sexual stimuli, arousal, desire, and enhanced intimacy.[5] While the mechanisms underlying the psychological aspects of the response cycle are not known, early studies investigating the relation between androgens and measures of sexuality suggest that testosterone may be the main driving force for sexual desire and motivation in the female.[6] However, it is well acknowledged that it is not hormonal influences alone that determine female sexual behavior. Contributions from social, emotional, cultural, and environmental forces are likely to be equally important, but are much more difficult to assess. It is clear from the evolution of sexual response models that female sexuality is multidimensional and difficult to characterize. Onset of the menopause introduces additional dimensions in these complex relationships, which are summarized in Figure 5.1.

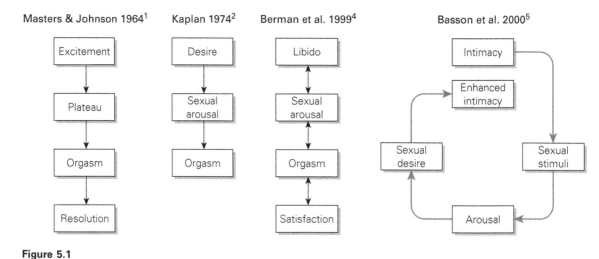

Figure 5.1

The evolution of models of female sexual response.

Female sexual dysfunction

While epidemiologic data on female sexual dysfunction are relatively sparse, the available reports suggest that it is a highly prevalent condition, affecting 25–63% of women.[7–9] A population-based cross-sectional study of 1749 women found that disturbances in sexual function are more common in women than men in the USA, affecting 43% of women and 31% of men aged 18–59.[10] The prevalence of sexual dysfunction increases among women who are not married, are less educated, or report feelings of unhappiness. Additionally, the presence of sexual dysfunction is highly associated with poor quality of life. Impairments in sexuality can lead to significant detriments in overall wellbeing, making this an extremely important area for research. Research, however, has been hampered by a lack of uniformity in assessing and defining sexual dysfunction.

Given the complex nature of normal sexuality in females, defining dysfunctional sexuality in women is a challenge. As defined by the American Psychiatric Association, sexual dysfunction is characterized by lack of desire as well as psychologic and physiologic changes associated with the sexual response cycle. Four classic categories of sexual disturbances were defined years ago in the DSM-IV:[3] sexual desire disorders; sexual arousal disorders; orgasmic disorders; and sexual pain disorders. Building upon these established categories,

the international consensus development panel on female sexual dysfunction convened and published revised classifications.[11] The current definitions specify psychogenic and organic causes of each of the original categories. The diagnoses are assigned subtypes as: A – lifelong versus acquired; B – generalized versus situational; and C – etiologic origin (organic, psychogenic, mixed, and unknown). An important concept, which is also incorporated in the refined definitions, is 'personal distress'. To shift the focus of the diagnosis away from the individual woman and to her relationship and surrounding environment, it has been recommended that additional descriptors detailing sources of distress be included. These are listed in Table 5.1, and their presence may have therapeutic implications.[12] It is important to recognize that there can be significant overlap and comorbidity among categories of sexual dysfunction, and they may be difficult to differentiate from one another. For example, desire disorders may arise as a result of arousal, response, or pain disorders.

Sexual desire disorders

Low sexual desire has become the most common sexual problem among women.[13] Hypoactive sexual desire disorders are characterized by the persistent or recurrent deficiency or absence of

Table 5.1 Additional descriptors for revised definitions of female sexual dysfunction[12]

- Negative upbringing/losses/trauma (physical, sexual, emotional), former interpersonal relationships, cultural/religious restrictions
- Current interpersonal difficulties, partner sexual dysfunction, inadequate stimulation, and unsatisfactory sexual and emotional contexts
- Medical conditions, psychiatric conditions, medications, or substance abuse

---

sexual fantasy and/or receptivity to sexual activity, which then leads to personal distress.[11] Newer terminology refers to 'women's sexual interest/desire disorder' which describes the absence of sexual thoughts or fantasy and a lack of responsive desire.[12] Pathologic loss of desire can be due to physiologic causes, such as states of hormonal deficiency, or psychologic causes, such as a history of sexual abuse or generalized depression. Often, sexual desire disorders can be attributed to a combination of physiologic and emotional factors.

Sexual arousal disorders

Sexual arousal disorder is defined by the persistent or recurrent inability to attain or maintain adequate sexual excitement, which causes personal distress.[11] The deficiency in sexual excitement may be subjective or can be illustrated by a lack of normal somatic responses associated with arousal, i.e. genital swelling or lubrication. Examples of arousal disorders include disturbances in clitoral or labial sensation, absent or diminished vaginal lubrication, or dysfunctional vaginal smooth muscle relaxation. Such problems can arise secondary to medications, pelvic surgery or trauma, or reduced vaginal and clitoral blood flow due to menopause. Psychosocial influences such as low self-esteem or stress can also play a role in inciting arousal disorders.

Orgasmic disorders

Orgasmic dysfunction is the persistent or recurrent difficulty, delay in, or absence of reaching orgasm

after sufficient sexual stimulation and arousal, which induces personal distress.[11] Orgasmic disorders are further classified into primary and secondary. Primary orgasmic dysfunction describes those women who have never achieved orgasm, and is commonly associated with psychologic factors, such as a history of sexual abuse or emotional trauma. Secondary disorders include all those women who were able at one time to attain orgasm but are no longer able. Physical events such as surgery, trauma, or hormonal disturbances are typical causes. Medications such as selective serotonin uptake inhibitors have also been associated with secondary orgasmic dysfunction.[14] Secondary conditions may be further divided into subtypes such as situational and coital orgasmic disorders. Situational orgasmic dysfunction refers to the patient who is able to reach sexual climax only under certain circumstances. For example, a patient who is able to achieve orgasm only with masturbation, and not in other situations, would be classified as situational. A variety of factors, both physiologic and emotional, can contribute to this type of disorder. It may often be a reflection of conflict in the patient's relationship with her partner. Coital orgasmic disorder is the inability to reach orgasm through coitus. This class of anorgasmia is common among women. However, it is important to note that the primary sensory trigger for female orgasm is clitoral rather than vaginal stimulation.[1] Studies investigating female orgasm have emphasized the role of clitoral stimulation before, during, and after intercourse. In questionnaires, women rated clitoral stimulation as at least somewhat more important than vaginal stimulation in achieving orgasm.[15] In the same study, only approximately 20% indicated that they did not require additional clitoral stimulation during intercourse. Many women believe that they should be able to reach orgasm through sexual intercourse, and failure to do so can result in distress, dissatisfaction, and relationship conflicts.[16]

Sexual pain disorders

This category of sexual dysfunction encompasses all disorders of pain due to intercourse and/or sexual stimuli.[11] Dyspareunia is defined as genital pain that occurs during intercourse. Vaginismus describes the condition of painful involuntary spasms of the lower third of the vagina. Noncoital sexual pain disorder is characterized by persistent genital pain caused by noncoital sexual stimulation. Anatomic causes of pain disorders, such as prior obstetrical trauma, vaginal atrophy, and fixation of pelvic organs secondary to endometriosis, are not unusual. Additionally, an association between pelvic floor disorders and sexual pain has been suggested by a recent cross-sectional study of women complaining of urinary incontinence or lower urinary tract symptoms. With the use of the Female Sexual Function Index and objective measures of urinary function in 227 women aged 19–66, sexual dysfunction in 46% of these patients was documented and sexual pain disorders were the most prevalent class of sexual dysfunction in women with urinary incontinence.[17] Psychologic elements of sexual pain have also been demonstrated, with up to one-third of dyspareunia cases reportedly due to interpersonal conflict.[18]

Sexual dysfunction and menopause

Reproductive aging is a process that occurs over time, and is associated with biologic, anatomic, and psychologic changes, which may negatively impact sexuality in the older woman. The menopausal transition is a period of hormonal flux. Ovarian function begins to decline and estrogen production decreases.[19] The state of relative estrogen deficiency leads to anatomic changes that influence sexual function.[20] Lack of estrogen also induces vasomotor symptoms and mood disorders, which can further impair the sexual experience.[21] For some women, the loss of reproductive capacity can be a source of severe emotional distress.[22] Additionally, the timing of the transition into menopause frequently coincides with the development of concomitant medical illnesses. These may exacerbate disturbances in sexuality.[23] Clearly, there are a multitude of factors associated with reproductive aging that influence female sexuality and may therefore predispose menopausal women to sexual dysfunction.

Epidemiologic studies vary widely in their reported prevalence of sexual dysfunction in menopausal women, likely because of differences in source populations and inconsistent

methods of assessing sexual function. Due to the accessibility of patients in the population of interest, a common setting for investigating sexuality and menopause is the menopausal clinic. One study of 185 women attending a menopause clinic, reported that 86.5% suffered some degree of psychosexual disturbance.[24] A more recent study of 355 women, also conducted in a menopause clinic setting, asked patients to rate sexual and nonsexual symptoms of menopause on a visual analog scale.[25] They found that approximately 30% of postmenopausal patients reported pain with intercourse and 20% were experiencing low libido. An estimated 46% reported lack of satisfaction. The intensity of the symptoms tended to be most severe if negative emotional feelings, poor physical health, or a genitourinary problem was present. The main limitation of studies conducted in menopause clinics is selection bias. It has been reported that only 20% of affected women will actually seek medical care for sex-related issues.[10] Therefore, it is unlikely that patients attending menopause clinics are representative of the overall population of menopausal women.

Several community-based studies have also aimed to determine the prevalence of sexual dysfunction in menopausal women. The Yale midlife study investigated sexual symptoms in 130 menopausal women recruited from the general community;[26] 77% reported decreased sexual desire, 58% complained of vaginal dryness and 39% had dyspareunia, illustrating a high prevalence of sexual dysfunction in menopausal women in the community. Lending support to these findings, another cross-sectional study of a cohort of 534 healthy women, recruited from a metropolitan health service,[27] had similar results. The study found a prevalence of 51.3% in women aged 40–64 and a threefold increase in sexual dysfunction associated with menopausal status (odds ratio 3.3, 95% CI 1.6 to 6.9).

Several groups have embarked upon population-based studies of sexuality in aging women. This is perhaps the best epidemiologic approach to accurately characterize sexual dysfunction in menopausal women. The Melbourne Women's Midlife Health Project prospectively evaluated a sample of 438 Australian women between 45 and 55 years of age, selected from the population via random telephone digit dialing.[28] Subjects were followed for 8 years and analyses were based upon annual face-to-face interviews using an abridged version of the validated Personal Experiences Questionnaire (PEQ). Dramatic decreases in sexual interest, responsivity, and frequency were associated with the menopausal transition. Even further decline in sexual responsivity, sex frequency, and libido were noted to occur with menopause. Significant increases in dyspareunia and sexual problems of the partner were also associated with menopausal status. Such findings suggest a propensity for disorders of sexual desire, arousal, and pain in perimenopausal and postmenopausal women.

The Massachusetts Women's Health Survey II, conducted by Avis and colleagues,[29] studied a population-based sample of 200 women aged 51–61 using a self-administered sexual activity questionnaire. The study aimed to elucidate the relation between menopause and various aspects of sexual functioning, and to determine the relative contributions of menopause and psychosocial variables to these aspects of sexuality. They excluded all women with a history of hormone replacement therapy within 2 years of the study, all those without a current partner, and all cases of surgical menopause. After controlling for multiple potential confounding factors, they found that postmenopausal women were significantly more likely to report decreased arousal when compared to premenopausal controls (adjusted odds ratio 2.25, 95% CI 1.14 to 4.45). The authors found no relation between menopausal status and dyspareunia, difficulty reaching orgasm, or sexual satisfaction. An important finding in this study is that, when controlling for multiple factors, the most consistent predictors of sexual activity were health and marital status. Women who reported better states of general health had higher levels of sexual frequency, interest, arousal, and satisfaction. Married women were five times more likely to report a decline in arousal (adjusted odds ratio 5.24, 95% CI 1.91 to 14.41) compared with unmarried women with current partners. These women also showed lower levels of interest and desire. These results contradicted those of the National Health and Social Life Survey[10] mentioned earlier in this chapter, which reported lower levels of sexual dysfunction in married women compared with unmarried women. The difference may be due to the fact that the latter study included a wide age range (18–59) and did not exclude unmarried

women without current partners. The findings of these and other epidemiologic studies emphasize the multifactorial nature of sexuality in the menopause. They underline the importance of controlling for confounders and disentangling effects of menopause per se versus other factors on sexual dysfunction.

Age and female sexual function

Perhaps the most important confounding factor in studying the association between menopause and sexual disorders is age. Masters and Johnson established that there are anatomic and physiologic changes in the female sexual response cycle that occur due to aging. These changes have the potential to negatively alter the sexual experience[1] (Table 5.2). Other investigators have evaluated the effects of age on measures of sexual function. Hartmann and colleagues[13] performed a cross-sectional study of women aged 20–45 years. One hundred and two women were recruited from the community and 52 were referred from a sexual medicine outpatient unit. Using a 28–item questionnaire, they determined that in both the patient-based and the community-based samples, age exerted little effect on sexual desire and other components of sexual function. However, they found that among the sexually dysfunctional women, the older women reported more severe problems than the younger women. Data from the National Health and Social Life Survey reported that the prevalence of sexual dysfunction actually decreased with increasing age in women aged 18–59.[10] This trend did not persist for women with lubrication problems. Neither of these studies addressed the impact of menopause on sexuality.

A Swedish population-based study of 800 women used discrete categories of age to determine the relative contributions of age and menopause to sexual functioning.[30] Women aged 38, 46, 50, and 54 were assessed by premenopausal, perimenopausal, and postmenopausal status. With menopausal status held constant, there was no significant relationship between age and sexual functioning. This study was limited by its cross-sectional design, which did not allow for adequate control for previous level of sexual functioning. A longitudinal analysis by Dennerstein's group found that, while controlling for menopausal

Table 5.2   Age-related changes in the sexual response cycle. Adapted from Masters & Johnson[1]

Sexual response phase	Physiologic change
Excitement phase: takes longer to achieve	Decreased vaginal blood flow and genital engorgement Decreased quantity and delay in lubrication
Plateau phase: prolonged	Reduced uterine elevation Decreased breast vasocongestion and nipple erection
Orgasm phase	Reduced number and intensity of vaginal contractions
Resolution phase	Prolonged resolution

Table 5.3   Anatomic changes due to decline in hormone levels. Adapted from Leiblum & Bachmann[31]

- Atrophy of vaginal epithelium
- Reduction of pubic hair
- Loss of fat and subcutaneous tissue from the mons pubis
- Atrophy of the labia majora
- Loss of elasticity and shortening of the vaginal vault
- Atrophy of the Bartholin glands

status, the only domain that decreased significantly with age was sexual responsivity.[28] While adjusting for age, these authors found that menopause was associated with a significant reduction in sexual responsivity, sexual frequency, and libido. Overall, while age appears to have some independent impact on sexuality, menopausal status seems to make a larger contribution.

Hormonal influences and female sexual function

Precise mechanisms for the effects of menopause on sexual functioning are difficult to elucidate, but are thought to be due at least in part to the associated decrease in hormone levels. A number of anatomic changes have been attributed to the hormonal declines in menopause. These are listed in Table 5.3.[31] In many women, these changes will alter the sexual experience. The major hormonal changes associated with the onset of menopause are the dramatic decline in circulating estradiol and a concomitant increase in the gonadotropins, luteinizing hormone (LH) and follicle stimulating hormone (FSH).[32] Whether or not there is also an age-related decline in androgen levels in

women remains controversial. Cross-sectional studies have reported lower levels of testosterone in postmenopausal women compared with premenopausal women,[33] while longitudinal studies have failed to show a significant change with age or time since the final menstrual period.[34] Nevertheless, there are potential roles for both estrogens and androgens in determining sexual function in menopause.

Estrogen and female sexual function

Until recently, estrogen was believed to be the primary regulator of female sexual function. Estradiol (E_2) has a vasodilating and vasoprotective effect on the genitourinary organs. It maintains vascularization and integrity of these organs at baseline, and facilitates increased blood flow during sexual excitement to allow for adequate thickening and lubrication of the vaginal epithelium. The decline in circulating serum levels results in a thinning of the vaginal epithelium and atrophy of the smooth muscle of the vaginal wall.[35] An increase in vaginal pH also arises secondary to estrogen deficiency, leading to an environment more conducive to vaginal infections, urinary tract infections, and sexual dysfunction.[26]

Estrogen influences sensation via both central and peripheral nervous systems. Primary mediators of sensation, such as nitric oxide and type 5 phosphodiesterase, which are localized in the nerve endings and smooth muscle of the clitoris and vagina, are thought to be regulated by estrogen.[36] In animal models, the administration of exogenous estrogen results in an expansion of sensory zones along the pudendal nerve.[35]

Similar effects are seen in postmenopausal women when estrogen replacement results in restoration of clitoral and vaginal vibration and pressure thresholds.[26]

Given the physiologic effects of estrogen decline, it would be expected that lower serum E_2 levels would be associated with greater degrees of sexual dysfunction. Indeed, some authors have reported a direct correlation between E_2 levels less than 50 pg/mL and increased sexual complaints.[26] Another study found that, after controlling for multiple factors, estradiol levels were related to sexual pain, but not to other components of sexual dysfunction.[29] In a longitudinal study of a population-based sample of women transitioning into menopause, lower serum estradiol levels were significantly associated with lower total scores in sexual functioning.[37] This study also assessed the relationship between androgens and sexual function. They measured total testosterone, free testosterone index and dehydroepiandrosterone sulfate (DHEAS) over time, and found that no aspect of sexual functioning correlated with serum levels of androgens. They concluded that the decline in female sexual functioning that occurs with natural menopause relates more to estradiol levels than androgen levels.

Androgens and female sexual function

The prevalent theory is that androgens regulate libido in women with normal sexual functioning. Androgen receptors have been identified in various regions of the central nervous system, including the cortex, pituitary, hypothalamus, thalamus, and amygdala.[33] Androgen-mediated effects in the brain include sexual behavior, libido, temperature control, sleep control, assertiveness, cognitive function, and learning capacities.[38] Androgens are thought to act directly by binding to their receptors, or indirectly through aromatization to estradiol. Physiologic components of female sexuality may also be influenced by androgens. Higher testosterone levels have been associated with higher orgasmic capacity[39] and less vaginal atrophy.[40] Ovarian androgen production begins to decline many years before the onset of menopause, and some investigators

believe that many of the changes in sexual behavior historically attributed to the lack of estrogen may actually be due to androgen deficiency.[41] Such beliefs are supported by studies evaluating the effects of androgen therapy on sexual symptomatology in menopausal women.[42] In a double blinded, randomized trial of 20 postmenopausal women, sexual desire, satisfaction, and frequency were improved significantly by combined estrogen–androgen therapy but not by estrogen or estrogen–progestin therapy. The authors concluded that androgens play a critical role in sexual function.[42] Furthermore, because they found relatively low circulating estrogen concentrations in the combined estrogen–androgen group, they proposed that estrogens are not a significant determinant of sexual drive or enjoyment.

The role of androgen deficiency in female sexual dysfunction is a topic of controversy. A correlation between low levels of testosterone and decreased libido has been shown in premenopausal women,[43] but the role in older menopausal women is less well established. A study of 105 women complaining of decreased sexual desire included 38 women who were postmenopausal.[44] They found lower levels of total and free testosterone in these women compared with age-matched historical controls. They also found significantly lower levels of DHEAS, suggesting a possible role for the adrenal gland in female libido. This study was limited by its use of historical controls and its cross-sectional design. Longitudinal studies to assess the impact of androgens on sexual functioning have failed to confirm the relationship.[37]

The diagnosis of androgen deficiency in women remains a challenge. It suffers from the lack of precise definitions and threshold values. Since the majority of commercial assays for total and free testosterone levels were developed to measure normal circulating levels in men, they lack the sensitivity to accurately quantify levels that are typical for women, and are even less precise in measuring the lowest levels which are characteristic of androgen deficiency.[45] Because of an accumulating number of studies supporting the beneficial effects of exogenous androgens on sexual function in surgically and naturally menopausal women,[46,47] evidence for the existence of androgen deficiency and its role in female sexuality grows stronger.

Psychologic impact of menopause

The existing literature supports an association between menopause and sexual dysfunction. However, not all menopausal women will experience sex-related problems. The manner in which a woman responds to changes brought about by menopause depends largely upon her individual psychic makeup and sociocultural factors.[22] Psychoanalytic reports have remarked that some women must properly mourn the loss of reproductive capacity to move forward successfully in their postmenopausal life.[22] The menopausal transition is a time of dramatic biologic change and, for many women, psychologic vulnerability. Depressive symptoms have been reported to increase significantly during the transition into menopause.[48] It is important to acknowledge these phenomena when considering sexuality in the aging female because depression as well as medications for depression can lead to sexual dysfunction.

Other psychologic, social, and cultural influences in menopause are also important and have been addressed in the literature. A study of 354 women enrolled in the Melbourne Women's Midlife Health Project found that the strongest predictor of sexual behavior was the woman's feelings for her partner.[49] These findings were reiterated in a more recent study of 102 women, which identified quality of the partnership as the most important factor in sexual satisfaction.[13] Another large study of 939 menopausal women reported that good self-esteem was one of the most influential variables in sexual satisfaction.[41]

Medical risk factors for sexual dysfunction

The timing of the menopause often coincides with the development of concomitant medical illnesses, which can contribute to female sexual dysfunction. Evidence suggests that up to 60% of sexual disorders can be attributed to an organic cause.[16] Medical conditions that have been associated with impaired sexuality are listed in Table 5.4.

Vascular conditions

Sexual dysfunction can occur due to diabetes mellitus, cardiovascular disease, hypertension,

Table 5.4 Medical conditions associated with sexual dysfunction. Adapted from Walsh & Berman[16]

Vascular

Diabetes mellitus
Artherosclerosis
Hypertension
Lipid disorders
Peripheral vascular disease

Hormonal

Hypogonadism
Hyperprolactinemia
Hypothyroidism
Hyperthyroidism

Neurogenic

Spinal cord injury
Multiple sclerosis

Musculogenic

Pelvic floor muscle hypertonocity or hypotonicity

Medications

Antihypertensive drugs
Central nervous system drugs
Chemotherapeutic drugs
Drugs affecting hormones

Psychogenic

Depression
Anxiety/obsessive–compulsive disorder
Social stressors
Religious inhibitions
Posttraumatic sexual experiences
Dysfunctional attitudes about sex

Other

Autoimmune disorders
Renal disease (dialysis)
Bowel disease (colostomy)
Bladder disease (urinary incontinence, cystitis)
Skin disorders (contact dermatitis, eczema)

peripheral vascular disease, and tobacco abuse.[16] Insufficient blood flow to the vagina and clitoris can result in vaginal dryness and dyspareunia. Type II diabetes has been associated with decreased libido, decreased lubrication, and reduced sexual activity.[50]

Hormonal conditions

Common primary endocrine causes of sexual dysfunction include natural or surgical menopause,

Table 5.5 Selected medications and their potential adverse effects on sexual function. Adapted from ACOG Technical Bulletin[57]

	Decreased libido	Delayed or absent orgasm	Painful clitoral tumescence
Bromocriptine			+
Cimetidine	+		
Clomipramine	+	+	
Diazepam		+	
Fenfluramine	+		
Fluoxetine		+	
Imipramine		+	
Methyldopa	+		
Phenelzine		+	
Propranolol	+		
Reserpine	+		
Spironolactone	+		
Timolol	+		
Trazadone			+

premature ovarian failure, and dysfunction of the hypothalamic–pituitary axis.[16]

Neurogenic conditions

Neurogenic sexual impairment occurs with spinal cord injury or any diseases affecting the central or peripheral nervous system. A study of 30 women with spinal cord injuries reported that <50% were able to achieve orgasm.[51] Additionally, upper motor neuron lesions can be associated with poor psychogenic lubrication.[52] Diabetic neuropathies may be related to complaints of increased vaginitis, decreased vaginal lubrication and increased time to reach orgasm.[53]

Musculogenic conditions

Hypotonicity of the muscles of the pelvic floor can result from trauma during childbirth, surgery or radiation or can be secondary to the aging process.[16] Such alterations can lead to loss in vaginal sensation, coital anorgasmia or urinary incontinence during intercourse. On the other hand, hypertonicity of these muscles can lead to pain disorders such as vaginismus or dyspareunia.[54]

Psychogenic conditions

In the presence or absence of other medical conditions, the psychologic aspects of sexuality are extremely important. Medical and emotional factors interact with one another and can induce stress in interpersonal relationships, causing further decline in sexual functioning. Additionally, mood disorders and psychologic stressors are known to negatively impact female sexuality.[55]

Medications

Many prescription medications have been reported to cause problems with sexual function, most of which are based on case reports or subjective evidence.[16] The three classes of medications that have been consistently implicated in causing sexual dysfunction are antihypertensives, antidepressants, and antipsychotic medications.[56] A list of selected medications and their potential adverse effects on sexual function are shown in Table 5.5.[57]

Hysterectomy and sexual functioning

Approximately 600 000 women undergo hysterectomy each year in the USA, making it the most common gynecologic procedure performed.[58] For many women, hysterectomy is accompanied by bilateral oophorectomy, resulting in immediate surgical menopause. Yet even when the ovaries are retained, removal of the uterus involves the definitive loss of reproductive capacity, which can lead to emotional distress in some women. Additionally, there is evidence that hysterectomy alone can lead to the onset of vasomotor symptoms, vaginal dryness, and quicker progression to natural menopause.[59,60] A population-based cross-sectional study of women aged 39–60 compared 986 women who had undergone hysterectomy with conservation of one or both ovaries to 5636 normal women with uterus and ovaries present. They found that hysterectomized women were 1.3–1.9 times more likely to report moderate to severe vasomotor symptoms and 1.3–4 times more likely to complain of vaginal dryness in a mailed questionnaire than their age-matched controls ($P<0.001$).[59] Anatomic sequelae of hysterectomy can include shortening of the vaginal vault and disruption of the uterovaginal nerve plexus, which may interfere with sensation and vaginal orgasmic potential. Given these events, there seems to be ample biologic and psychologic basis for the belief that hysterectomy might result in increased sexual dysfunction.

The impact of hysterectomy on sexual function has been investigated and the issue remains controversial. The estimated prevalence of deterioration of sexual function after hysterectomy ranges from 13 to 37%.[61–63] These studies were largely retrospective and based on self-report measures of sexuality, which are often limited by recall bias, particularly if the patients inaccurately recall their presurgical level of sexual functioning.

The Maryland Women's Health study elegantly assessed the effect of hysterectomy on sexual functioning in a prospective uncontrolled study of 1101 women undergoing hysterectomy for benign indications.[64] They interviewed patients using a series of validated questions about sexual behavior shortly before surgery and at 3, 6, 12, 18, and 24 months after surgery. Interestingly, for each component of sexuality, the strongest predictor of a problem after hysterectomy was the presence of the problem before hysterectomy. Overall, they found that sexual function improved on all measures after hysterectomy. The frequency of sexual relations, frequency of orgasm, and libido increased significantly after hysterectomy. They also reported a significant decrease in frequency of vaginal dryness and dyspareunia after hysterectomy. Notably, prehysterectomy depression was associated with a significantly increased risk of posthysterectomy dyspareunia (odds ratio 2.28; 95% CI 1.09 to 4.76) and posthysterectomy low libido (odds ratio 2.83; 95% CI 1.28 to 6.23). The main limitation of this study is that prehysterectomy sexual function might have been negatively influenced by the presence of gynecologic pathology or anxiety about the upcoming surgery, biasing the results of the study in favor of posthysterectomy status.

Another group examined both subjective and objective measures of sexual arousal in two groups with gynecologic pathology.[65] They compared 15 women with benign uterine fibroids who had undergone hysterectomy with 17 women with fibroids who had not undergone hysterectomy. They used several validated instruments, including the Beck Depression Inventory, the Body Satisfaction Scale, the Female Sexual Function Index, and the Index of Sexual Satisfaction, as well as a daily diary to assess subjective measures of sexual function. Women who had and had not undergone hysterectomy did not differ significantly on any of these measures. They used vaginal photoplethysmography to obtain vaginal pulse amplitude (VPA) as a physiologic measure of sexual arousal during exposure of the women to neutral and erotic films. They found that the hysterectomy group had significantly lower VPA responses to both neutral and erotic stimuli than the group that had not undergone hysterectomy. They concluded that, while there was no difference between groups in subjective and self-reported measures of sexuality, their findings did support a potential impairment of physiologic sexual arousal after hysterectomy. Further research on the impact of hysterectomy on sexual function is needed to resolve this issue.

Evaluation and treatment

There is adequate evidence of an association between menopause and a decline in sexual function independent of age. The relationship is complex, and is influenced by biologic, psychologic, and social factors. Evaluation of the menopausal patient who reports symptoms of sexual disturbance should always begin with a thorough history, which may uncover past or current psychosocial stressors. Certain 'psychosexual red flags' have been identified which should prompt referral of the patient to a specialist trained in sex therapy. These are listed in Table 5.6.[16]

The history should be followed by a complete physical examination to assess for signs of

Table 5.6   Psychosexual red flags. Adapted from Walsh & Berman[16]

- Symptoms are lifelong rather than acquired
- Symptoms are situational (e.g. disappear when source of stress removed)
- History of sexual abuse or trauma
- Psychiatric history
- Current or past history of depression and/or anxiety
- The couple experiences relationship conflict (e.g. overt conflict, lack of intimacy)
- The partner has a sexual dysfunction

coexisting medical problems as well as signs of hormonal imbalance. The external genitalia examination should assess the perineal muscle tone and the posterior fourchette to investigate for causes of vaginismus or dyspareunia. Skin texture and turgor and pubic hair distribution should also be inspected to gain information suggestive of vaginal atrophy. A speculum examination should be done to inspect the vaginal mucosa and assess for vaginal discharge or uterine prolapse, which can contribute to sexual dysfunction. This should be followed by careful palpation of the internal pelvic organs and the rectovaginal surface. This part of the examination can further identify potential causes for sexual pain disorders.

The recommended baseline hormonal evaluation includes serum levels of FSH, LH, estradiol, total and free testosterone, sex hormone binding globulin and prolactin.[16] A relationship between estradiol deficiency and sexual dysfunction has been established, while the impact of androgen deficiency on sexuality remains controversial. Improvements in sexual function achieved with estrogen replacement seem to be further enhanced by the addition of testosterone.[38] The impact of hormonal therapy on sexual function is discussed elsewhere in this volume.

References

1. WH Masters, VE Johnson. Human Sexual Response. 1966. Boston: Little Brown.
2. HS Kaplan. Disorders of Sexual Desire. 1979. New York: Brunner/Mazel.
3. American Psychiatric Association. Diagnostic and Statistical Manual of Mental Disorders, 4th ed. 1994. Washington, DC: American Psychiatric Press.
4. Berman JR, Berman L, Goldstein I. Female sexual dysfunction: incidence, pathophysiology, evaluation, and treatment options. Urology 1999; 54:385–391.
5. Basson R. The female sexual response: A different model. J Sex Marital Ther 2000; 26:51–65.
6. Myers LS, Dixen J, Morrisette D et al. Effects of estrogen, androgen, and progestin on sexual psychophysiology and behavior in postmenopausal women. J Clin Endocrinol Metab 1990; 70:1124–1131.
7. Frank E, Anderson C, Rubenstein D. Frequency of sexual dysfunction in 'normal' couples. N Engl J Med 1978; 299:111–115.
8. Spector IP, Carey MP. Incidence and prevalence of the sexual dysfunctions: a critical review of the empirical literature. Arch Sex Behav 1990; 19:389–408.
9. Rosen RC, Taylor JF, Leiblum SR, Bachmann GA. Prevalence of sexual dysfunction in women: results of a survey study of 329 women in an outpatient gynecological clinic. J Sex Marital Ther 1993; 19:171–188.
10. Laumann EO, Paik A, Rosen RC. Sexual dysfunction in the United States: Prevalence and predictors. JAMA 1999; 281:537–544.
11. Basson R, Berman J, Burnett A et al. Report of the international consensus development conference on female sexual dysfunction: Definitions and classifications. J Urol 2000; 163:888–893.
12. Basson R, Leiblum S, Brotto L et al. Definitions of women's sexual dysfunction reconsidered: advocating expansion and revision. J Psychosom Obstet Gynecol 2003; 24:221–229.
13. Hartmann U, Philippsohn S, Heiser K et al. Low sexual desire midlife and older women: personality factors, psychosocial development, present sexuality. Menopause 2004; 11:726–740.
14. Clayton AH, Pradko JF, Montano CB et al. Prevalence of sexual dysfunction among newer antidepressants. J Clin Psychiatry 2002; 63:357–366.
15. Fisher S. Female orgasm: an interview with Seymour Fisher, PhD. Med Aspects Hum Sex 1973; 7:81–84.
16. Walsh KE, Berman JR. Sexual dysfunction in the older woman: An overview of the current understanding and management. Drugs Aging 2004; 21:655–675.
17. Salonia A, Zanni G, Rosella N et al. Sexual dysfunction is common in women with lower urinary tract symptoms and urinary incontinence: Results of a cross-sectional study. Eur Urol 2004; 45:642–648.
18. Fry RP, Crisp AH, Beard RW. Sociopsychological factors in chronic pelvic pain, a review. J Psychosom Res 1997; 42:1–15.
19. Bachmann GA. The changes before 'the change': strategies for the transition to the menopause. Postgrad Med 1994; 95:113–115.
20. Bachmann GA. Influence of menopause on sexuality. Int J Fertil Menopausal Stud 1995; 40:16–22.

21. Joffe H, Hall JE, Soares CN et al. Vasomotor symptoms are associated with depression in peri-menopausal women seeking primary care. Menopause 2002; 9:392–398.

22. Bemesderfer S. Psychoanalytic aspects of menopause. J Am Psychoanal Assoc 1996; 44:631–638.

23. Palacios S, Tobar AC, Menendez C. Sexuality in the climacteric years. Maturitas 2002; 43:S69–S77.

24. Sarrel PM & Whitehead MI. Sex and menopause: defining the issues. Maturitas 1985; 7:217–224.

25. Nappi RE, Verde JB, Polatti F et al. Self-reported sexual symptoms in women attending menopause clinics. Gynecol Obstet Invest 2002; 53:181–187.

26. Sarrel PM. Sexuality and menopause. Obstet Gynecol 1990; 75:26S–30S.

27. Castelo-Branco C, Blumel JE, Araya H et al. Prevalence of sexual dysfunction in a cohort of middle-aged women: influences of menopause and hormone replacement therapy. J Obstet Gynaecol 2003; 23:426–430.

28. Dennerstein L, Dudley E, Burger H. Are changes in sexual functioning during midlife due to aging or menopause? Fertil Steril 2001; 76:456–460.

29. Avis NE, Stellato R, Crawford S et al. Is there an association between menopause status and sexual functioning? Menopause 2000; 7:297–309.

30. Hallstrom T. Sexuality in the climacteric. Clin Obstet Gynaecol 1977; 4:227–239.

31. Leiblum SR, Bachmann GA. The sexuality of climacteric women. In: BA Eskin (Ed.). The Menopause: Comprehensive management, 3rd ed. 1994:137. New York: McGraw-Hill, Inc.

32. Burger HG. The endocrinology of the menopause. Maturitas 1996; 23:129–136.

33. Padero MM, Bhasin S, Friedman TC. Androgen supplementation in older women: too much hype, not enough data. J Am Geriatr Soc 2002; 50:1131–1140.

34. Burger HG, Dudley EC, Cui J et al. A prospective longitudinal study of serum testosterone, dehydro-epiandrosterone sulfate, and sex hormone-binding globulin levels through the menopause transition. J Clin Endocrinol Metab 2000; 85:2832–2838.

35. Berman JR, Bassuk J. Physiology and pathophysiology of female sexual function and dysfunction. World J Urol 2002; 20:111–118.

36. Bachmann G, Leiblum S. The impact of hormones on menopausal sexuality: a literature review. Menopause 2004; 11:120–130.

37. Dennerstein L, Randolph J, Taffe J et al. Hormones, mood, sexuality, and the menopausal transition. Fertil Steril 2002; 77:S42–S48.

38. Sarrel PM. Psychosexual effects of menopause: role of androgens. Am J Obstet Gynecol 1999; 180:S319–S324.

39. Penteado SRL, Fonseca AM, Bagnoli VR et al. Sexuality in healthy postmenopausal women. Climacteric 2003; 6:321–329.

40. Leiblum S, Bachmann G, Kemmann E et al. Vaginal atrophy in the postmenopausal woman. The importance of sexual activity and hormones. JAMA 1983; 249:2195–2198.

41. Sarrel PM. Androgen deficiency: menopause and estrogen-related factors. Fertil Steril 2002; 77: S63–S67.

42. Sarrel PM, Dobay B, Wiita B. Estrogen and estrogen-androgen replacement in postmenopausal women dissatisfied with estrogen-only therapy. Sexual behavior and neuroendocrine responses. J Reprod Med 1998; 43:847–856.

43. Guay AT. Decreased testosterone in regularly menstruating women with decreased libido: A clinical observation. J Sex Marital Ther 2001; 27: 513–519.

44. Guay AT, Jacobson J. Decreased free testosterone and dehydroepiandrosterone-sulfate (DHEA-S) levels in women with decreased libido. J Sex Marital Ther 2002; 28:S129–S142.

45. Sinha-Hikim I, Arvaer S, Beall G et al. The use of sensitive equilibrium dialysis method for the measurement of free testosterone levels in healthy, cycling women and in human immunodeficiency virus-infected women. JCEM 1998; 83:1312–1318.

46. Shifren JL, Braunstein GD, Simon JA et al. Transdermal testosterone treatment in women with impaired sexual function after oophorectomy. N Engl J Med 2000; 343:682–688.

47. Davis SR, McCloud P, Strauss BJG, Burger H. Testosterone enhances estradiol effects on postmenopausal bone density and sexuality. Maturitas 1995; 21:227–236.

48. Freeman EW, Sammel MD, Liu L et al. Hormones and menopausal status as predictors of depression in women in transition to menopause. Arch Gen Psychiatry 2004; 61:62–70.

49. Dennerstein L, Lehert P, Burger H, Dudley E. Factors affecting sexual functioning of women in the mid-life years. Climacteric 1999; 2:254–262.

50. Schreiner-Engel P, Schiavi RC, Vietorsz D et al. The differential impact of diabetes type on female sexuality. J Psychosom Res 1987; 31:23.

51. Sipski ML, Alexander CJ, Rosen RC. Sexual response in women with spinal cord injuries: implications for our understanding of the able-bodied. J Sex Marital Ther 1999; 25:11–22.

52. Sipski ML. Sexual response in women with spinal cord injury: neurologic pathways and recommendations for the use of electrical stimulation. J Spinal Cord Med 2001; 24:155–158.

53. LeMone P. The physical effects of diabetes on sexuality in women. Diabetes Educ 1996; 22: 361–366.

54. Shafik A, El-Sibai O. Study of the pelvic floor muscles in vaginismus: a concept of pathogenesis. Eur J Obstet Gynecol Reprod Biol 2002; 105:67–70.

55. Meston CM. The psychophysiologic assessment of female sexual function. American Association of Sex Educators, Counselors, and Therapists, Inc (AASECT). J Sex Educ Ther 2000; 25:6–16.

56. Finger WW, Lund M, Slagle MA. Medications that may contribute to sexual disorders: a guide to assessment and treatment in family practice. J Fam Pract 1997; 44:33–43.

57. ACOG Technical Bulletin, Number 211. Sexual Dysfunction. Int J Gynecol Obstet 1995; 51:265.

58. Lepine LA, Hills SD, Marchbanks PA et al. Hysterectomy surveillance in the United States, 1980–1993. MMWR Morb Mortal Wkly Rep 1997; 46:1–15.

59. Oldenhave A, Jaszmann LJB, Everaerd WT, Haspels AA. Hysterectomized women with ovarian conservation report more severe climacteric complaints than do normal women of similar age. Am J Obstet Gynecol 1993; 168:765–771.

60. Siddle N, Sarrel P, Whitehead M. The effect of hysterectomy on the age of ovarian failure: identification of a subgroup of women with premature loss of ovarian function after hysterectomy. Fertil Steril 1987; 47:94–100.

61. Dennerstein L, Wood C, Burrows GD. Sexual response following hysterectomy and oophorectomy. Obstet Gynecol 1977; 49:92–96.

62. Nathorst-Boos J, van Schoultz B. Psychological reactions and sexual life after hysterectomy with and without oophorectomy. Gynecol Obstet Invest 1992; 34:97–101.

63. Helstrom L, Lundberg PO, Sorbom D, Backstrom T. Sexuality after hysterectomy: a factor analysis of women's sexual lives before and after subtotal hysterectomy. Obstet Gynecol 1993; 81:357–362.

64. Rhodes JC, Kjerulff KH, Langenberg PW, Guzinski GM. Hysterectomy and sexual functioning. JAMA 1999; 282:1934–1941.

65. Meston CM. The effects of hysterectomy on sexual arousal in women with a history of benign uterine fibroids. Arch Sex Behav 2004; 33:31–42.

Chapter 6

Effects of combined estrogen–androgen preparations on sexual function in postmenopausal women

Barbara B Sherwin

Summary

Animal studies have shown that testosterone receptors are found in areas of the brain important for sexual behavior and that proceptive behavior (solicitation of sexual attention) is diminished following ovariectomy and restored by testosterone administration. Some studies in postmenopausal women have found that decreases in aspects of sexual functioning are associated with low testosterone levels. The most compelling evidence comes from the prospective, randomized controlled trials (RCTs) where estrogen and either an oral, intramuscular, or transdermal testosterone preparation were administered to surgically menopausal women. These RCTs consistently found that both but not estrogen-alone, estrogen and androgen, enhanced sexual desire, interest, and satisfaction in surgically menopausal women. The relatively low doses of testosterone used to effect these changes in sexual behaviour may be without significant side effects. It would therefore seem that the use of combined preparations presents a safe and effective treatment strategy for complaints of reduced sexual desire, interest, and satisfaction in a select group of surgically menopausal women.

Introduction

At the present time, there is considerable information on the effects of estrogen on various organ systems in postmenopausal women which provide protection against diseases such as osteoporosis and improvement in symptoms such as hot flashes and atrophic vaginitis. Although androgen production decreases in women during their forties, before spontaneous menopause has usually occurred,[1] relatively little is known of the biologic effects of this sex steroid in postmenopausal women and of its potential to enhance their quality of life. This chapter will review the evidence from randomized clinical trials and cross-sectional studies of the efficacy of combined estrogen–androgen (E-A) preparations on sexual functioning in postmenopausal women.

Testosterone and the central nervous system

Autoradiographic studies have demonstrated that neurons containing specific receptors for testosterone are predominantly found in the preoptic area of the hypothalamus, with smaller concentrations in the limbic system (amygdala and hippocampus) and the cerebral cortex.[2] Therefore, testosterone can exert effects on behavior by binding to the androgen receptor in these brain areas. Importantly, some proportion of testosterone is converted to estradiol in the brain.[3] Hence it is sometimes difficult to distinguish in studies that do not have an estrogen-alone group as comparison, whether the observed behavioral change is directly due to the testosterone in combined E-A preparations or to the estradiol to which the testosterone had been converted. Added to this complexity is the fact that estrogen increases sex hormone binding globulin (SHBG) while androgen reduces it[4] so that a dose of estrogen-alone equal to that in a combined E-A drug will result in different concentrations of bioavailable serum estradiol.

Animal studies

Effects of testosterone on various components of mating behavior have been studied intensively in nonhuman female primates. On the whole, these studies show that the administration of testosterone to an ovariectomized rhesus monkey increased proceptive behavior (i.e. increased attempts to solicit mounts from the male) which signifies her increased interest in sex. Implantation of minute amounts of testosterone into the anterior hypothalamus of estrogen-treated ovariectomized and adrenalectomized unreceptive female rhesus monkeys also resulted in restoration of only proceptivity but not other aspects of sexual function such as attractivity.[5]

These studies on testosterone and sexual behavior in nonhuman female primates serve to underline two points. First is that there is a specificity of action of testosterone on components of sexual behavior such that it enhances proceptivity (the animal's motivation to engage in sexual behavior) but has no effect on its attractivity or its receptivity to males. Second, the fact that a very small dose of testosterone implanted into the hypothalamus was effective in restoring sexual desire in rhesus monkeys[5] suggests that testosterone exerts its affect on sexual desire directly on the brain rather than by influencing peripheral tissues.

Testosterone and sexuality in postmenopausal women

Cross-sectional studies

Several cross-sectional studies have investigated whether associations occur between circulating levels of the sex steroids and aspects of sexual behavior in postmenopausal women. Leiblum et al.[6] reported that levels of both estradiol and testosterone failed to discriminate between sexually active and inactive untreated postmenopausal women but sexually active women had less vaginal atrophy than the inactive women. However, because these postmenopausal women were untreated, their endogenous sex hormone levels were, of course, very low. In a longitudinal study of perimenopausal women, plasma testosterone levels were positively associated with coital frequency.[7] Moreover, a positive correlation occurred between testosterone levels and sexual desire and sexual arousal in premenopausal women over the age of 40 years.[8] Other epidemiologic studies that have investigated changes in sexual functioning in perimenopausal and postmenopausal women failed to measure circulating levels of hormones.[9,10] One population-based study in middle-aged women failed to find an association between testosterone levels and any aspect of sexual functioning.[11] These findings were subsequently confirmed in another report of 40–60-year-old untreated women in whom endogenous androgen levels failed to predict scores on any of the measures of sexuality.[12] On the other hand, findings from a longitudinal, community-based study of women aged 45–55 years at baseline and followed for 9 years provided evidence that decreases in sexual functioning occurred during the menopausal transition in the majority of women.[13] Specifically, these women reported a decrease in sexual desire, sexual responsivity, and in sexual frequency as they transitioned through the menopause although age and relationship factors also played an important role. These findings serve to underline the fact that aspects of sexual functioning are negatively impacted by the transition through menopause in the majority of women although they do not establish a causal relationship between the behavior and the changes in sex hormone production at that time.

Treatment studies

By now, evidence is available from numerous treatment studies carried out in Europe and North America on the efficacy of combined E-A preparations on sexual functioning in postmenopausal women. Because different products are available in different countries and because the route of administration may influence behavioral and metabolic effects of these drugs, they will be categorized and reviewed according to their routes of administration.

Subcutaneous hormone pellet implants

In Britain and Australia, subcutaneous implantation of pellets containing estradiol and testosterone has been used as a treatment for menopausal symptoms for several decades. This route of sex-steroid administration results in a slow, constant release of the sex hormones over a period of at least 6 months. In a single blind study, a mixed group of 17 surgically and naturally menopausal women who complained of loss of libido despite treatment with estrogen received subcutaneous implants of 40 mg estradiol and 100 mg testosterone.[14] By the third month following implantation, the patients reported a significant increase in libido, in enjoyment of sex, and in the frequency of orgasm and initiation of sexual activities. Whereas the normal range of total testosterone levels for cycling women was 1–3 nmol/L in the assay used in that study, the mean baseline level of these women was 2.3 ± 1.2 nmol/L and rose to 4.2 ± 1.8 nmol/L 3 months postimplantation. Therefore, the improvements in sexual functioning experienced by these postmenopausal women occurred coincident with an increase in their serum total testosterone to supraphysiologic levels. One woman developed very mild hirsutism and another had a change in her voice range.

These findings gained support from a double-blind study of women complaining of loss of libido despite treatment with oral estrogens and progestins that adequately relieved other symptoms such as hot flashes and vaginal dryness.[15] They randomly received a subcutaneous implant containing either estrogen 40 mg or estrogen 40 mg plus testosterone 50 mg. After 6 weeks, the loss of libido in the estrogen-alone implant group remained whereas the combined estrogen-testosterone group experienced significant symptomatic relief. The mean peak testosterone concentrations after implantation of the combined pellet slightly exceeded the upper limit of the normal female range (3 nmol/L) reaching 3.5 nmol/L in the combined pellet group.

In a prospective, 2-year, single blind randomized trial, 34 postmenopausal women, none of whom had complained of low libido at the time of recruitment, received subcutaneous implantation of pellets containing either estradiol 50 mg or estradiol 50 mg plus testosterone 50 mg administered every 3 months.[16] Although all sexual behaviors (measured by the Sabbatsberg Sexual Self-rating Scale) improved in both treatment groups, women in the combined E-A group reported a significantly greater improvement in sexual activity, satisfaction, pleasure, and orgasm compared to the estrogen-alone group. Mean serum testosterone levels rose from 1.2 ± 0.55 nmol/L at baseline to 2.7 ± 1.39 nmoL at 6 months postimplantation in women treated with the combined estrogen + testosterone pellets so that the improvements in aspects of sexual functioning occurred under the influence of testosterone values within the normal female physiologic range (1.0–2.8 nmol/L) throughout the treatment period.

Although all these implant studies were single blind, in two of them,[14,15] patients had been preselected on the basis of loss of libido that had been unresponsive to treatment with estrogen-alone and one study[16] contained an estrogen-alone group as a basis for comparison. Even bearing in mind their methodologic flaws, the findings of these studies serve to point out that the addition of testosterone to an estrogen replacement regimen reversed the loss of libido in postmenopausal women that had not been alleviated with an equivalent dose of estrogen-alone.

Intramuscular E-A preparations

Perhaps the most powerful research paradigm for investigating the role of testosterone in women involves administering hormone therapy to women who have just undergone total abdominal hysterectomy (TAH) and bilateral salpingo-oophorectomy (BSO). When both ovaries are removed from premenopausal women, circulating testosterone levels decrease significantly within the first 24–48 h postoperatively.[17] The fact that these women are deprived of ovarian androgen production following this surgical procedure has provided a rationale for administering both estrogen and androgen as replacement therapy.

During the past two decades, several prospective, controlled studies of psychologic, metabolic, and sexual effects of a combined E-A intramuscular preparation in surgically menopausal women were carried out in our laboratory. One milliliter of the combined preparation we used contains testosterone enanthate 150 mg, estradiol dienanthate 7.5 mg, and estradiol benzoate 1.0 mg. At the time, the recommendation for the treatment of postmenopausal women was for the administration of 1 mL of this preparation intramuscularly every 28 days. Since the marketing of this drug predated the development of radioimmunoassay techniques for measuring hormone levels in serum, it was not known at the time these studies were undertaken, what serum levels of testosterone this dose would induce. The premenopausal women who participated in these prospective, controlled studies provided data on preoperative baseline performance, and then had surgery for benign conditions (uterine myomas or endometriosis). All of the women were in good general health, not taking any medications, and were in stable, long-term marital relationships. They were tested before surgery and then, again, 3 months following random assignment to either a combined E-A group, to an estrogen-alone group (E), to an androgen-alone group (A), or to a placebo group (PL).[18] Women in the E-alone and A-alone groups received amounts of estradiol valerate or testosterone enanthate equivalent to those found in 1 mL of the combined drug administered intramuscularly every 28 days. During the fourth postoperative month, all women received an injection of placebo (sesame oil) following which they were crossed-over to a treatment they had not received during treatment phase 1 for an additional 3 months. A fifth group of premenopausal women who underwent TAH, but whose ovaries were retained, served as a control group for the surgical procedure itself. Women who received either the E-A or A drugs following surgery had higher scores on energy level and sense of wellbeing than those who received E or PL. Administration of the androgen-containing preparations (A or E-A) were also associated with lower somatic and psychosomatic symptom scores than E or PL. Moreover, all women treated with hormones following surgery had more positive mood than those who had randomly received placebo.[19] Whereas total testosterone levels were a mean of 81.1±5.3 ng/dL at preoperative baseline when these women were cycling normally, they rose to 133.1±12.4 ng/dL by the third to fifth postinjection day following the administration of the combined E-A drug.

Androgenic effects on sexual behaviors were also investigated in these women. They monitored several aspects of their sexual behavior daily for the 8-month duration of the study. Women who received either of the androgen-containing preparations postoperatively reported an enhancement of sexual desire and arousal, and an increase in the number of sexual fantasies compared with those who received treatment with E or PL during both treatment phases.[20] Interestingly, ratings of sexual behavior of these surgically menopausal women treated with androgen did not differ from those of the TAH control group whose ovaries were retained and who were approximately 10 years younger than the women who had undergone BSO. Sherwin and Gelfand subsequently confirmed these findings on the androgenic enhancement of aspects of sexual behavior when the E-A combined drug was administered long-term for 2–4 years and sexual functioning was compared with that of a group of postmenopausal women treated with E-alone long term and a third group that had remained untreated following their TAH and BSO at least 2 years earlier.[21] In these women treated long term for 2 years with a combined E-A intramuscular drug, serum total testosterone reached peak, supraphysiologic levels at day 8 postinjection (2.85±0.04 ng/mL) and declined slowly across the next 3 weeks as the drug was being metabolized.[22] Therefore, while the average level of total testosterone induced by the intramuscular E-A preparation used was at the upper level of the normal female range of testosterone values when averaged over the entire 28 day period, levels were above the normal range when blood was sampled on day 8 postinjection. The findings from these studies clearly demonstrated that the addition of testosterone to an estrogen treatment regimen enhanced sexual desire, interest, and fantasy in surgically menopausal women.

Transdermal preparations

Recently, findings were reported on the efficacy of a transdermal testosterone patch for the treatment of postmenopausal women. Seventy-five healthy women who had undergone TAH and BSO approximately 5 years earlier were selected because they reported impaired sexual functioning despite receiving at least 0.625 mg conjugated equine estrogen (CEE) daily for at least 2 months before entry into the study.[23] Sexual behavior was quantified by means of the 22-item Brief Index for Sexual Functioning for Women (BISFW) at screening and again, after 12 weeks of treatment with their usual dose of CEE and, in random order, placebo, 150 μg of testosterone, and 300 μg testosterone per day transdermally for 12 weeks each. Despite a considerable placebo response, the 300 μg, but not the 150 μg dose of testosterone resulted in further increases in scores for frequency of sexual activity and pleasure-orgasm as measured by the BISFW. Again, at the higher, but not at the lower dose of transdermal testosterone, the percentages of women who had sexual fantasies, masturbated, or engaged in sexual intercourse at least once a week increased two to three times compared to baseline. Positive wellbeing, depressed mood, and composite scores of the Psychological General Well-Being Index also improved significantly in women when they were receiving the 300 μg testosterone patch compared to the placebo patch. It is noteworthy that mean bioavailable testosterone levels were 2.0 ± 1.4 ng/dL at pretreatment (normal female range 1.6–12.7 ng/dL), rose to 7.1 ± 4.1 ng/dL with the 150 μg patch and to 11.4 ± 9.5 ng/dL with the 300 μg testosterone patch. Therefore, the enhancement of sexual behavior reported by women who received treatment with the 300 μg testosterone patch was achieved when the serum levels of bioavailable testosterone it induced were at the upper limit of the normal female range.

Two recent large, multicenter, randomized, controlled trials have provided further support for these finding using the same transdermal testosterone patch. In a double blind, placebo controlled trial, healthy women who had developed low sexual desire following TAH and BSO and who had been receiving oral estrogen therapy were randomly given either a placebo, a 150 μg/day, a 300 μm/day, or a 450 μg/day testosterone patch for 24 weeks in addition to oral estrogen.[24] Women who received the 300 μg/day testosterone patch but not those who received the 150 μg or 450 μg patches experienced greater increases in sexual desire and in frequency of satisfying sexual activity than those treated with placebo. In the second study, 533 estrogen-treated surgically menopausal women with hypoactive sexual desire disorder randomly received treatment with either a placebo or a 300 μg/day testosterone patch for 24 weeks.[25] Once

again, the 300 μg testosterone patch significantly increased satisfying sexual activity and sexual desire while decreasing personal distress. Taken together, these studies on the efficacy of the transdermal patch provide strong support for the conclusion that 300 μg/day of testosterone administered transdermally increases sexual desire and the incidence of satisfying sexual encounters in surgically menopausal women.

A recent study investigated whether a transdermal testosterone cream administered to premenopausal women complaining of low libido would have a beneficial effect. Thirty-four women (mean age 39 years) who had normal cycles and were complaining of low libido were randomized to receive either testosterone cream (10 mg) or placebo cream daily for two double blind, 12-week treatment periods separated by a single blind, 4-week washout period.[26] Scores on the Sabbatsberg Sexual Self-Rating Scale increased significantly with the testosterone cream but not with placebo cream. Total testosterone levels were within the lower third of the normal female range before treatment and the Free Androgen Index (FAI) increased to values above the upper limit of the normal female range after treatment with the testosterone cream. However, no increased incidence of acne or hirsutism appeared to result from these high testosterone levels. These findings suggest that testosterone cream may be a safe and efficacious treatment for complaints of low libido in premenopausal women although more information is needed on this drug.

Oral E-A preparations

In the USA, an oral E-A combined drug has been available for several decades and evidence of its efficacy on sexual functioning in postmenopausal women is available. Twenty postmenopausal women (40% of whom were surgically menopausal) dissatisfied with their estrogen therapy were monitored for 2 weeks while still on estrogen-alone (baseline).[27] Then, all of the women received a placebo in single blind fashion for 2 weeks following which they were randomly assigned to treatment with either 1.25 mg esterified estrogen or to 1.25 mg esterified estrogen plus 2.5 mg methyltestosterone daily for 8 weeks. Sexual functioning was measured by means of a 10-item Sexual Activity and Libido Scale.

Combined ratings of sexual sensation and desire increased significantly in the group treated with the combined oral E-A drug after 4 and 8 weeks of treatment in comparison to both their pretreatment scores on estrogen-alone and to the postplacebo baseline assessments. In addition, an increase in the frequency of sexual intercourse occurred by week 4 of treatment in the combined group but was no longer significant by week 8. No changes in any aspect of sexual behavior occurred in the group treated with estrogen-alone despite the fact that effects of both drugs on vaginal cytology did not differ.

Two randomized trials that used oral hormone preparations provide additional information on testosterone and sexual functioning in women. Forty-four women who had undergone a TAH and BSO (mean age 54 years) and who were not specifically complaining of sexual dysfunction were randomly assigned to receive either oral estradiol valerate 2 mg plus testosterone undecanoate 40 mg or estradiol valerate 2 mg (E-alone) plus placebo daily for 24 months.[28] Then the women were crossed over to the other treatment for an additional 24 weeks. Those who received the combined E-A preparation reported a significant increase in enjoyment of sex, frequency of sexual activity, and interest in sex compared to the E-alone plus placebo. Both regimens improved psychological wellbeing and self-esteem equally. However, there was considerable variability in serum levels of total testosterone and free testosterone in the women and values exceeded the upper limit of normal female values in 57% of the participants following 24 weeks of treatment. In the second study, 218 naturally or surgically postmenopausal women (mean age 53 years) who were complaining of loss of libido despite treatment with estrogen for at least 3 months prior to their recruitment were randomly treated with esterified estrogens (EE) 0.625 mg and methyltestosterone (MT) 1.25 mg or with EE 0.625 mg alone for 16 weeks.[29] The combined EE+MT preparation increased the concentration of bioavailable testosterone, suppressed sex hormone binding globulin, and significantly enhanced scores on sexual desire and frequency of desire compared to the women's own baseline scores and also to the posttreatment scores of the placebo group. Moreover, there were no differences in hirsutism or acne scores between the groups by the end of the study; markedly abnormal hepatic enzymes were not detected in any of the women treated with EE and MT.

Possible side-effects of E-A replacement therapy

The possibility that exogenous testosterone could induce symptoms of virilization in women has long been a concern. Although we did not use an objective measure of hirsutism in our studies of the injectible E-A preparation,[20–22] our clinical experience with this drug suggests that approximately 20% of women who receive 150 mg testosterone enanthate plus estradiol intramuscularly every 28 days will develop mild hirsutism manifested by an increased growth of hair on the chin and/or upper lip. When the dose is reduced to 75 mg testosterone per 28 days (the dose currently recommended), less than 5% of women develop hirsutism and, when they do, the symptom is reversible when they are withdrawn from the combined drug and given estrogen-alone. This suggests that variability in response to the potential virilizing effects of testosterone exists between women and that the occurrence of these symptoms is likely also dose dependent. From 5 to 20% of women treated with subcutaneous pellet implants of estrogen and testosterone developed hirsutism although, once again, this was not evaluated systematically.[14–16] In a safety surveillance of oral esterified estrogen and methyltestosterone,[30] the risk of hirsutism was less than 5%, and in another safety study of the same oral preparation, the incidence of hirsutism with the addition of methyltestosterone was not different from that of women who received estrogen-alone.[31] Neither did the hirsutism scores change significantly in women treated with transdermal testosterone plus estrogen,[23,25] although the mean facial depilation rate increased slightly but not significantly during treatment with 300 µg of testosterone per day. Acne and deepening of the voice were reported rarely or not at all in these reports.

There is some evidence that oral E-A preparations modify the lipoprotein lipid profile. Oral methyltestosterone plus estrogen resulted in a decrease in high-density lipoprotein (HDL) cholesterol by up to 20% compared to baseline.[23] However, low-density lipoprotein (LDL) cholesterol is reduced to a similar extent as with estrogen-alone and triglycerides, which tend to increase with oral estrogen-alone, actually decreased by approximately 15% when methyltestosterone was added.[32,33] Moreover, testosterone may be beneficial for dilating coronary arteries[34] and does not negatively influence coronary vasodilation in Cynomolgus monkeys.[35] Neither did the combined intramuscular preparation,[36] the E-A pellet implants,[37] or the transdermal testosterone patch[23,24] cause changes in the lipoprotein lipid profile compared to treatment with estrogen-alone. Clearly, route of administration of sex hormones modulates metabolic responses to hormone therapy and the available data suggest that nonoral routes of administration of testosterone do not have significant negative side effects on lipid metabolism, at least in the doses and regimens tested. Since the addition of testosterone to an estrogen replacement regimen does not mitigate against endometrial hyperplasia,[38] a progestational agent needs to be added to the hormone regimen when treatment with a combined drug is administered to women with intact uteri.

Finally, it is clear that when testosterone is administered via the subcutaneous implantation of pellets, it metabolizes very slowly and, often, levels are still supraphysiologic 4 months postimplantation.[14–16] Therefore it is necessary to assess serum levels of testosterone prior to reimplantation of the pellets in women receiving chronic therapy.

Conclusion

Taken together, the randomized controlled trials of both naturally and surgically postmenopausal women who were administered either subcutaneous implants of estrogen and testosterone, an intramuscular E-A preparation, an oral E+MT drug or, more recently, an oral estrogen (CEE) combined with a transdermal testosterone patch have consistently shown that combined treatment with estrogen and testosterone induces a greater sense of energy levels and wellbeing and is associated with fewer somatic and psychologic symptoms compared with the administration of estrogen-alone. Furthermore, E-A preparations increased motivational aspects of sexual behavior (such as desire and fantasies) as well as the

frequency of orgasm and of sexual intercourse. We have shown that levels of sexual desire and interest vary with plasma testosterone levels throughout a treatment month as the intramuscularly administered drug is being metabolized. The fact that, in several studies, this enhancement of sexual functioning occurred in women who complained of deficits in their sexual function while being treated with estrogen-alone underlines the fact that, while estrogen is necessary for the integrity of reproductive tissues, it does not otherwise contribute towards the maintenance of a variety of sexual behaviors in postmenopausal women. Rather, the demonstration in these randomized controlled trials that sexual complaints in estrogen-treated postmenopausal women responded to the addition of testosterone to their estrogen regimen provides compelling evidence that testosterone is critical for the maintenance of sexual desire/interest in women. It is also noteworthy that combined E-A drugs seem to be equally effective in naturally and in surgically postmenopausal women although there is some suggestion from the literature that younger women who have had BSO and therefore experienced an abrupt decrease in their testosterone levels may be both more highly symptomatic and more highly responsive to combined estrogen–testosterone therapy.

Sufficient evidence is now available from well controlled studies to inform decisions regarding the use of combined E-A drugs for the treatment of postmenopausal women. The extant findings show that combined preparations enhance energy level, wellbeing, and sexual desire and/or interest to levels over and above those that may be induced by treatment with estrogen-alone. Therefore, women currently being treated with estrogen whose symptoms of fatigue and impaired sexual functioning are enduring may benefit by the addition of testosterone to their estrogen regimen. However, it is also important to acknowledge that human sexuality is very complex and has multiple determinants; it is clear that personality factors, psychologic factors, relationship factors as well as hormonal factors all play a role in determining the quality of sexual functioning in the individual woman. The most clear-cut indication for combined E-A therapy is for complaints of decreased sexual desire whose onset occurred during the peri or postmenopause in a woman who reports a satisfactory sexual history during her premenopausal years. In these cases, there is a greater likelihood that the perimenopausal decrease in sexual desire is due to endocrine factors and a greater probability that exogenous testosterone will reverse it. When the history is complicated by concurrent life stress, physical illness or previous sexual dysfunctions, then it is unlikely that combined E-A therapy alone will reverse the symptoms and sexual counseling should also be sought.

Because different combined preparations are available in Canada, the USA and Europe, it is not useful to recommend specific products or doses. In general, the frequency of virilizing side effects were rare in the randomized controlled trials reviewed above and, when they occurred, appeared to be dose dependent. Indeed, in the studies that used a dose of testosterone that induced levels within the normal female range, these side effects did not occur. Although the efficacy of the oral combined preparation on sexual complaints has been demonstrated, parenteral routes of administration of testosterone would appear to have fewer metabolic side effects.

Acknowledgements

The preparation of this chapter was supported by research funds associated with the Canadian Institutes for Health Research Distinguished Scientist Award given to BB Sherwin.

References

1. Burger HG, Dudley EC, Cui J et al. A prospective longitudinal study of serum testosterone dehydroepiandrosterone sulphate, and sex hormone-binding globulin levels through the menopause transition. J Clin Endocrinol Metab 2000; 85: 2832–2838.
2. McEwen BS. The brain as a target organ of endocrine hormones. In: DT Kreiger, JS Hughes (Eds.). Neuroendocrinology, 1989: 33–42. Sutherland, MA: Sinauer Assoc.
3. Celotto F, Melcangi RC, Negri-Cesi P et al. Testosterone metabolism in brain cells and membranes. J Steroid Biochem Mol Biol 1991; 40:673–678.
4. Anderson DCP. Sex hormone binding globulin. Clin Endocrinol 1974; 3:69–74.
5. Everitt BJ, Herbert J. The effects of implanting testosterone propionate in the central nervous system on the sexual behavior of the female rhesus monkeys. Brain Res 1975; 86:109–120.
6. Leiblum S, Bachmann G, Kemmann E et al. Vaginal atrophy in the postmenopausal woman: the importance of sexual activity and hormones. JAMA 1984; 249:2195–2198.
7. McCoy N, Davidson J. A longitudinal study of the effects of menopause on sexuality. Maturitas 1985; 7:203–210.
8. Flöter A, Nathorst-Böös J, Carlstrom K et al. Androgen status and sexual life in perimenopausal women. Menopause 1997; 4:95–100.
9. Dennerstein L, Smith AMS, Morse CA et al. Sexuality and the menopause. J Psychosom Obstet Gynaecol 1994; 15:59–66.
10. Hallstrom T. Sexuality in the climacteric. Clin Obstet Gynecol 1977; 4:227–239.
11. Dennerstein L, Dudley EC, Hopper JL et al. Sexuality, hormones and the menopausal transition. Maturitas 1977; 26:83–93.
12. Cawood EHH, Bancroft J. Steroid hormones. The menopause, sexuality and well-being of women. Psychol Med 1996; 26:925–936.
13. Guthrie JR, Dennerstein L, Taffe JR et al. The menopause transition: the Melbourne Women's Midlife Health Project. Climacteric 2004; 7:375–389.
14. Burger HG, Hailes J, Menelaus M et al. The management of persistent menopausal symptoms with oestradiol testosterone implants: Clinical, lipid and hormonal results. Maturitas 1984; 6:351–358.
15. Burger HG, Hailes J, Nelson J et al. Effects of combined implants of estradiol and testosterone on libido in postmenopausal women. Br Med J 1987; 294:936–937.
16. Davis SR, McClaud P, Strauss BJG et al. Testosterone enhances estradiol's effects on postmenopausal bone density and sexuality. Maturitas 1995; 21:227–236.
17. Longcope C. Metabolism clearance and blood production rates of estrogen in postmenopausal women. Am J Obstet Gynecol 1981; 111:779–785.
18. Sherwin BB, Gelfand MM. Differential symptom response to parenteral estrogen and/or androgen administration in the surgical menopause. Am J Obstet Gynecol 1985; 151:153–160.
19. Sherwin BB. Affective changes with estrogen and androgen replacement therapy in surgically menopausal women. J Affective Dis 1988; 14: 177–187.
20. Sherwin BB, Gelfand MM, Brender W. Androgen enhances sexual motivation in females: A prospective cross-over study of sex steroid administration in the surgical menopause. Psychosom Med 1985; 7:339–351.
21. Sherwin BB, Gelfand MM. The role of androgen in the maintenance of sexual functioning in oophorectomized women. Psychosom Med 1987; 49:397–409.
22. Sherwin BB. Changes in sexual behavior as a function of plasma sex steroid levels in post-menopausal women. Maturitas 1985; 7:225–233.

23. Shifren JL, Braunstein GD, Simon JA et al. Transdermal testosterone treatment in women with impaired sexual function after oophorectomy. N Engl J Med 2000; 343:682–688.
24. Braunstein GD, Sundwall DA, Katz M et al. The safety and efficacy of a testosterone patch for the treatment of hypoactive sexual desire disorder in surgically menopausal women: a randomized, placebo-controlled trial. Arch Intern Med, in press.
25. Buster JE, Kingsberg SA, Aguirre O et al. Testosterone patch for low sexual desire in surgically menopausal women: a randomized trial. Obstet Gynecol, in press.
26. Goldstat R, Esther B, Tran J et al. Transdermal testosterone therapy improves well-being, mood and sexual function in premenopausal women. Menopause 2003; 10:390–398.
27. Sarrel P, Dobay B, Wiita B. Estrogen and estrogen-androgen replacement in postmenopausal women dissatisfied with estrogen-alone therapy. J Reprod Med 1998; 43:847–856.
28. Flöter A, Nathorst-Böös J, Carlstrom K et al. Addition of testosterone to estrogen replacement therapy in oophorectomized women: effects on sexuality and well-being. Climacteric 2002; 5: 357–365.
29. Lobo RA, Rosen RC, Yang HM et al. Comparative effects of oral esterified estrogens with and without methyltestosterone on endocrine profiles and dimensions of sexual function in postmenopausal women with hypoactive sexual desire. Fertil Steril 2003; 79:1341–1352.
30. Phillips E, Bauman C. Safety surveillance of esterified estrogens-methyltestosterone (Estratest and Estratest HS) replacement therapy in the United States. Clin Ther 1997; 19:1070–1084.
31. Barrett-Connor E, Timmons C, Young R et al. Interim safety of a two-year study comparing oral estrogen-androgen and conjugated estrogens in surgically menopausal women. J Women's Health 1996; 5:593–602.
32. Watts NB, Notelovitz M, Timmons MC et al. Comparison of oral estrogens and estrogens plus androgen on bone mineral density, menopausal symptoms and lipid-lipoprotein profiles in surgical menopausal women. Obstet Gynecol 1995; 85: 529–537.
33. Hickok LR, Toomey C, Speroff L. A comparison of esterified estrogens with and without methyltestosterone: Effects on endometrial histology and serum lipoproteins in postmenopausal women. Obstet Gynecol 1993; 82:919–924.
34. Yue P, Chatterkee K, Beale C. Testosterone relaxes rabbit coronary arteries and aorta. Circulation 1995; 91:1154–1160.
35. Honoré EH, Williams JK, Adams MR et al. Methyltestosterone does not diminish the beneficial effects of estrogen replacement therapy on coronary artery reactivity in cynomolgus monkeys. Menopause 1996; 3:20–26.
36. Sherwin BB, Gelfand MM, Schucher R et al. Postmenopausal estrogen and androgen replacement and lipoprotein lipid concentrations. Am J Obstet Gynecol 1987; 156:414–419.
37. Farish E, Fletcher CD, Hart DM et al. The effect of hormone implants on serum lipoproteins and steroid hormones in bilaterally oophorectomized women. Acta Endocrinol 1984; 106:116–123.
38. Gelfand MM, Ferenczy A, Bergeron C. Endometrial response to estrogen-androgen stimulation. In CB Hammond, FB Haseltine, I Seniff (Eds.). Menopause Evaluation, Treatment and Health Concerns. 1989; 29–40. New York: Alan R Liss.

Chapter 7

Transdermal testosterone treatment in women

Livia Rivera-Woll and Susan R Davis

Summary

Recently the transdermal route for delivery of reproductive steroids has been developed for the delivery of testosterone at low doses in androgen-deficient women. Clinical studies evaluating physiologic doses have shown benefits in sexual function and mood in both postmenopausal and premenopausal androgen-deficient women. Many of the available preparations have not been specifically designed and are not formulated in the appropriate doses required for use in women. Achieving physiologic free testosterone levels by transdermal delivery appears to be the best approach for minimizing the adverse effects of androgens. New innovative transdermal agents designed to deliver testosterone for specific use in women are being developed and are now becoming available.

Introduction

The transdermal route for delivery of reproductive steroids has been used for at least two decades in women with one of the earliest reports of use of a transdermal patch delivery system for estradiol published in 1983.[1] More recently this mode of delivery has been developed for the delivery of testosterone with the use of the testosterone patch. Transdermal patches and gels are a generally accepted measure of androgen replacement in men. This form of androgen replacement has been developed at lower doses for use in androgen-deficient women. The testosterone matrix patch is currently in phase III clinical trials for the treatment of low libido in oophorectomized and naturally menopausal women. A novel form of transdermal delivery of testosterone, a metered dose transdermal testosterone spray is also currently in phase II clinical trial in premenopausal and postmenopausal women with symptomatic androgen deficiency.

Clinical studies for transdermal testosterone treatment in women

Clinical studies evaluating the use of transdermal testosterone have shown benefits in sexual function and mood in both postmenopausal and premenopausal androgen-deficient women. Initial studies evaluated pharmacologic doses, which result in supraphysiologic testosterone levels. More recently physiologic doses which result in free testosterone levels within the normal range for healthy young women have been studied and found similar benefits.

Results in postmenopausal women

Initial studies assessing the use of supraphysiologic doses of testosterone treatment in oophorectomized and naturally menopausal women have shown improvements in sexual function. In a prospective, cross-over study of 53 surgically menopausal women, those treated with supra-physiologic doses of intramuscular testosterone or testosterone–estradiol combined had significant improvements in sexual desire, fantasies, and arousal compared with women treated with estradiol alone or placebo.[2] The dose of testosterone enanthate administered in this study was 150 mg per month, which is a dose producing full virilization when given to hypogonadal males.

Sherwin and Gelfand showed that the addition of intramuscular testosterone to estrogen replacement in oophorectomized women resulted in improvements in sexual motivation behaviors, namely desire, fantasy, and arousal as well as increases in coital frequency and orgasm, with the improvements due to testosterone and not estrogen.[3] Treatment with testosterone resulted in improved wellbeing and increased energy levels than in those who received estrogen alone.

Burger et al. treated 17 women with decreased libido not adequately relieved by oral estrogen (conjugated equine estrogen (CEE) 1.25 mg daily or estradiol valerate 4 mg daily) with combined subcutaneous implants of estradiol (40 mg) and testosterone (100 mg).[4] Following treatment with combined estradiol–testosterone implants, significant improvements were noted in libido, enjoyment of sex, and tiredness ($P<0.01$). There were no significant changes in flushes, sweats and depression. At 3 months libido increased in all assessable women from a mean basal level of 13.5 to a maximum of 86.1 (on an analog scale with a maximum score of 100). Symptomatic improvement was maintained for 4–6 months. Total testosterone plasma concentration rose from 2.3 nmol/L (measured at the point of discontinuing oral estrogen) to 6.7 nmol/L at 1 month and returned to baseline at 5 months. This dose of the testosterone can be considered pharmacologic.

The same authors undertook a single blind, controlled study with lower dose testosterone implants in 20 postmenopausal women complaining of loss of libido, unresponsive to adequate estrogen replacement.[5] The women were treated with implants of either estradiol alone (40 mg) or estradiol in combination with testosterone (50 mg) at concentrations raising the total testosterone level to just above the upper limit of normal (3.5–3.7 nmol/L). Women receiving combined implants showed a marked improvement in the various sexual measures recorded along with an improvement in general wellbeing. The women receiving estradiol implants alone showed no improvement in sexual function after 6 weeks but were subsequently shown to have marked improvement in sexual functioning following treatment with combined implants. The dose of testosterone used here could be considered to be in the high physiologic or low pharmacologic range.

Davis et al. conducted a single blind, randomized trial of 34 postmenopausal women not identified as having sexual dysfunction over a 2-year period.[6] Women received either estradiol implants 50 mg alone or estradiol 50 mg with testosterone 50 mg. The combined treatment increased serum testosterone concentrations to high in the normal range and improved all parameters of sexual function measured using the Sabbatsberg Sexual Self-rating Scale as compared with estradiol alone.

Shifren et al. conducted a study of physiologic testosterone therapy in 75 women who experienced decreased libido following hysterectomy and oophorectomy despite treatment with CEE in a dose of at least 0.625 mg daily.[7] The women were treated with transdermal testosterone matrix patches delivering 150 μg/day or 300 μg/day or placebo, each for 12 weeks, in a cross-over, randomized controlled trial. The higher dose testosterone patch produced circulating free testosterone concentrations close to the upper end of the normal female range. Although there was a considerable placebo response, women receiving the higher testosterone dose experienced significant increases in the frequency of sexual activity and pleasure-orgasm. At this dose the percentages of women who had sexual fantasies or engaged in sexual activity at least once a week increased two to threefold over baseline. A post-hoc analysis showed that in contrast to the younger subjects in the study (under the median age of 48 years), the 'older half' of the population had a much smaller placebo response and exhibited significant improvements in sexual function parameters at both doses of testosterone (150 μg/day or 300 μg/day). Positive wellbeing and depressed mood (measured by the Psychological General Well Being Index) also improved significantly in the group receiving the higher testosterone dose. Although use of the 300 μg patch increased mean serum total testosterone levels into the supraphysiologic range (102 ng/dL; normal range 14–54 ng/dL), mean serum free and bioavailable testosterone levels remained within the high-normal range (5.9 pg/mL; normal range 1.3–6.8 pg/mL).

Results in premenopausal women

Although the clinical evidence for testosterone use in premenopausal women is limited the available evidence has shown benefit in this group of women as well. In a placebo controlled, randomized trial with a cross-over design of 45 premenopausal women presenting with low libido demonstrated that transdermal testosterone cream (10 mg/day) significantly improved sexual motivation, fantasy, frequency of sexual activity, pleasure, orgasm, and satisfaction ($P=0.001$).[8] In addition to the positive effects on sexual function, the women receiving testosterone showed a significant improvement in the total score and all subscale scores of the Personal General Wellbeing Index ($P=0.003$) as well as an improvement in mood as measured by the Beck Depression Inventory ($P=0.06$). The mean free androgen index was just above the proposed upper limit for young women, although no true range has been formally established for this estimate of free testosterone. A number of ongoing studies are assessing the use of testosterone in premenopausal women.

Methods of androgen administration

A variety of preparations are available for the administration of testosterone. However, many have not been specifically designed for use in women and are therefore not formulated in the appropriate doses required for use in women. The following is a list of testosterone preparations currently being used in clinical practice or in investigational research protocols for the treatment of low libido in women with low testosterone levels:

- Testosterone products designed for use in men that are used off-label at lower doses in women:
  - intramuscular T-ester depot formulations
  - subcutaneous testosterone implants
  - oral testosterone undecanoate (TU)
  - transdermal testosterone reservoir patches
  - transdermal testosterone gels

- Oral methyltestosterone (MT) combined with CEE
- A transdermal 1% testosterone cream for women available off-label in Australia
- An investigational transdermal testosterone matrix patch designed for use in women
- An investigational testosterone gel for women
- An investigational transdermally absorbed metered dose testosterone spray designed for use in women.

In the USA, the oral combination of MT and CEE is used with the MT given in lower doses than those used in men. Oral MT is not ideal for long-term administration as it is subject to first pass hepatic metabolism and is associated with a reduction in circulating levels of sex hormone binding globulin (SHBG),[9] thyroxine binding globulin,[10] and high-density lipoprotein (HDL) cholesterol levels.[11] Moreover, supraphysiologic doses of oral MT have been associated with hepatotoxicity.[12]

Oral TU, available in Europe and Canada, is a capsule designed for use in men. It is absorbed via the intestinal lymphatics which although avoids hepatic first pass metabolism, has been shown to lead to unpredictable absorption with variable and short-lived serum testosterone concentrations.[13] It is not recommended for use in women, as neither efficacy data nor safety data for this therapy in women are available and available doses have been shown to result in supraphysiologic serum testosterone levels.[12]

Intramuscular mixed testosterone esters at doses of 50 mg to 100 mg have been used at 4–6 weekly intervals but the use of this agent is empirical and not supported by clinical data. T-ester injections are associated with supraphysiologic peak levels; as such the potential for adverse effects is high. Long-term use of injectable T-esters (in combination with injectable estrogens) at doses of 150 mg every 2–4 weeks has been shown to result in virilization in women.[14] This form of testosterone administration is not suitable for long-term use in women.

Transdermal testosterone

Achieving physiologic free testosterone levels by transdermal delivery appears to be the best approach for minimizing the adverse effects of androgens. Unlike oral testosterone therapy, transdermal testosterone therapy avoids hepatic first pass metabolism and does not result in a reduction in SHBG, thyroxine binding globulin, or HDL.[7] Transdermal administration of testosterone with subcutaneous implants, transdermal patches and gels at doses comparable to premenopausal hormone production, has not been associated with virilization, polycythemia, abnormal carbohydrate metabolism, or adverse effects on the liver in the published short-term studies[7] and longer-term data (up to 12 months) from subsequent unpublished studies.[15]

Subcutaneous testosterone implants

In the UK and Australia, testosterone is commonly administered in the form of a fused crystalline subcutaneous implant.[6] Subcutaneous testosterone implants are approved for use in post-menopausal women in the UK. The T-implant is inserted subcutaneously in the lower anterior abdominal wall under local anesthetic using a trochar and cannula. The dose commonly initiated is 50 mg. This is achieved by halving a 100 mg implant, which is specifically formulated for use in men. These slow-release implants remain effective for a period of 4–6 months at which time a low free T or total T with SHBG should be confirmed prior to repeat implantation. The dose can be increased in increments of 25 mg to achieve clinical efficacy. However, it is recommended that doses do not exceed 100 mg, as this dose has been shown to result in supraphysiologic serum testosterone levels for at least the first 1–2 months[12] and virilizing side effects are more likely to occur above this dose.[16] A therapeutic trial of a topical 1% T cream applied daily is often given for 4–6 weeks prior to inserting a T-implant. If there is a positive response, with no adverse effects a T-implant may be inserted.

Compounded topical preparations containing MT and dihydrotestosterone (DHT) have also been suggested for use in women, as neither is aromatizable to estrogen. However, their use is not recommended as the dose of testosterone available in these preparations is not standardized and evidence for the safety of these preparations in women is limited.

Innovative agents designed for specific use in women

Testosterone matrix patch

Daily testosterone production rate in women is about 5% of that in men. Healthy, premenopausal women produce approximately 250 µg/day of testosterone and this decreases to approximately 180 µg/day in post-menopausal women.[17] Subsequently, an alcohol-free transdermal T matrix patch has been developed for specific use in women. The T matrix patch has been formulated in two doses, which deliver approximately 150 µg or 300 µg/day of testosterone and is applied twice weekly to the abdomen. These smaller patches are generally associated with much less local skin side effects than the T reservoir patches used in men. The T matrix patch delivers testosterone to the systemic circulation by passive diffusion through the skin where it is absorbed through the dermal capillaries.

Unlike testosterone subcutaneous implants, the transdermal testosterone matrix patch has been shown to provide relatively stable testosterone concentrations with little within- and between-subject variability.[12] The currently available patch doses have been shown to result in physiologic increases in serum free testosterone levels. In a pharmacokinetic study conducted by Mazer, the 150 µg/day T patch was shown to elevate serum testosterone levels by approximately 1 nmol/L (28 ng/dL).[18] In this study, a 150 µg/day testosterone patch was applied for 4 days in 11 oophorectomized women who had a normal SHBG levels and had discontinued estrogen therapy for at least 6 weeks. While wearing the patch, testosterone levels increased into the middle and upper half of the normal range and remained relatively stable for 96 hours. The mean time-averaged increments above baseline for total and free testosterone were 27.6 ± 13.1 ng/dL and 2.7 ± 0.9 pg/mL, respectively. Following removal of the patch, testosterone levels returned to baseline within 12–24 h. Although the 300 µg/day T patch has been associated with higher serum total testosterone levels, serum free testosterone levels were in the high normal range.[7]

The dermal activity of aromatase[19] and 5α-reductase[20] is minimal in nongenital skin. As such, the dermal conversion of testosterone to estradiol (E_2) and DHT, respectively, is expected to be minimal with the use transdermal testosterone applied to the abdominal skin. In Mazer's study,[18] the DHT:T ratio attained with application of the T patch was shown to be greater than the DHT:T ratio attained in women by systemic conversion alone.[21] This suggests that a small degree, approximately 6%,[22] of dermal conversion of testosterone to DHT by 5α-reductase occurs with transdermal testosterone delivery through nongenital skin. In contrast, there appeared to be negligible dermal aromatisation of T to E_2. With the use of the testosterone patch, the E_2:T ratio was not significantly different from the known systemic conversion of testosterone to E_2 in women. Therefore, plasma levels of E_2 and DHT measured while using the T matrix patch are predominantly reflective of systemic aromatase and 5α-reductase activity, respectively.

The testosterone matrix patch is currently in phase III clinical trials in postmenopausal women. To date the investigational matrix patches have been well tolerated and local androgenic effects on the skin have not been reported. Providing that circulating androgen concentrations are kept within or close to the upper limit of the normal physiologic range, masculinizing effects are extremely unlikely.[7] The major side effect encountered has been allergy to the patch adhesive with an erythematous reaction at the patch site.[7] The site reaction is usually mild and can be minimized by rotating the patch site on each application. However, evidence of systemic sensitization requires discontinuation of therapy.

The patch should be applied to clean, dry skin over the abdomen twice a week. To avoid skin irritation, when the patch is changed the new patch should be applied at a different site. Bathing while wearing the patch is allowable but women should not apply oil-based products or cosmetics on or around the patch. Additional advantages associated with the use of the T patch include rapid onset and termination of action following removal of the patch, and patches are noninvasive and can be self-administered.

Although studies of the T matrix patch have reported only minimal adverse effects, this needs to be verified in long-term studies, as there may be a duration effect. Long-term safety with the use of the T matrix patch is currently being evaluated in phase III clinical trials.

Testosterone metered dose transdermal spray

The testosterone metered dose transdermal spray (MDTS®) comprises a single phase solution of testosterone and enhancer which is designed to dry rapidly, leaving an invisible water-resistant depot in the skin from which testosterone is slowly absorbed into the dermal capillaries. This provides sustained delivery of testosterone to the systemic circulation. It is applied onto clean, dry skin on the abdomen and allowed to dry for 2 minutes before covering with clothing and for 30 minutes before wetting the area. After this women can bathe and swim. Additional advantages include ease of use, dosage flexibility, cosmetic acceptability, and low risk of skin irritation, as there is no adhesive.

Pharmacokinetic studies assessing the MDTS in postmenopausal women have been completed. Initial studies in five oophorectomized women taking oral estrogen therapy allowed determination of the dose required to increase serum steady-state free testosterone levels into the high normal range for premenopausal women.[23] In a subsequent study, 11 naturally menopausal and three surgically menopausal women receiving transdermal estradiol therapy ($50\,\mu g$/day) with low serum testosterone levels applied $2 \times 91\,\mu L$ sprays of the MDTS for 5 days.[23] This dose was found to increase average serum free testosterone concentrations into the mid-to-high normal range for premenopausal women. Steady-state serum concentrations of free and total testosterone concentrations were attained on day 5. Average and maximum serum concentrations of free and total testosterone were significantly higher after application to the forearm compared to the abdomen. SHBG levels did not change significantly over the dosage intervals.

A phase II clinical trial evaluating the efficacy of the MDTS has been completed in premenopausal women with low testosterone levels and symptoms of androgen insufficiency.[23] This is a placebo controlled, randomized trial in which 261 women were randomized to one of four treatment groups for a 16-week period. The four groups comprised $2 \times 90\,\mu L$ sprays daily of the MDTS; $1 \times 90\,\mu L$ spray daily of the MDTS; $1 \times 56\,\mu L$ spray daily of the MDTS and a placebo group using one or two sprays daily of a placebo spray. The data will be published in 2006 and will provide yet another promising, noninvasive form of transdermal testosterone delivery for use in women.

Testosterone cream

There is a 1% testosterone cream available as an off-label prescription in Australia, which has been shown to be effective in treating symptoms of low libido in premenopausal women as discussed previously.[8] This mode of testosterone administration requires daily application to the skin over the thigh or abdomen. It must be applied after bathing and be allowed to dry for 30 minutes. Serum free testosterone and SHBG levels should be checked 4 weeks after commencing therapy and every 6 months thereafter ensuring that the calculated free testosterone levels are maintained within the normal range.

Testosterone gel

A testosterone gel is currently being designed for specific use in women and is in early phase clinical trials.

Compounded topical testosterone gel and buccal troches

Some pharmacists prepare compounded testosterone products for administration as topical gels containing micronized testosterone or buccal troches. This form of testosterone therapy is not recommended as the doses prescribed are empirical, there are no published safety data or efficacy studies to validate this method of administration and pharmacokinetic studies are preliminary. In a pharmacokinetic study by Slater et al.,[24] 10 oophorectomized women taking estrogen therapy were randomized to 14 days of treatment with either 1mg testosterone gel applied topically daily to the inner thigh or a 1mg testosterone propionate lozenge applied daily to the buccal mucosa. Treatment with the buccal lozenge at this dose resulted in a rapid but brief increase in testosterone concentration with levels approximating the upper limit of the normal male range. Treatment with the testosterone gel resulted in a more prolonged increase in testosterone concentration to supraphysiologic levels well above the normal range for premenopausal women. The doses used in this study were excessive for both modes of administration and buccal administration was associated with a large and erratic increase in testosterone levels. These formulations cannot be recommended for the administration of testosterone at this time.

Conclusions

There is clinical evidence that transdermal testosterone therapy provides effective treatment of low libido in women with low testosterone levels with minimal adverse effects. The safety issues associated with testosterone treatment depend on the dose and hormone levels attained, the duration of treatment, the type of androgenic agent and its route of administration, and the woman's skin sensitivity. Ultimately, the decision to institute any hormonal therapy must be individualized and the patient adequately informed about risks and benefits. Further studies are required to assess the long-term efficacy and safety of transdermal testosterone therapy and these studies are currently underway.

References

1. Laufer LR, DeFazio JL, Lu JK et al. Estrogen replacement therapy by transdermal estradiol administration. Am J Obstet Gynecol 1983; 146:533–540.
2. Sherwin BB, Gelfand MM, Brender W. Androgen enhances sexual motivation in females: a prospective, crossover study of sex steroid administration in surgical menopause. Psychosom Med 1985; 47:339–351.
3. Sherwin BB, Gelfand MM. The role of androgen in the maintenance of sexual function in oophorectomized women. Psychosom Med 1987; 49:397–409.
4. Burger HG, Hailes J, Menelaus M. The management of persistent symptoms with estradiol-testosterone implants: clinical, lipid and hormonal results. Maturitas 1984; 6:351–358.
5. Burger HG, Hailes J, Nelson J, Menelaus M. Effect of combined implants of estradiol and testosterone on libido in postmenopausal women. Br Med J 1987; 294:936–937.

6. Davis SR, McCloud PI, Strauss BJG, Burger HG. Testosterone enhances estradiol's effects on post-menopausal bone density and sexuality. Maturitas 1995; 21:227–236.

7. Shifren JL, Braunstein G, Simon J et al. Transdermal testosterone treatment in women with impaired sexual function after oophorectomy. N Engl J Med 2000; 343:682–688.

8. Goldstat R, Briganti E, Tran J et al. Transdermal testosterone improves mood, well being and sexual function in premenopausal women. Menopause 2003; 10:390–398.

9. Simon JA. Safety of estrogen/androgen regimens. J Reprod Med 2001; 46(3 Suppl):281–290.

10. Arafah BM. Decreased levothyroxine requirement in women with hypothyroidism during androgen therapy for breast cancer. Ann Intern Med 1994; 121:247–251.

11. Watts NB, Notelovitz M, Timmons MC et al. Comparison of oral estrogens and estrogens plus androgen on bone mineral density, menopausal symptoms, and lipid-lipoprotein profiles in surgical menopause. Obstet Gynecol 1995; 85:529–537.

12. Westaby D, Ogle SJ, Paradinas FJ et al. Liver damage from long-term methyltestosterone. Lancet 1977; 2:262–263.

13. Buckler HM, Robertson WR, Wu FCW. Which Androgen Replacement Therapy for Women? J Clin Endocrinol Metab 1998; 83:3920–3924.

14. Urman B, Pride SM, Yuen HB. Elevated serum testosterone hirsutism and virilism associated with combined androgen-estrogen hormone replacement therapy. Obstet Gynecol 1991; 77:595–598.

15. Simon J, Davis SR, Watts NB et al. Safety and tolerability of transdermal testosterone therapy versus placebo in surgically menopausal women receiving oral or transdermal estrogen. Menopause 2002; 9:Abstract P-87-503.

16. Davis SR, Tran J. Testosterone influences libido and wellbeing. Trends Endocrinol Metab 2001; 12:33–37.

17. Adashi EY. The climacteric ovary as a functional gonadotropin-driven androgen-producing gland. Fertil Steril 1994; 62:20–27.

18. Mazer NA. Testosterone deficiency in women, etiologies, diagnosis and emerging treatments. In J Fertil Womens Med 2002; 47:77–86.

19. Svenstrup B, Brunner N, Dombernowsky P et al. Comparison of the effect of cortisol on aromatase activity and androgen metabolism in two human fibroblast cell lines derived from the same individual. J Steroid Biochem 1990; 35:679–687.

20. Griffin JE, Allman DR, Durrant JL, Wilson JD. Variation in steroid 5 alpha-reductase activity in cloned human skin fibroblasts. Shift in phenotypic expression from high to low activity upon subcloning. J Biol Chem 1981; 256:3662–3666.

21. Longcope C. Androgen and estrogen conversion rations in aging women. Maturitas 1980; 2:13–17.

22. Mazer NA, Shifren JL. Transdermal testosterone for women: a new physiological approach for androgen therapy. Obstet Gynecol Surv 2003; 58: 489–500.

23. Acrux Australia, PTY Ltd. (Data on file.)

24. Slater CC, Souter I, Zhang C et al. Pharmacokinetics of testosterone after percutaneous gel or buccal administration. Fertil Steril 2001; 76:32–37.

Chapter 8

Tailoring menopausal hormone therapy: role of antiandrogens

Hermann PG Schneider and Hermann M Behre

Summary

Antiandrogenic progestins such as cyproterone acetate, dienogest, and drospirenone differ in their structure, metabolites, and pharmacodynamic actions. It is inappropriate to consider their various actions as a class effect. They have beneficial effects on skin disorders related to hormonal deficiency and imbalance, and they do not counteract estrogen effects on lipid metabolism. Drospirenone with its unique antialdosterone properties can control and lower blood pressure in hypertensive women. Such beneficial effects offer a novel potential for reducing cardiovascular disease in postmenopausal women; they are also associated with reduced incidence of postmenopausal nonvertebral fractures. Continuous-combined hormone replacement therapy (HRT) with antiandrogenic progestins appears to have excellent mental tonic effects.

HRT with antiandrogenic progestins preserves metabolic estrogenicity and eliminates the counteracting effects of progestogen on estrogen. Alternative antiandrogenic progestins such as chlormadinone acetate do not have the same clinical advantages.

Introduction

Women experiencing menopausal hot flushes or vaginal atrophy can obtain relief with estrogens. In the past decade, the objective of HRT has changed from short-term treatment to long-term prevention. As life expectancy increases, there will be more postmenopausal women. HRT is usually given to estrogen-deficient women in late perimenopause and to postmenopausal women for a period of approximately 5 years. Administration of hormones to asymptomatic women is called hormone therapy or late therapy, and includes women of more than 5 years post menopause.[1] These defining terms to describe menopausal hormone treatment (MHT) have emerged from the epidemiologic confusion of the past few years.

Healthy tissue is required for an effective response to estrogen and maintenance of health. Evidence from experimental on monkeys and studies in women indicates that when endothelial cells become involved with atherosclerosis and neurons become affected with the pathologic process of Alzheimer, the beneficial responses to estrogen diminish.[2–4] Maximal benefit requires early onset of hormone treatment, near the time of menopause (HRT). The accepted indications for HRT include relief of vasomotor and urogenital symptoms, prevention of osteoporosis and related fractures, as well as prevention of atrophy of connective tissue and epithelia.[1]

As part of MHT, progesterone and progestins are only required for the protection of the endometrium.[1] However, additional roles of available progestins are continuously emerging. The basic structure of the 21-carbon progestins is the pregnane nucleus. The 19-carbon series includes all the androgens and is based on the androstane nucleus. The synthetic progestins used in clinical practice are derived either from testosteron

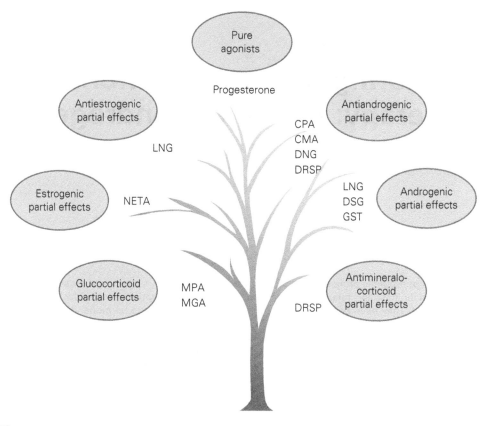

Figure 8.1

The 'progestogen tree'.[5] CMA, chlormadinone acetate; CPA, cyproterone acetate; DNG, dienogest; DRSP, drospirenone; DSG, desogestrel; GST, gestodene; MGA, megestrol acetate; LNG, levonorgestrel; MPA, medroxyprogesterone acetate; NETA, norethisterone acetate.

(19-nortestosterone derivatives) or from progesterone (17-OH-progesterone derivatives). In addition, there are more recently synthesized nonpregnanes constituting 19-norprogesterone derivatives: nestorone, nomegestrol acetate, promegestone, and trimegestone. The 'progestogen tree' identifies and categorizes steroid hormones derived from progesterone, the pure agonist and mother compound, which is represented by the trunk of the tree (Figure 8.1).[5] A great variety of nonprogesterone partial effects of progestins is apparent. Among these, levonorgestrel is known for its antiestrogenicity, while norethisterone acetate exerts estrogenic partial effects. Medroxyprogesterone acetate and megestrol acetate have partial glucocortical effects, while drospirenone (DRSP) is antimineralocorticoid. Levonorgestrel, desogestrel and gestodene are known for their androgenic partial effects. On the other hand, cyproterone acetate (CPA), chlormadinone acetate, dienogest (DNG) and drospirenone have documented antiandrogenicity. The latter may be of particular interest in hormone treatment of postmenopausal women. The androgen-dominant hormonal status of the climacteric is associated with adverse metabolic effects as well as clinical signs of androgenization such as seborrhea, acne, and hirsutism. The management of such biologic changes in postmenopausal women is an important consideration. In practice, the main problems relate to hirsutism and whether the prevalent alopecia is of androgenetic origin.

Hirsutism is the development of male pattern body hair growth in women. This is a frequent cause of psychologic distress because the affected individual erroneously feels as if gender is changing. The extent of problematic body hair growth varies, and depends on the amount of normal body hair among racial groups or sub-groups. Hirsutism includes terminal hair on the face, chest, or back. It is often associated with an endocrine abnormality of the adrenals or ovary causing raised androgens and is frequently associated with polycystic ovarian syndrome. Some women have no obvious underlying disorder and this is termed 'idiopathic' hirsutism. The assumption that idiopathic hirsutism is due to a greater sensitivity of the follicles to normal androgens is suggested by the observation of asymmetrically occurring hirsutism.[6]

The skin is a target organ of numerous neuro-endocrine signals and corresponding receptors.[7] These include cholinergic, adrenergic, and serotonergic receptors and also receptors for histamine, glutamate, growth hormone, propiomelanocortin, cortisol, parathyroid hormone, vitamin D, androgens, estrogens, progesterone, calcitonin gene-related peptide, prolactin, and triiodothyronine.[8] Thus, the skin may react to stress situations and changes in the immune system (inflammation, allergy) and the hormonal environment. Cellular repair and differentiation impaired in skin by age and in chronic inflammation such as acne. Treatment with antiandrogenic progestins, therefore, is not merely a cosmetic therapy, but has a more general impact on women's health.[8]

Androgenetic alopecia has also been described in women, but the pattern of expression is normally different. Women generally do not show frontal recession, they retain the frontal hairline and exhibit thinning of the vertices which may lead to balding.[6] Postmenopausal women may exhibit the masculine pattern.[9] The progression of balding in women is normally slow and a full endocrinologic investigation is recommended if a rapid onset is seen.[10] The female pattern of hair loss frequently occurs in association with hyperandrogenism; other women, however, will not present any signs of androgen abnormality. Therefore, it remains unclear whether androgen is responsible for loss in women.[11]

Antiandrogens and women's health

Clinical aspects of menopausal transition

Interest in progestogens treatment started in 1934 when substitution therapy was first administered to ovariectomized women. This was followed by treatment of oligomenorrhea and hypomenorrhea (1937), anovulation (1938), menorrhagia (1953), and endometriosis (1960). In addition, contraceptive pills containing norethynodrel was developed in 1956. The past three decades have seen the development of oncologic indications (1970s), postmenopausal hormone replacement (1980s), and male contraception (1990s). The first antiandrogen, CPA was synthesized in Berlin in the late 1950s and introduced into clinical practice in the 1960s.[12] In order to elucidate the particular clinical importance of antiandrogens, a close look into the varying hormonal balance of the climacteric is warranted. The total amount of testosterone produced after menopause is decreased because of reduced peripheral conversion of androstenedione, the primary source. The early postmenopausal circulating level of androstenedione approximately 62% is less than in young adult life.[13] A prospective longitudinal study from Australia, looking at serum testosterone, dehydroepiandrosterone sulfate and sex hormone binding globulin (SHBG) levels from 5 years before menopause to 7 years after, did not show any change of circulating levels of testosterone.[14] Because of a decrease in the SHBG the Australian authors reported an increase in free androgens. Nonetheless, some clinicians argue that androgen treatment may be indicated in the postmenopausal period. The potential benefits of such androgen treatment include improvement in psychologic wellbeing and an increase in sexually motivated behavior.

Any balance of androgens must consider their unwanted effects: in particular acne, alopecia, seborrhea, and hirsutism, as well as a negative impact on the cholesterol–lipoprotein profile. Decreases in levels of high-density lipoprotein cholesterol (HDL-C) and increases in levels of low-density lipoprotein cholesterol (LDL-C) and free fatty acids, for example, shift the lipid status of the climacteric towards atherogenicity. Other effects include loss of insulin receptors, which leads to incremental insulin resistance, hyperinsulinemia and increased ovarian androgen production.[15] Later in the postmenopausal years, circulating androgen levels are mostly derived from the adrenal gland. Women with more than 12 years post menopause and complete adrenal insufficiency have no circulating androgens and no intraovarian testosterone or androstenedione.[16] The androgen/estrogen ratio changes drastically after menopause because of the more marked decline in estrogen. Mild hirsutism is common, reflecting this marked shift in the sex hormone ratio. With increasing postmenopausal age, circulating levels of dehydroepiandrosterone sulfate and dehydroepiandrosterone decrease whereas the circulating postmenopausal levels of androstenedione, testosterone, and estrogen remain relatively constant.[17,18]

Pharmacology of antiandrogens

Marketed products

The most widely used antiandrogens in clinical practice are CPA, DNG and DRSP. CPA is a derivative of 17-hydroxy-progesterone, has 100% bioavailability, a short half-life (2–8 h), and an elimination time of 60 h. It is mostly bound to albumin and is metabolized by 15β-hydroxylation, which distinguishes it from other hydroxyprogesterones (Table 8.1).

DNG is a 19-norprogestin with high bioavailability, and a short half-life (0.24 h) and elimination time (6.3 h). Serum level after doses of 2–3 mg is approximately 50 ng/mL. It is 90% albumin bound and, in contrast to other nortestosterones, is not bound by SHBG or corticosteroid binding globulin (CBG) (Table 8.1). DNG has a 17α-cyanomethyl group instead of the 17α-ethinyl group typical of the common 19-nortestosterone derivatives.

DRSP is a derivative of 17α-spirolactone. It has progestogenic, antiandrogenic, and antialdosterone properties with a bioavailability of up to 85%. Its elimination half-life is between 35 and 39 h.[1] After oral administration, serum DRSP levels decrease with a mean terminal half-life of about 35–39 h. DRSP does not bind to SHBG or CBG, but it binds to other plasma proteins. The free fraction of DRSP in the plasma is approximately 3–5%. DRSP is extensively metabolized after oral or intravenous administration. At least 20 different metabolites have been observed in the urine and feces, but only trace amounts are excreted unchanged. The renally excreted drospirenone metabolites do not exhibit pharmacologic activity. The total clearance of DRSP is 1.2–1.5 mL/min/kg. Impaired renal function would cause a slight increase in serum DRSP concentration as creatinine clearance decreases. This apparently lacks clinical relevance in view of the excellent tolerability of DRSP.

Basic clinical investigations

CPA is a highly progestogenic compound that produces excellent endometrial transformation and good bleeding control. The latter is seen with CPA in a sequential regimen consisting of 11 days of 2 mg estradiol valerate, 10 days of 2 mg estradiol valerate with 1 mg CPA, followed by a 7-day drug-free interval (Climen®). Good bleeding control does not hold, however, in a continuous-combined formulation. The sequential regimen protects the endometrium, reduces menopausal symptoms, and may also protect the mammary glands. In addition, the antiandrogenic properties of CPA have proved to be highly beneficial in androgen-related disorders such as acne, seborrhea, and androgenic alopecia.[19]

Unfavorable androgen-related effects on lipid and nonlipid cardiovascular risk factors may contribute to the increased incidence of cardiovascular disease seen in menopausal women. A sequential regimen with CPA lowers total cholesterol and LDL-C and may increase HDL-C and triglyceride levels.[20,21] Due to the lack of androgenic properties, CPA does not alleviate the metabolic effects of the estrogen component in a relevant fashion. This beneficial effect seems to be more pronounced in women with a significant atherogenic lipoprotein pattern.[19]

Administration of high doses of CPA during the hormone-sensitive differentiation phase of the genital organs (approximately day 45 of pregnancy) could lead to feminization in male fetuses. In one study observation of male newborns who had been exposed *in utero* to CPA did not show any signs of feminization. However, pregnancy is the only absolute contraindication for the use of CPA preparations.[22]

Table 8.1 Hydroprogesterones and nortestosterones (modified from Schneider[5])

	Bioavailability (%)	Serum (ng/mL)*	Half-life α/β (h) Binding protein	Metabolism
Hydroxyprogesterones				
Chlormadinone acetate	**100**	**4**	**2.4/89 albumin**	**Reduction 3-keto hydroxylation**
Medroxyprogesterone acetate	100	12	2.2/33 albumin	Hydroxylation $C_{6\beta}$ and C_{12}
Cyproterone acetate	**100**	**11**	**2–8/60 albumin**	**15β-Hydroxylation**
Megestrol acetate	100	7–42	–	Hydroxylation
Medrogesterone	100	10–15	4/36 albumin	Hydroxylation
Dydrogesterone	100	1.5–2.0	5–7/77	20-Keto-hydroxylation No reduction 3-keto and Δ^4 No 17α-hydroxylation
Nortestosterones				
Norethisterone	5–77	Oral 5–10	2.5/8	Ring A reduction
Norethisterone acetate	~100	Transdermal 0.5–1	36% SHBG 61% albumin	Aromatization (0.35%)
Levonorgestrel	100	3.5	1/24	Reduction
DL-Norgestrel	D–N = inactive	0.1–0.2	48% SHBG 50% albumin	3-Keto and Δ^4
Dienogest	**High**	**50**	**0.24/6.3 90% albumin No SHBG/CBG**	**Reduction 3-keto 17α cyanomethyl hydroxylation Δ^4**
Tibolone	Prodrug of 7α-methylnorethisterone $3\alpha_1\beta$ OH tibolone	1	45 (β)	Ring A aromatization No Δ^4 reduction
17α spirolactone	**76–85**	**10–35**	**35–39 (β) no SHBG/CBG**	**20 different metabolites**
Drospirenone			**90% albumin 4–5% free fraction**	**Cytochrome P450 enzymes not involved**

*Following application of standard dosages.

DNG is a hybrid progestogen (Table 8.2) which has been investigated as a monophasic estrogen–progestogen combination. DNG contains estradiol valerate and dienogest in a ratio of 2 : 2 mg (Climodien). In a pivotal study for endometrial safety, Climodien was administered for 12 cycles in a blinded fashion with Kliogest® (a widely used continuous–combined preparation of 2 mg estradiol and 1 mg norethisterone acetate) serving as control.[23] Biopsies were obtained before and at the end of treatment. The incidence of atrophic proliferative and secretory endometrium was similar with both treatments (Figure 8.2). A total of 85–87% of women had an atrophic endometrium,

there were few proliferative and secretory changes, but there were no cases of hyperplasia. In addition, fewer days of bleeding occurred during 12 cycles of treatment with Climodien compared with Kliogest. The incidence of adverse events with Climodien was similar to that with Kliogest. The most common adverse events reported were breast problems, vaginal bleeding/dysmenorrhea, and central nervous system/sensory events.

The efficacy of DNG in combination with estrogen is comparable to various formulations containing estradiol, estradiol valerate or conjugated estrogens in combination with different progestogens.[24] Climodien caused a profound and rapid

Table 8.2 Dienogest: a 'hybrid' progestogen[5]

Similarities to 19-norprogestins	Similarities to progesterone derivatives	Specific properties of dienogest
Short plasma half-life	Weak antigonadotropic properties	No interaction with specific transport proteins (SHBG, CBG)
Good cycle control if used in oral contraceptives	Antiandrogenic partial action	Weak influence on drug metabolizing enzymes
High transformatory effect on endometrium	Antiproliferative effects (breast in vitro)	High concentration of unbound substance in serum
	Dosages in milligram range	

SHBG, sex hormone binding globulin; CBG, corticoid binding globulin.

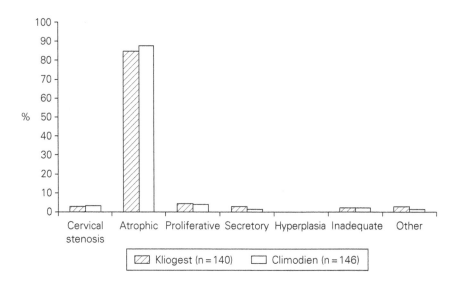

Figure 8.2

Results of endometrial biopsies after 12 cycles of treatment.[5]

improvement of vasomotor symptoms and a precipitous drop of the Kupperman Index from 20/24 to 9 within one cycle and to 6 after six cycles.

The pharmacodynamic profile of DRSP is similar to that of endogenous progesterone. This is consistent with theoretical modeling of molecular electron densities in three dimensions, by which considerable similarities between the binding regions of DRSP and progesterone are seen.[25] Like progesterone, DRSP displays antialdosterone and antiandrogenic properties, but is devoid of any estrogenic, androgenic, glucocorticoid, or antiglucocorticoid activity. The antiandrogenic properties of DRSP have been demonstrated in the classical Hershberger test, which is based on the ability of test compounds to inhibit the effects of testosterone on the growth of seminal vesicles and the prostate in castrated rats. DRSP performed well when compared with the highly antiandrogenic CPA. Depending on the route of administration, the antiandrogenic potency of DRSP is approximately three to nine times lower

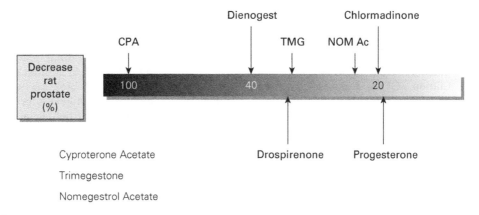

Figure 8.3

Antiandrogenic potency.[8,26,27] CPA, cyproterone acetate; TMG, trimegestone; NOM Ac, nomegestrol acetate.

than that of CPA, and is equal to or approximately three times higher than that of spirolactone.[26] Figure 8.3 gives an estimate of relative antiandrogenic properties of various progestins.[8] This information has partially been derived from in vivo data when DRSP was administered orally or subcutaneously in preclinical studies.[26,27] Animal studies have demonstrated that the antiandrogenic potency of DRSP is about a third of CPA; this marked antiandrogenic activity, but no androgenic potential.[27]

Clinical profiles of antiandrogens as hormone replacement therapy

Continuous–combined hormone therapy with estrogens in combination with a progestin is intended to cause endometrial atrophy. The atrophy reduces frequency and severity of the withdrawal bleeding that is associated with sequential combined regimens and which many women find unacceptable. Although spotting and bleeding are often seen early in the first 3–6 months of continuous–combined HRT, these effects tend to decrease over time.[28] The risk of irregular bleeding among women receiving continuous–combined MHT appears to be related with the dose and type of progestin.[28] Bleeding problems are the main reasons for discontinuing hormone therapy.[29] Therefore, adequate

combinations of estrogen with proper type and dose of a progestin are needed. Many progestogens have androgenic activities, which counteract the effects of estrogen. One major challenge of hormone therapy has been to find a progestin which closely matches endogenous progesterone and is devoid of estrogenicity. Antiandrogenicity benefits skin and hair, and causes favorable changes in the serum lipid profiles. These observations stimulated clinical studies to investigate the potential of antiandrogens for HRT.

Cyproterone acetate

The first HRT product combining CPA, a well defined antiandrogenic progestin, with estradiol valerate (E_2V) in a sequential combined fashion is Climen. This has been on the market since September 1996. In a double blind, randomized, multicenter study of 594 women during menopausal transition, Climen was compared to Cyclo-Progynova®.[30] Hot flushes, insomnia, depression, headaches, and acne lesions were effectively reduced by both treatments. Climen offered rapid relief such that hot flushes were reduced by about one-third after only one cycle. More than 70% of patients kept their body weight constant through the 12 month study period, with 20% gaining more than 2 kg; there was no difference between the treatment groups. Climen did not influence

HDL-C levels unlike the reduction seen with Cyclo-Progynova by the third month. The percentage of patients reporting seborrhea in the Climen group decreased as treatment progressed. LDL-C plasma levels were significantly reduced by Climen. Other less specific complaints were also seen to improve (e.g. insomnia, depression, headaches, skin changes).[30]

In an attempt to characterize Climen and its effect on menopause-specific symptoms both with regard to profile and intensity of the symptoms, our original 10-item Menopause Rating Scale (MRS) was applied in a large postmarketing surveillance study of Climen.[31] A total of 10 904 premenopausal and postmenopausal women presented with a pretreatment profile of menopausal complaints was divided into four independent subscores with the factors: hot flushes, atrophy, and psychologic and somatic symptoms. Current or previous HRT did not alter the factorial profile of this self-rating scale. After 6 months of treatment with Climen, the factorial loading of all specific scores dropped significantly. Climen was confirmed to have a wide spectrum of activity in all aspects of a menopause-specific rating scale.

A global psychiatric symptom index and anxiety scores improved significantly after 12 months of Climen compared with a control group.[32] The applied self-administered questionnaire did not indicate any change in sexual parameters.

An earlier study evaluated the effects of climen on bone mass, serum lipids, and lipoproteins, bleeding pattern, blood pressure and climacteric symptoms. This was done in a double blind, placebo controlled fashion in 65 healthy early postmenopausal women, allocated to 2 years of treatment.[33] Bone mass at forearm, spine, and total skeleton remained unchanged from initial values in the Climen group. The placebo group values declined to 95% of baseline at 2 years. Total cholesterol and LDL-C serum levels were reduced in the Climen group. Serum triglycerides increased during HRT with CPA. HDL-C levels remained stable during the first 6 months, increasing slightly thereafter. Body weight and blood pressure remained unchanged with Climen. Most women experienced a regular bleeding pattern.

By examining the effect of Climen and low-dose vitamin D supplementation on the prevention of bone loss in nonosteoporotic early postmenopausal women, Komulainen's group, confirmed the beneficial effects of antiandrogenic HRT on BMD.[34] Vitamin D has only a minor effect in preventing osteoporosis in the above population with no additional antiosteoporotic benefit of Climen alone. In another study on the incidence of new nonvertebral fractures during Climen and low-dose vitamin D_3 supplementation, the authors confirmed the beneficial effect of Climen in preventing peripheral fractures in nonosteoporotic menopausal women. In this study, lumbar (L1–L4) and femoral neck bone mineral density were examined before and after 2.5 and 5 years of treatment in a group of 464 randomly assigned postmenopausal women.[35] The estimated risk of new nonvertebral fractures was 0.29 (CI 0.10 to 0.90) for Climen versus 0.47 (CI 0.20 to 1.14) for vitamin D.

Randomized studies proved that antiandrogenic HRT with CPA is highly effective in relieving the classic climacteric symptoms, and induced full secretory changes similar to those observed during the luteal phase of the menstrual cycle. No endometrial hyperplasia was observed. In addition bone loss was prevented, and CPA did not significantly modify the favorable changes in lipid and lipoprotein metabolism induced by estrogen.[36] Thus, the combination of estradiol valerate and CPA has many of the properties of an ideal HRT estrogen–progestogen combination.

Increased body weight, particularly increased central distribution of body fat, is recognized as an independent predictor of coronary heart disease in women.[37–40] The early postmenopausal period is associated with a progressive increase in body weight and body fat, and a shift to a more central, android body fat distribution. Changes in body weight are an important concern for menopausal women.[29] The effect of Climen on body weight and body fat distribution (determined by dual-energy X-ray absorptiometry) was first investigated by Gambacciani and colleagues in Italy.[41] A comparison with the effect of oral calcium (500 mg per day) revealed a significant increase in body weight after 12 months in those women on oral calcium but not in women who received Climen. The weight changes were from 61.8 ± 2.1 kg to 63.3 ± 1.9 kg for oral calcium ($P < 0.05$), and from 62.2 ± 1.6 kg to 62.7 ± 1.6 kg for Climen (not significant). Total body fat mass and fat mass in the trunk and arms were also significantly increased in the controls, but not in the women who received Climen (Figure 8.4). The

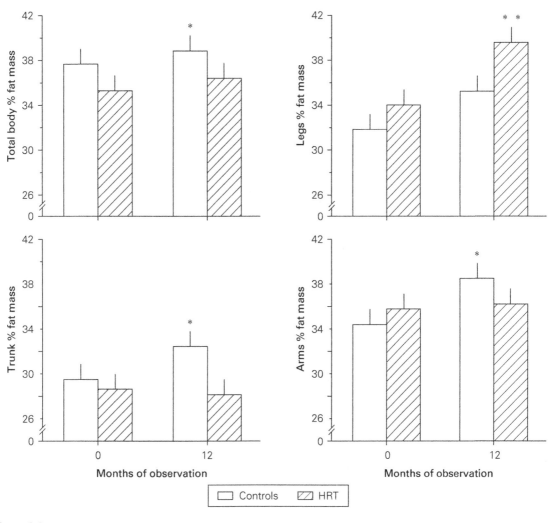

Figure 8.4

Body fat distribution with Climen compared with controls[41] (mean±SE) in women treated with calcium (controls; n = 12) or with estradiol valerate and cyproterone acetate (HRT; n = 15). *$P<0.01$; **$P<0.005$ (vs. corresponding basal value).

reverse was true for fat mass in the upper thighs. Thus, Climen can partially counteract the increase in body weight and body fat observed in post-menopausal women, and prevent the shift to a distribution of central, android body fat. The observed stabilization of body weight and body fat distribution may be interpreted as a protective effect of antiandrogenic HRT against coronary heart disease. In addition, a 3-year HRT program with Climen, evaluating appendicular lean tissue mass in early postmenopausal women aged 45–54 years, suggested no significant effect on the appendicular lean tissue, representing skeletal muscle mass.[42] During the third year of this study, a catabolic rather than anabolic effect became apparent. Larger studies measuring lean tissue mass and bioavailable testosterone simultaneously will provide a more conclusive answer regarding the existence of potential reverse effects of long-term HRT.

Estrogen therapy reduces the internal carotid artery pulsatility index (PI).[43] The improvement in carotid PI following HRT has been proposed as a marker of the cardioprotective effect of estrogen therapy. Cyclical progesterone in addition to ERT partially antagonized the reduction on the carotid artery PI. Androgens have been shown to decrease arterial vasodilatation and carotid PI in menopausal women, and androgen supplementation during HRT partially counteracts the beneficial effects of estrogen on cerebral blood flow.[44] In one study 15 postmenopausal women on Climen were compared with another 15 ovariectomized women who received estradiol hemihydrate (2 mg) for 3 months. In both groups, Doppler ultrasound was performed before the start and at the end of therapy. The investigated PI as indicator of impedance to blood flow downstream demonstrated that estradiol hemihydrate and estradiol valerate plus CPA lead to similar improvement in carotid artery response and thereby potentially reduce the incidence of cerebral vascular disease in postmenopausal women.[45]

Dienogest

There are mechanisms other than receptor binding which may be responsible for the antiandrogenic property of DNG. As 19-norprogestogens such as levonorgestrel and norethindrone compete with testosterone for the same binding site on the SHBG molecule, it has been suggested that owing to its unique structure, DNG may not compete with testosterone in the same manner. As mentioned above, DNG is neither bound by CBG (like progesterone) nor by SHBG (like the norprogestogens). Promegestone, which also does not interfere with SHBG, has the same 4,9-diene structure element. The antiandrogenic effect of DNG rather resides in its decremental effect on the local formation of dihydrotestosterone by competitive inhibition of 5α-reductase in the skin. The comparative antiandrogenicity of DNG to CPA may be reflected by their potencies in the Hershberger test (see Figure 8.3).

Climodien® is a continuous-combined oral product. Its estrogen component of 2 mg estradiol valerate in combination with 2 mg DNG produced optimal endometrial and bleeding effects. Climodien has been studied in many clinical trials, which included the combinations DNG 2 mg with 30–50 µg of ethinyl estradiol as oral contraceptives. All of these products have shown good tolerability. The benefits of Climodien can be summarized as follows:

- quick and safe relief of climacteric symptoms
- reliable continuous-combined efficacy with approved breakthrough bleeding control in comparison to Kliogest
- constant blood coagulation, body weight, and blood pressure
- protection against long-term risk of osteoporosis as suggested by data on markers of bone metabolism
- reliable endometrial protection (see Figure 8.2).

Climacteric symptoms were evaluated by the use of a modified Kupperman Index,[20] symptoms recorded were hot flushes, paresthesias, insomnia, nervousness, melancholia, vertigo, fatigue, arthralgias/myalgias, headache, palpitations and formications (sensation of crowling under the skin). A maximum possible index of 51 was found to be either 25.6 for Climodien or 24.4 for the comparator Kliogest at study entry. After 12 cycles, the scores were reduced to 5.6 and 6.4, respectively.

Estrogens may affect structure and function of brain areas known to be involved in memory. Experimental evidence indicates that estrogen promotes neuronal outgrowth, prevention of neuronal atrophy, regulates of synaptic plasticity, influence on neurotransmitter metabolism, and increases cerebral blood flow, and expression of neurotropic factors.[46] Estrogen deficiency has an important role in memory deficits of postmenopausal women.

Austrian investigators studied electroencephalographic (EEG) mapping in postmenopausal women versus premenopausal controls and documented an association of low peripheral estradiol levels with a loss of neurophysiologic correlates of vigilance; at the same time, depression and climacteric symptomatology were more frequent.[47,48] Such deficits in vigilance and cognitive function can be alleviated by MHT. In a prospective, randomized, double blind study of postmenopausal women treated with continuous-combination of estradiol valerate plus DNG, psychophysiologic and psychopathologic parameters were investigated.[49] This combination treatment led to improvement of behavior, which was objectively demonstrated by rating and self-rating scales, by clinical observation, and by psychometric testing. After 2 months of treatment, the most important EEG

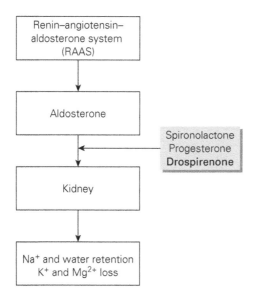

- Estrogen stimulates synthesis of angiotensinogen, which increases aldosterone and promotes Na^+ and water retention.

- Progesterone acts as an aldosterone antagonist to prevent Na^+ retention. Postmenopausal women secrete insufficient progesterone to counteract estrogen-induced Na^+ retention.

- Drospirenone, unlike other synthetic progestins, mimics progesterone as an aldosterone antagonist, thus promoting Na^+ excretion and preventing water retention.

Figure 8.5

Effect of drospirenone on the renin–angiotensin–aldosterone system.[25,51] Rübig A. Climacteric. 2003; 6(Supp 3):49–54. Oelkers W. Mol Cell Endocrinol. 2004; 217:255–261.

changes were an increase in absolute power of all frequency bands, but predominantly in the fast alpha band, which is typical of enhanced vigilance. The improvement in speed and amount of cognitive resources was extrapolated from changes in evoked potentials, especially in the latency and amplitude of the P300 wave. The reduction of latency reached similar proportions in postmenopausal women on estradiol valerate alone and on estradiol valerate plus DNG; however, an incremental amplitude was only seen in women on the combination treatment.[49] By looking at the various EEG patterns, estradiol valerate did improve the stimulus evaluation time (e.g. classification speed), and DNG enhanced cognitive information-processing capacity. These data points to a DNG-associated potential of improving the neurophysiologic effects of estradiol, based on the assumption that estrogen has a stimulatory and progesterone a sedative effect on the brain. Continuous-combined HRT with DNG (e.g. Climodien) therefore has protective mental tonic effects and may represent an elective HRT in postmenopausal women with mood defects.

The vasodilation mediated by estradiol via nitric oxide (NO) and prostaglandin $F_{1\alpha}$ ($PGF_{1\alpha}$) is not antagonized by DNG, as documented by biochemical markers of vascular function. Cyclic guanoside monophosphate and 5-hydroxyindolacetic acid were measured in an open, randomized, parallel group study comparing Climodien with 2 mg estradiol valerate over a period of 3 months in postmenopausal women.[50] Overall, this study indicates that DNG does not significantly alter the vasorelaxation effects of estradiol valerate. A combination product like Climodien can therefore be considered to have vasorelaxant effects.

Drospirenone

The affinity of DRSP for the mineralocorticoid receptor results in antagonism to aldosterone (Figure 8.5).[25,51] Aldosterone has been implicated in the pathogenesis of progressive cardiovascular disease. The latter has been associated with postmenopausal estrogen deficiency. Consequently, HRT with DRSP has emerged as a potentially promising strategy for reducing cardiovascular events while maintaining favorable effects on vasomotor symptoms and bone wasting. Most clinical trials of standard formulations of HRT have not confirmed the predictive benefit in reducing cardiovascular disease in older postmenopausal

Table 8.3 Effect on ambulatory blood pressure in hypertensive postmenopausal women receiving enalapril[55]

	Baseline (mmHg)	After 14 days' treatment (mmHg)
Enalapril 10 mg bid + placebo (n = 12)	139/83 (± 12/8)	139/83(±11/9)
Enalapril 10 mg bid + DRSP 3 mg/E$_2$ 1 mg (n = 12)	139/80 (± 19/7)	130*/75**(±9/6)

Data shown as mean SBP/DBP (±SD). bid, twice daily.
*P = 0.006; **P = 0.003 for baseline-adjusted decline versus placebo.

women.[1] The development of new generations of progestins with improved selectivity profile has recently culminated with the introduction of DRSP. Endometrial transformation, inhibition of ovulation, and antimineralocorticoid effects together with mild antiandrogenicity were observed in women in the dose of 0.5–4.0 mg/day.[52]

Studies in postmenopausal women have demonstrated that an oral, daily continuous combination of 1 mg 17β-estradiol plus 2 mg DRSP significantly decreases the mean number of hot flushes per week within 2–4 weeks of treatment.[53] In an intent-to-treat population of 149 participants taking this combination regimen, only one case of simple endometrial hyperplasia without atypia was observed, and no cases of complex hyperplasia or endometrial cancer.[54] Endometrial atrophy was observed in more than 85% of the subjects treated for up to 2 years, with a resultant more than 80% amenorrhea within the first year.[25] Adverse events were seen in 14 of 52 participants, ranging from breast pain (n = 4) to headache (n = 2) and nausea (n = 1).[53] The cardiovascular issue was investigated in a double blind, randomized, two parallel group studying comparing the effects of 3 mg DRSP combined with 1 mg estradiol versus placebo on 24-h ambulatory blood pressure in postmenopausal hypertensive women treated with 10 mg of enalapril maleate (ENA) twice daily.[55] Twenty-four nonsmoking postmenopausal women received 10 mg of ENA twice a day before the study and were then randomized to either DRSP/E$_2$ plus ENA (n = 12) or placebo plus ENA (n = 12) for 14 days. Compared with the group receiving placebo, the estradiol plus DRSP group had a significant decrease in 24-h mean baseline ambulatory blood pressure (139/83 mmHg) in both systolic blood pressure (−9±5 mmHg, P = 0.014) and diastolic blood pressure (−5±4 mmHg, P = 0.007); no change in blood pressure was observed in the placebo group (Table 8.3, Figure 8.6).[55]

According to the investigators, the implications of this study are twofold. First, the mean DRSP/E$_2$ blood pressure lowering effect in the presence of angiotensin-converting enzyme inhibition was associated with a concomitant increase in serum aldosterone that approached statistical significance. This is consistent with an antimineralocorticoid effect. Second, assuming a DRSP/spirolactone potency ratio of 7, the above combination of DRSP/E$_2$ would be expected to have an aldosterone antagonist activity roughly equivalent to 25 mg of spirolactone. In view of a growing body of evidence supporting an independent role for aldosterone in mediating chronic cardiovascular and renal disease, the antimineralocorticoid effect of DRSP may confirm cardiovascular protective properties beyond its effects as HRT in postmenopausal women (Figure 8.7).[25,51,56]

In confirmation of such novel potential mechanisms, the effect on ambulatory blood pressure in postmenopausal women with systolic hypertension was studied.[57] DRSP 3 mg/E$_2$ 1 mg (n =110) resulted in a highly significant reduction of systolic blood pressure at week 2 up to week 12 of treatment compared to placebo (n =102). Favorable effects on lowering total cholesterol, LDL-C, and triglycerides with a combination of 2 mg DRSP/1 mg estradiol plus improved oral glucose tolerance would add to the potential cardiovascular benefits of the DRSP/E$_2$ product for HRT.[25,58]

Estrogen deficiency in postmenopausal women contributes significantly to the problems of hypertension, and subsequently cardiovascular disease. Once women enter the menopause, their risk of hypertension doubles when adjusted for age and body mass index; and hypertension is a well-documented antecedent of congestive heart failure.[58] The favorable profile of DRSP/E$_2$ HRT is complemented by the reduction in body weight, which was shown in an endometrial safety study.[54] When comparing DRSP 2 mg

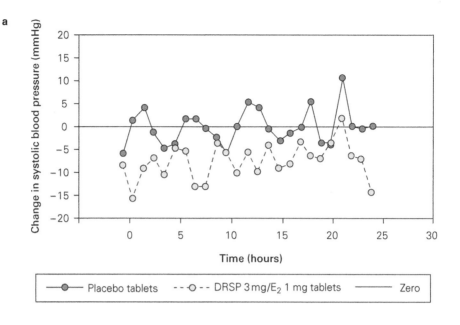

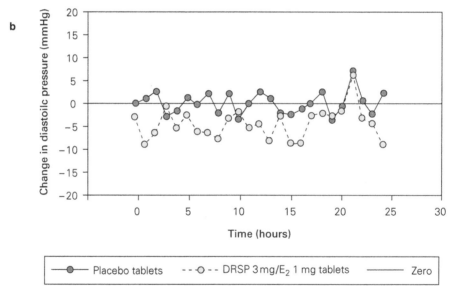

Figure 8.6

Mean change from baseline for 24-h systolic (A) and diastolic (B) blood pressure on treatment day 14.[55]

combined with 17β-estradiol 1 mg (n = 221) to 17β-estradiol 1 mg (n = 22), a clear-cut reduction in body weight was evident in cycle 3 to cycle 13 of treatment.

The antiandrogenic activity of DRSP is superior to that of chlormadinone but inferior to that of CPA (Figure 8.8).[59] The effect on body composition, lipid parameters, insulin resistance, and hair growth as

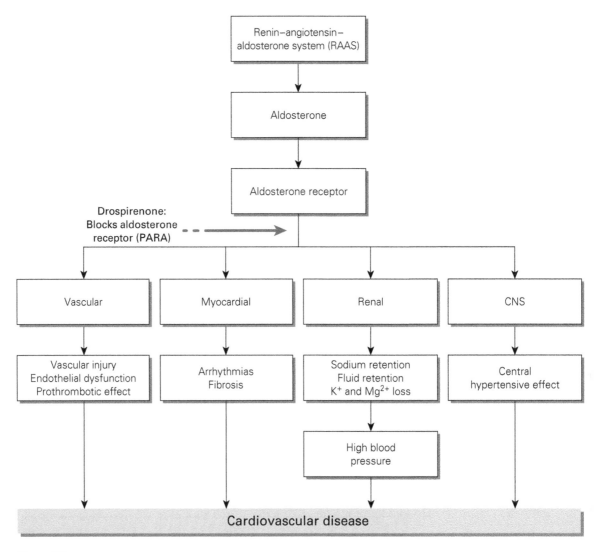

Figure 8.7

Pharmacologic and clinical effects of aldosterone and antialdosterone action of drospirenone.[25,51,56]

described above may, to a larger extent, reside in the antiandrogenic activity of DRSP.

The DRSP/E$_2$ combination was also prospectively investigated in a total of 180 healthy postmenopausal women ages 45–65 for 2 years.[60] Bone mass density at the lumbar spine, hip, and total body increased significantly. All markers such as serum osteocalcin, serum bone-specific alkaline phosphatase, serum cross-linked N- and C-telopeptides decreased accordingly. Thereby,

DRSP/E$_2$ is a new HRT which is safe and well tolerated; the incidence of adverse events is similar to other HRT preparations.[61] DRSP/E$_2$ prevents postmenopausal osteoporosis, provides endometrial protection and maintains amenorrhea in the majority of women. Also, sodium and water retention are prevented, negating estrogen-related side effects (e.g. weight gain), thus improving compliance. DRSP/E$_2$ has a positive influence on blood pressure, lipid parameters,

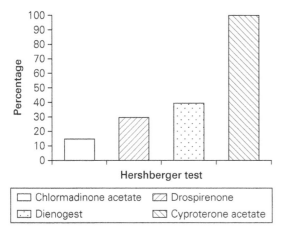

Figure 8.8

The clinical antiandrogenicity of dienogest and some other synthetic progestogens, according to the Hershberger test.[59,61]

insulin resistance and hair growth and thereby offers novel potential mechanisms for individual risk profile adapted HRT.

Other products presenting antiandrogenic potential – chlormadinone acetate, spirolactone, flutamide, finasteride

Chlormadinone acetate is a derivative of 17α-hydroxyprogesterone also known as pregnanes. The endometrial response in postmenopausal women treated with a sequential hormone preparation of estradiol and either chlormadinone acetate or micronized progesterone (MP) was determined.[62] On weakly estradiol-primed endometrium, chloramidone acetate 10 mg per day is a powerful progestin compared with MP 200 mg per day. The endometrium in both groups varied in intensity due to the length of progestative impregnation; predecidualization occurred later in the chloramidone acetate group. Chloramidone acetate as well as MP give a molecule-specific histologic aspect with a good endometrial safety.[62] As shown in Figure 8.8, chloramidone acetate is the weakest of all antiandrogenic progestins in clinical practice.[59] It is also partially antiestrogenic, a fact which might be important with cyclical HRT in the presence of higher-dosed estrogens with longer-standing application. However, this

antiestrogenic effect does not compare with that of 19-nortestosterone derivatives such as norgestrel and norethisterone.

Finasteride inhibits 5α-reductase activity, thus blocking conversion of testosterone into dihydrotestosterone. Finasteride, used to treat prostate cancer, inhibits both isoenzymes of 5α-reductase, but its potency for the treatment of hirsutism and alopecia is limited because it is less active against the type-I enzyme found in skin. A dose of 5 mg per day (Proscar®) decreases hirsutism without side effects.[63] Propecia®, containing a smaller dose of 1 mg finasteride, is available for the treatment of hair loss in men. Finasteride, flutamide, and spirolactone (100 mg daily) have been compared in randomized clinical trials and were found to be equally effective.[64,65] However, one randomized clinical trial found a dose of 100 mg daily of spirolactone to be more effective than finasteride.[66] Finasteride is less potent than either flutamide or a reversed sequential regimen with estrogen and CPA.[67] Both the 1 mg and 5 mg dose of finasteride has not been found to be effective on alopecia in postmenopausal women.[68]

Spirolactone treatment of hirsutism is dose related and has a better effect with 200 mg daily.[69,70] After some period of treatment, a maintenance dose of 25–50 mg daily appears adequate. As with progestational agents, the response is relatively slow; a maximal effect will appear only after 6 months of treatment.[71] Side effects such as diuresis in the first few days and occasional complaints of fatigue are minimal. Spirolactone should be used with caution in elderly women who are diabetic because of the possibility of hyperkalemia. Combined treatment with an estrogen-progestin contraceptive may produce better clinical effects. However, spirolactone in combination with HRT has, to our knowledge, not been investigated.

References

1. Naftolin F, Schneider HPG, Sturdee DW. Guidelines for hormone treatment of women in the menopausal transition and beyond. Position Statement of the Executive Committee of the International Menopause Society. Climacteric 2004; 7:333–337.
2. Mikkola TS, Clarkson TB. Estrogen replacement therapy: atherosclerosis, and vascular function. Cardiovasc Res 2002; 53:605–619.

3. Herrington DM, Espeland MA, Crouse JR III. et al. Estrogen replacement and brachial artery flow-mediated vasodilatation in older women. Arterioscl Thromb Vasc Biol 2001; 21:1955–1961.

4. Zandi PP, Carlson MC, Plassman BL et al. Hormone replacement therapy and incidence of Alzheimer disease in older women. The Cache County Study. JAMA 2002; 288:2123–2129.

5. Schneider HPG. The role of antiandrogens in hormone replacement therapy. Climacteric 2000; 3(Suppl 2):21–27.

6. Jenkins JS & Ash S. The metabolism of testosterone by human skin in disorders of hair growth. J Endocrinol 1973; 59:345–351.

7. Slominski A, Wortsman J. Neuroendocrinology of the skin. Endocr Rev 2000; 21:457–487.

8. Sitruk-Ware R. Role of progestins with partial antiandrogenic effects. Climacteric 2004; 7:238–254.

9. Ludwig E. Classification of the types of androgenetic alopecia (common baldness) occurring in the female sex. Br J Dermatol 1977; 97:247–254.

10. Venning VA, Dawber R. Patterned androgenic alopecia. J Am Acad Dermatol 1988; 18:1073–1077.

11. Dawber R, Van Neste D. Hair and Scalp Disorders. 1995 London: Martin Dunitz.

12. Neumann F, Berswordt-Wallrabe R. Effects of the androgen antagonist cyproterone acetate on the testicular structure, spermatogenesis and accessory sexual glands of testosterone-treated adult hypophysectomized rats. J Endocrinol 1966; 35:363–371.

13. Labrie F, Bélanger A, Cusan L et al. Marked decline in serum concentrations of adrenal C19 sex steroid precursors and conjugated androgen metabolites during aging. J Clin Endocrinol Metab 1997; 82: 2396–2402.

14. Burger HG, Dudley EC, Cui J et al. A prospective longitudinal study of serum testosterone, dehydroepiandrosterone sulfate, and sex hormone-binding globulin levels through the menopause transition. J Clin Endocrinol Metab 2000; 85: 2832–2838.

15. Sitruk-Ware R. Progestogens in hormonal replacement therapy: new molecules, risks and benefits. Menopause 2002; 9:6–15.

16. Couzinet B, Meduri G, Lecce MG et al. The postmenopausal ovary is not a major androgen-producing gland. J Clin Endocrinol Metab 2001; 86:5060–5066.

17. Jiroutek MR, Chen M-H, Johnston CC et al. Changes in reproductive hormones and sex hormone-binding globulin in a group of postmenopausal women measured over 10 years. Menopause 1998; 5:90–94.

18. Meldrum DR, Davidson BJ, Tataryn IV et al. Changes in circulating steroids with aging in postmenopausal women. Obstet Gynecol 1981; 57:624–628.

19. Husmann F. Klinische Erfahrungen mit Climen® bei Peri- und Postmenopausalen Frauen. Zentralbl Gynakol 1997; 119:123–127.

20. Gambacciani M, Spinetti A, Orlandi R et al. Effects of a new estrogen/progestin combination in the treatment of postmenopausal syndrome. Maturitas 1995; 22:115–120.

21. Alwers R, Urdinola J, Onatra W et al. Changes in normal lipid profile of menopausal women with combined hormone replacement therapy. Comparative clinical trial of two hormonal combinations (conjugated estrogen/medroxyprogesterone acetate versus estradiol valerate/cyproterone acetate). Maturitas 1999; 32:41–50.

22. Jahn A, Blode H, Günzel P. Developmental toxicology data of cyproterone acetate – their relevance for clinical safety assessment. Teratology 1996; 53:31A.

23. Gräser T, Koytchev R, Römer T et al. Dienogest as a progestin for hormone replacement therapy. Drugs Today 1999; 35(Suppl C):115–126.

24. Udoff L, Langenberg P & Adashi EY. Combined continuous hormone replacement therapy: a critical review. Obstet Gynecol 1995; 86:306–316.

25. Rübig A. Drospirenone: a new cardiovascular-active progestin with antialdosterone and antiandrogenic properties. Climacteric 2003; 6(Suppl 3):49–54.

26. Muhn P, Krattenmacher R, Beier S et al. Drospirenone: a novel progestogen with antimineralocorticoid and antiandrogenic activity. Contraception 1995; 51:99–110.

27. Krattenmacher R. Drospirenone: pharmacology and pharmacokinetics of a unique progestogen. Contraception 2000; 62:29–38.

28. Archer DF, Pickar JH. Hormone replacement therapy: effect of progestogen dose and time since menopause on endometrial bleeding. Obstet Gynecol 2000; 96:899–905.

29. Strothmann A, Schneider HPG. Hormone therapy: the European women's perspective. Climacteric 2003; 6:337–346.

30. Schneider HPG, Schmidt-Gollwitzer K. Clinical experiences with a non-androgenic progestogen in an estradiol-valerate-containing regimen for hormone replacement therapy. In: HPG Schneider, AR Genazzani (Eds.). A New Approach in the Treatment of Climacteric Disorders. New Developments in Biosciences 7. 1992:17–28. Berlin: Walter de Gruyter.

31. Schneider HPG, Rosemeier HP, Schnitker J et al. Application and factor analysis of the menopause rating scale (MRS) in a post-marketing surveillance study of Climen®. Maturitas 2000; 37:113–124.

32. Chatel A, Fugère P, Bissonnette F et al. Psychological distress and sexuality in a group of women attending a menopause clinic: Effect of hormonal replacement therapy. Menopause 1996: 3:165–171.

33. Christiansen C. Cyproterone acetate in hormone replacement therapy. In: HPG Schneider, AR

Genazzani (Eds.). A New Approach in the Treatment of Climacteric Disorders. New Developments in Biosciences 7. 1992:1–8 Berlin: Walter de Gruyter.

34. Komulainen M, Tuppurainen MT, Kröger H et al. Vitamin D and HRT: no benefit additional to that of HRT alone in prevention of bone loss in early post-menopausal women. A 2.5–year randomized placebo-controlled study. Osteoporos Int 1997; 7:126–132.

35. Komulainen MH, Kröger H, Tuppurainen MT et al. HRT and vitamin D in prevention of non-vertebral fractures in postmenopausal women: a 5 year randomized trial. Maturitas 1998; 31:45–54.

36. Koninckx PR, Schmidt-Gollwitzer K. Use of estradiol valerate in combination with cyproterone acetate to control menopausal symptoms: A review of efficacy, influence on endometrium, on bone metabolism and cardiovascular risk factors. Eur Menop J 1997; 4:49–59.

37. Evans DJ, Hoffman RG, Kalkhoff RK et al. Relationship of body fat topography to insulin sensitivity and metabolic profiles in postmenopausal women. Metabolism 1983; 33:68–75.

38. Evans DJ, Hoffman RG, Kalkhoff RK et al. Relationship of androgenic activity to body topography, fat cell morphology and metabolic aberrations in premenopausal women. J Clin Endocrinol Metab 1983; 57:304–310.

39. Lapidus L, Bengtsson C, Larsson B et al. Distribution of adipose tissue and risk of cardiovascular disease and death: a 12 years follow up of participants in the population study of women in Gothenburg, Sweden. Br Med J 1984; 289: 1257–1261.

40. Haarbo J, Hassager C, Schlemmer A et al. The influence of smoking, body fat distribution, and alcohol consumption on serum lipids, lipoproteins, and apolipoproteins in early postmenopausal women. Atherosclerosis 1990; 84:239–244.

41. Gambacciani M, Ciaponi M, Cappagli B et al. Body weight, body fat distribution, and hormonal replacement therapy in early postmenopausal women. J Clin Endocrinol Metab 1997; 82:414–417.

42. Tankó LB, Movsesyan L, Svendsen OL et al. The effect of hormone replacement therapy on appendicular lean tissue mass in early postmenopausal women. Menopause 2002; 9:117–121.

43. Gangar KF, Vyas S, Whitehead M et al. Pulsatility index in internal carotid artery in relation to transdermal oestradiol and time since menopause. Lancet 1991; 338:839–842.

44. Penotti M, Sironi L, Cannata L et al. Effects of androgen supplementation of hormone replacement therapy on the vascular reactivity of cerebral arteries. Fertil Steril 2001; 76:235–240.

45. De Leo V, la Marca A, Orlandi R et al. Effects of estradiol alone or in combination with cyproterone acetate on carotid artery pulsatility index in postmenopausal women. Maturitas 2003; 46: 219–224.

46. Genazzani AR (Ed.). Hormone Replacement Therapy and the Brain: the Current Status of Research and Practice. 2003 New York: CRC Press.

47. Anderer P, Semlitsch HV, Saletu B et al. Effects of hormone replacement therapy on perceptual and cognitive event-related potentials in menopausal insomnia. Psychoneuroendocrinology 2003; 28:419–445.

48. Saletu B, Anderer P, Gruber D et al. Hormone replacement therapy and vigilance: double-blind, placebo-controlled EEG-mapping studies with an estrogen-progestogen combination (Climodien, Lafamme) versus estrogen alone in menopausal syndrome patients. Maturitas 2002; 43:165–181.

49. Saletu H. Sleep, vigilance and cognition in postmenopausal women: placebo-controlled studies with 2 mg estradiol valerate, with and without 3 mg dienogest. Climacteric 2003; 6(Suppl 2):37–45.

50. Mueck AO, Seeger H, Ludtke R et al. Effect on biochemical vasoactive markers during postmenopausal hormone replacement therapy: estradiol versus estradiol/dienogest. Maturitas 2001; 38: 305–313.

51. Oelkers W. Drospirenone, a progestogen with antimineralocorticoid properties: a short review. Mol Cell Endocrinol 2004; 217:255–261.

52. Elger W, Beier S, Pollow K et al. Conception and pharmacodynamic profile of drospirenone. Steroids 2003; 68:891–905.

53. Schürmann R, Holler T, Benda N. Estradiol and drospirenone for climacteric symptoms in postmenopausal women: a double-blind, randomized, placebo-controlled study of the safety and efficacy of three dose regimens. Climacteric 2004; 7:189–196.

54. Archer D, Thorneycroft I, Foegh M et al. A multicenter trial of the efficacy and safety of drospirenone-estradiol combinations when used for hormone therapy. Menopause 2005, in press.

55. Preston RA, Alonso A, Panzitta D et al. Additive effect of drospirenone/17–β-estradiol in hypertensive postmenopausal women receiving enalapril. Am J Hypertens 2002; 15:816–822.

56. Pitt B, Zannad F, Remme WJ et al. The effect of spironolactone on morbidity and mortality in patients with severe heart failure. N Engl J Med 1999; 341:709–717.

57. White WB, Pitt B, Foegh M et al. Drospirenone with estradiol lowers blood pressure in postmenopausal women with systolic hypertension. Obstet Gynecol 2004; 103(Suppl):26S.

58. Levy D, Larson ME, Vosan RS et al. The progression from hypertension to congestive heart failure. JAMA 1996; 275:1557–1562.

59. Stölzner W, Kurischko A, Freund R et al. Tierexperimentell-endokrinologische Charakterisierung des Gestagens Dienogest (STS 557). II. Antigonadotrope, gestagene, androgene und anti-androgene Wirkungen. III Jenaer Symposium Zur hormonale Kontrazeption 10–11 April 1984, JAMA 1985:165–182.

60. Warming L, Ravn P, Nielsen T et al. Safety and efficacy of drospirenone used in a continuous combination with 17 beta-estradiol for prevention of postmenopausal osteoporosis. Climacteric 2004; 7:103–111.

61. Teichmann A. Pharmacology of estradiol valerate/dienogest. Climacteric 2003; 6(Suppl 2):17–23.

62. Jondet M, Maroni M, Yaneva H et al. Comparative endometrial histology in postmenopausal women with sequential hormone replacement therapy of estradiol and, either chlormadinone acetate or micronized progesterone. Maturitas 2002; 41:115–121.

63. Birch MP, Lalla SC, Messenger AG. Female pattern hair loss. Clin Exp Dermatol 2002; 727:383–388.

64. Tolino A, Petrone A, Sarnacchiaro F et al. Finasteride in the treatment of hirsutism: new therapeutic perspectives. Fertil Steril 1996; 66:61–65.

65. Wong IL, Morris RS, Chang L et al. A prospective randomized trial comparing finasteride to spironolactone in the treatment of hirsute women. J Clin Endocrinol Metab 1995; 80:233–238.

66. Moghetti P, Tosi F, Tosti A et al. Comparison of spironolactone, flutamide, and finasteride efficacy in the treatment of hirsutism: a randomized, double blind, placebo-controlled trial. J Clin Endocrinol Metab 2002; 85:89–94.

67. Erenus M, Yücelten D, Durmusoglu F et al. Comparison of finasteride versus spironolactone in the treatment of idiopathic hirsutism. Fertil Steril 1997; 68:1000–1003.

68. Venturoli S, Marescalchi O, Colombo FM et al. A prospective randomized trial comparing low dose flutamide, finasteride, ketoconazole, and cyproterone acetate-estrogen regimens in the treatment of hirsutism. J Clin Endocrinol Metab 1999; 84: 1304–1310.

69. Price VH, Roberts JL, Hordinsky M et al. Lack of efficacy of finasteride in postmenopausal women with androgenic alopecia. J Am Acad Dermatol 2000; 43:768–776.

70. Lobo RA, Shoupe D, Serafini P et al. The effects of two doses of spironolactone on serum androgens and anagen hair in hirsute women. Fertil Steril 1985; 43:200–205.

71. Barth JH, Cherry CA, Wojnarowsaka F et al. Spironolactone is an effective and well tolerated systemic anti-androgen therapy for hirsute women. J Clin Endocrinol Metab 1989; 68:966–970.

Chapter 9

Is there a role for androgens in premenopausal women?

Camille Sylvestre and William Buckett

Summary

The natural history of production and role of androgens will be reviewed across the different reproductive phases of the woman. Specific cases such as surgical oophorectomy and declining ovarian production of androgens will be addressed. Finally, the benefits and potential risks of testosterone therapy will be discussed based on the available studies.

Introduction

Androgens are produced by adrenal glands and ovaries, and circulating levels of testosterone decline with age. Androgen deficiency could be a consequence of normal aging, ovarian insufficiency, adrenal insufficiency, or a combination of these causes. Androgen deficiency can also be a result of iatrogenic ovarian or adrenal insufficiency.

Symptoms of androgen deficiency are mainly loss of libido and sexual desire, but there may also be diminished wellbeing and depressed mood.[1] Symptoms are more pronounced in premenopausal women because androgens levels steadily decrease with increasing age and in the forties are about 50% levels typically found in the twenties. However, once menopausal, the androgen levels do not acutely change.[2]

This review will cover androgen production by the ovaries and adrenal glands and the occurrence of clinical androgen deficiency in premenopausal women. The possible role of androgen therapy will be discussed in relation to androgen deficiency.

Ovarian androgen production and ovarian function

The major androgens produced by the ovary are dehydroepiandrosterone (DHEA) and androstenedione, with a small amount of direct testosterone secretion. Androgens are secreted by stromal tissue derived from theca cells, although half the total DHEA is produced in peripheral tissue. Excessive accumulation of stromal tissue (or even an androgen-producing tumor) can lead to significant secretion of testosterone.

The rate of production of testosterone in normal women is 0.2–0.3 mg/day, and 50% arises from peripheral conversion of androstenedione (and small amounts of DHEA) to testosterone by the enzyme 17β-hydroxysteroid dehydrogenase. A further 25% is secreted directly by the ovary and the remaining 25% by the adrenal gland. All androgens are then common precursors of estrogens. Testosterone is aromatized to estradiol and androstenedione is aromatized to estrone, which can then be converted to estradiol. The major androgens are excreted in the urine as 17-ketosteroids. Aside from aromatization, testosterone is also bound to the sex hormone binding globulin (SHBG). The androgenic effects of these circulating androgens are therefore dependent upon the unbound fraction which can move freely from the vascular compartment into the target cells.

Dihydrotestosterone (DHT) levels are one-tenth of circulating testosterone levels, but DHT is the active androgen in tissue after conversion of testosterone by the enzyme 5α-reductase. In women, because the production of androstenedione is so much greater than testosterone, blood DHT is primarily derived from androstenedione and partly from DHEA, thus peripheral production of DHT is mainly influenced by circulating androstenedione levels.

Measures of endocrine parameters around menopause show a gradual increase in the gonadotrophins follicle stimulating hormone (FSH) and luteinizing hormone (LH) during 3 years before and subsequent stabilization 1 year after the menopause. Ovarian estradiol (E_2) and estrone (E_3) production starts to decrease steadily 3 years before menopause, and in the postmenopausal state, E_3 is primarily derived from aromatization of androstenedione in peripheral tissue. Therefore in the postmenopausal state, most of circulating E_2 is a result of E_3 conversion.

The androgen-producing capacity of the ovary is not completely compromised at menopause and actually there is a slight increase in testosterone production just at menopause,[3] secondary to the increased level of gonadotrophins. The level of androstenedione is about one-half that seen prior to menopause. Overall though, testosterone and androstenedione start to decrease 3 years before menopause, and have fallen about 15% by the postmenopausal years. This diminution is due to the decreased activity of follicular theca cells. After menopause, they are produced by the stromal and hilar cells and the decline stabilizes.

Adrenal gland androgen production

Under normal conditions, adrenal production of sex steroids is less than ovarian production of androgens and estrogens. As noted earlier, half of the daily production of DHEA and androstenedione comes from the adrenal gland, the other half of androstenedione comes from the ovary, and the other half of DHEA is split between the ovary and peripheral tissue; 25% of total daily testosterone is produced by the adrenal gland. Dehydroepiandrosterone sulfate (DHEAS) is derived almost exclusively from the adrenal gland. It is therefore a direct measure of adrenal androgen activity.

Adrenal gland androgens – DHEA and DHEAS – show a gradual age-dependent decrease after age 40 and the exact regulation of the adrenal production is unknown.[3] Most of the postmenopausal androstenedione is derived from the adrenal gland, with only a small amount secreted by the ovary. The total amount of testosterone produced after menopause is therefore decreased because the primary source, peripheral conversion of androstenedione, is reduced.

Changes in androgens with oophorectomy

The effects of a sudden drop in estradiol on androgens levels were assessed in premenopausal women by De Leo et al.[4] Androgen levels were measured before and 8 days after oophorectomy with a corticotrophin releasing hormone test. Basal levels of DHEAS, androstenedione, testosterone, and 17-hydroxyprogesterone were significantly lower after the oophorectomy. The androgens measured have a weak binding to SHBG, thus the decrease cannot be solely imputable to an estrogen-dependent change in the level of binding proteins. It was postulated that the decrease in androgens after oophorectomy is not only the direct consequence of the cessation of ovarian androgen production, but also that the acute deficiency of estrogens may affect adrenal steroidogenesis.[4]

In summary, total and free testosterone decline with age so that premenopausal women in their forties have half of the level of women in their twenties. The levels remain fairly stable across the perimenopausal years, although there are some increases followed by a decrease, and then remain fairly stable or very slowly decline with declining adrenal androgen production associated with increasing age. In the decade preceding the menopause, there is a loss of the midcycle surge of free testosterone and androstenedione.

Thus the clinical manifestations of androgen insufficiency – namely loss of libido, lowered mood, and fatigue – may precede menopause and not be a consequence of natural menopause. The published data demonstrating beneficial effects of androgen therapy on sexual function, mood, and wellbeing in premenopausal women will be reviewed.

Benefits of androgen therapy

With the aforementioned consequences of androgen decline with age, theoretical advantages of testosterone therapy are increased libido and greater sense of wellbeing. Several androgens have been tried but none is currently approved by the US Food and Drug Administration specifically for female sexual dysfunction – either in premenopausal or postmenopausal women.

DHEA has gained some publicity as a dietary supplement which could potentially be an 'antiaging' medication and restore wellbeing and libido. This drug is widely available over the counter. Two studies have analyzed DHEA administration. The first study was comparing oral micronized, nonmicronized (crystaline) and vaginal DHEA administration in a double blind, placebo controlled randomized single-dose comparison. In a previous study by Mortola and Yen,[5] when DHEA was given in high dose (1600 mg/day), there was a decrease in SHBG and an increase in testosterone level, but also there was an adverse lipid profile and increased insulin resistance. There was a decline of 11.3% in serum cholesterol and 20% in high-density lipoprotein within the first week, as well as a nonsignificant downward trend in low-density lipoprotein, very–low-density lipoprotein and triglycerides. There were no adverse clinical effects. By giving a lower dose, the hypothesis was that there would be a slight increase in testosterone without the adverse atherogenic effects. In this study, 150 mg were used and still supraphysiologic elevations were seen of DHEA, DHEAS, and testosterone. Calculations were made that a 50 mg oral dose of micronized or nonmicronized DHEA once a day to premenopausal women with low endogenous adrenal androgens may be adequate to increase serum DHEAS to upper normal range, with only a slight increase in testosterone. The comparison of oral micronization and the vaginal

delivery of DHEA showed that there was an advantage in avoiding the hepatic first pass metabolism in terms of metabolic side effects, however, there was also a decrease in bioconversion into testosterone.[6]

The second study on DHEA was a double blind, placebo controlled randomized trial of a dose of 50 mg orally for 3 months given to 60 premenopausal symptomatic women (altered mood and wellbeing). They measured an increase in DHEAS and testosterone levels, but a decrease in cortisol, high-density lipoprotein (HDL) cholesterol and lipoprotein A. There was no improvement in libido or wellbeing compared to placebo.[7]

Androgens have also been thought to play a role in hot flashes occurring during the perimenopausal years. The flashes occur when there are variations in the estrogen levels. Estrogen and androgen receptors are present in the central nervous system areas related to hot flashes. Some women will continue to have hot flashes despite adequate estrogen levels. In this case, estrogens are thought to increase SHBG and therefore free androgen and free estrogen levels are low. Thus a combination of estrogens and testosterone (for example esterified estrogen 0.625 mg and methyltestosterone 1.25 mg daily) supplementation might be efficient because it will decrease SHBG, increase the bioavailability of estrogens and testosterone and alleviate menopausal symptoms.[8] This specific combination was proved in a placebo controlled trial to be superior to estrogen alone to reduce hot flashes, night sweats, and vaginal dryness after 3 months of treatment.[8]

One of the major problem affecting menopausal women and which begins sometimes in premenopausal years is the stress urinary incontinence (SUI). Well known studies such as the HERS trial (2001), the Nurses' Study (2004) and the Women's Health Initiative trial (2005) all demonstrated that hormonal replacement therapy worsens both the incidence and severity of SUI by roughly 50%. On the other hand, almost all randomized clinical trials of androgens in women and animals show that it improves skeletal muscle. There is no trial in humans which specifically addresses SUI and androgen treatment, but animal trials[9] indicate that androgens plays a major role in female continence, in bladder relaxation to increase capacity, as well as perineal muscle support. Even in elderly men, androgen replacement has been shown to increase skeletal muscle strength and bulk more than placebo, so it should also help prevent and treat muscle atrophy bladder and bowel incontinence in females.

An interesting recent randomized trial of androgens in women with anorexia nervosa was performed. The hypothesis was that transdermal testosterone (Intrinsa 150 µg or 300 µg, Procter and Gamble Pharmaceuticals, Cincinnati, OH, USA) would improve bone formation and depressive symptoms in those patients.[10] At the end of a 3-week treatment, depressed patients receiving testosterone improved from severely depressed to moderately depressed; the placebo group was unchanged. Spatial cognition was also improved in the testosterone group. It may also prevent decreased bone formation in patients with, anorexia nervosa but because testosterone did not affect all markers of bone formation studied, further data are needed.

One of the main roles of testosterone therapy is in female sexual dysfunction (FSD), which is thought to affect up to 43% of women aged from 18 to 59 in the USA. FSD consists mainly of decreased libido, but also decreased arousal, difficulty achieving orgasm, and dyspareunia. The treatment of FSD must address underlying psychologic and medical problems, adjustment of medication and lifestyle, counseling and sex therapy. Androgen therapy should be oriented towards women with low androgens as in aging, hypopituitarism, oophorectomy, adrenal insufficiency or taking drugs which increase SHBG. Products which have been assessed include oral methyltestosterone and DHEA (as already noted), topical testosterone gel 2% vaginally, testosterone pellets 50 mg inserted subcutaneously every 3 months, and testosterone esters 25–50 mg injected intramuscularly every 4–6 weeks. Those products in physiologic dosing increase libido and sexual function but there are no data on long-term efficacy.[11] The subcutaneous implants are often a combination of estradiol and testosterone which not only alleviate the climacteric symptoms but also at the same time, a more favorable lipid profile is obtained. If the uterus is still in place, progesterone must be added to the treatment.[12]

A double blind, placebo controlled, randomized trial using a testosterone cream 10 mg 1% daily on the thighs specifically analyzed the effects in premenopausal women with low libido using questionnaires. Testosterone therapy improved wellbeing, mood, and sexual function in those women.[13]

Most of these studies have been done on small numbers of women for a short duration, and the effects are very subjective. Further studies are needed to evaluate the benefits in the long term. Nevertheless, based on the current available evidence, testosterone therapy seems to be beneficial in premenopausal women with decreased libido.

Potential risks of androgen therapy in premenopausal women

Adverse effects of androgen therapy include hirsutism, acne, irreversible deepening of the voice, and adverse changes in liver function, lipids (decrease in high-density lipoprotein) and lipoprotein (decrease in lipoprotein A).[11,14] Androgens have also been shown to decrease plasminogen activator inhibitor 1, and thus increasing fibrinolysis.[14] The risks and benefits of androgen therapy for all women are discussed elsewhere in this volume. Oral androgens have more effects on lipids because they decrease high-density lipoprotein cholesterol, whereas parenteral (transdermal, implants, and injections) or vaginal androgens would avoid hepatic first pass metabolism and are therefore lipid neutral.

In a woman of reproductive age, virilization of a female fetus would be a potential risk of androgen therapy. Also, as most androgens are aromatized to estrogens, other risks to premenopausal women would be the same as giving estrogens – namely thromboembolic diseases and estrogen-dependent cancer – except breast cancer which seems to be decreased.[15] Potential risks are thought to be more likely with supraphysiologic doses of androgens. As noted earlier, most studies on premenopausal women have been too small or lacked sufficient follow-up to determine the long-term risks of androgen therapy.

Conclusions

Sexual dysfunction in premenopausal women is a prevalent problem and could be a consequence of declining androgen levels with aging and ovarian function. After underlying psychologic and medical problems have been assessed and corrected, and after appropriate counseling, androgen treatment could be considered. Data so far indicates an improvement in libido, mood, and wellbeing. The dose should be adjusted individually and be ideally within the physiologic limits to avoid side effects. Nevertheless, further studies are warranted to determine the efficacy and safety of long-term use.

References

1. Shifren JL. Is there a role for testosterone therapy in premenopausal women? Menopause 2003; 10: 383–384.
2. Davis SR. When to suspect androgen deficiency other than at menopause. Fertil Steril 2002; 77(Suppl 4): S68–S71.
3. Overlie I, Moen MH, Morkrid L et al. The endocrine transition around menopause-a five years prospective study with profiles of gonadotropines, estrogens, androgens and SHBG among healthy women. Acta Obstet Gynecol Scand 1999; 78:642–647.
4. De Leo V, La Marca A, Talluri B et al. Hypothalamo-pituitary-adrenal axis and adrenal function before and after ovariectomy in premenopausal women. Eur J Endocrinol 1998; 138:430–435.
5. Mortola JF, Yen SS. The effects of oral dehydro-epiandrosterone on endocrine-metabolic parameters in post-menopausal women. J Clin Endocrinol Metab 1990; 71:696–704.
6. Casson PR, Straughn AB, Umstot ES et al. Delivery of dehydroepiandrosterone to premenopausal women: Effects of micronization and nonoral administration. Am J Obstet Gynecol 1996; 174:649–653.
7. Barnhart KT, Freeman E, Grisso JA et al. The effect of dehydroepiandrosterone supplementation to symptomatic perimenopausal women on serum endocrine profiles, lipid parameters, and health-related quality of life. J Clin Endocrinol Metab 1999; 84:3896–3902.
8. Notelovitz M. Hot flashes and androgens: a biological rationale for clinical practice. Mayo Clin Proc 2004; 79(Suppl):S8–S13.
9. Ho MH, Bhatia NN, Bhasin S. Anabolic effects of androgens on muscles of female pelvic floor and lower urinary tract. Curr Opin Obstet Gynecol 2004; 16:405–409.
10. Miller K, Grieco K, Klibanski A. Testosterone administration in women with anorexia nervosa. J Clin Endocrinol Metab 2005; 90:1428–1433.
11. Shifren JL. The role of androgens in female sexual dysfunction. Mayo Clin Proc 2004; 79(Suppl): S19–S24.
12. Jones MS. Subcutaneous estrogen replacement therapy. J Reprod Med 2004; 49:139–142.
13. Goldstat R, Briganti E, Tran J et al. Transdermal testosterone therapy improves well-being, mood, and sexual function in premenopausal women. Menopause 2003; 10:390–398.
14. Winkler UH. Effects of androgens on haemostasis. Maturitas 1996; 24:147–155.
15. Dimitrakakis C, Jones RA, Liu A et al. Breast cancer incidence in menopausal women using testosterone in addition to usual hormone therapy. Menopause 2004; 11:531–535.

Chapter 10

Treatment of osteoporosis in postmenopausal women: is there a place for androgens?

László B Tankó and Claus Christiansen

Summary

Estrogen/hormone replacement therapy increases circulating sex hormone binding globulin (SHBG) and cortisol binding globulin, which in turn limit the bioavailability of circulating testosterone and dihydrotestosterone. The increases in SHBG can be effectively countered by the combination of HRT with androgens, which in turn can reverse the decreases in bone formation markers and result in greater increases in bone mass density compared with those induced by HRT only. The benefits at the hip are particularly noteworthy. Parallel effects on skeletal muscle mass may also have implications for hip fracture prevention, since it contributes to decreased risk of falls. Low-dose or parenteral androgen replacement is safe and well tolerated. The ability of combined estrogen plus androgen therapy to evoke considerable increases in BMD at both the hips and spine is particularly important and warrants randomized clinical trials to assess the clinical potentials in terms of fracture prevention.

Introduction

Osteoporosis remains a major epidemiologic and socioeconomic problem in the industrialized countries of the world. Moreover, the increasing longevity and thereby relative number of the elderly population in these countries forecast an increasing rather than decreasing prevalence in the upcoming decades.[1] Despite major advances in the understanding of the pathogenesis, diagnosis, and clinical management of osteoporosis, curative treatments are still not available for wide scale use. Currently available drugs used for prevention provide 'only' a 50–60% decrease in risk for fractures, and very few, except for hormone replacement therapy (HRT), has been consistently shown to provide effective protection against nonvertebral fractures.[2-4] In light of the fact that hip fractures remain the most feared complication of osteoporosis due to 10–20% excess mortality in

the first year,[5,6] the ability of HRT to decrease the risk should not be neglected, but rather taken as the ground basis for continuing research aiming the definition of how to use this therapeutical option adequately.[7]

Estrogen deficiency has an established role in the pathogenesis of osteoporosis in postmenopausal women, whereas the indirect and direct implications of androgens for bone metabolism is still a growing field of research.[8-10] Although no precipitous drop in androgen production is apparent at the time of the natural menopause, androgens do decrease slowly and progressively from early adulthood until old age.[11-14] In contrast, surgical menopause induced by bilateral removal of the ovaries is associated with not only a sudden and complete loss of ovarian estrogens, but also a similar drop in circulating androgens.[15,16] The notion that the two sex steroids both participate in the modulation of bone turnover is emphasized by an earlier and more accelerated bone loss of surgical menopausal women.[17] Another clinical situation associated with a marked drop in bio-available androgens is HRT itself.[18] HRT restores circulating estradiol to premenopausal levels and decelerates osteoclast-mediated bone resorption. Yet a somewhat delayed and slowly emerging parallel inhibition of bone formation narrows the window of positive calcium balance and thereby the therapeutical window. Indeed, long-term studies indicate that after 2–3 years HRT the gain in bone mass density (BMD) reaches plateau after which no further increases can be elicited with prolongation of the therapy.[19] It is tempting to hypothesize that this phenomenon might involve, at least in part, the impact of oral HRT on circulating sex hormone binding globulin (SHBG) limiting the bioavailability of androgens, and thereby their anabolic impact on osteoblast-mediated bone formation.

The present chapter summarizes the experimental and clinical findings arguing for due consideration of androgen supplementation to HRT, which might considerably increase the efficacy of HRT for the prevention of osteoporotic fractures, and in particular hip fractures.

Rational for considering androgens

Androgen receptors: localization and effects

Androgen receptors are expressed in the nuclei of all three bone cells – osteoblasts, osteoclasts, and osteocytes – testosterone, dihydrotestosterone, and dehydroepiandrostendione (DHEA) having their own specific binding receptors.[20] The highest density of receptors is present in osteoblasts, particularly those present at the site of active bone formation. Importantly, receptor expression is more dense in the cortical compared with the trabecular compartment of bone tissue. Experimental studies indicate that androgen receptors are upregulated by androgens in bone.[20]

Androgens may act via receptors in the nucleus (genomic effects) or via a more rapid mechanism involving receptors in the cytoplasmic membrane (nongenomic effects). Androgens can directly stimulate proliferation and differentiation of osteoblasts

as well as the synthesis of extracellular matrix proteins (e.g. type 1α1 collagen, osteocalcin, and osteonectin). Thus, androgens have critical implications for the regulation of bone matrix production, organization, and even mineralization.

Skeletal effects of androgens in animal models

Studies support the contention that estrogens and androgens are both required for normal skeletal health in males and females. In support, the administration of flutamide, a specific androgen receptor antagonist, to female rats results in osteopenia.[21] Moreover, Lea et al.[22] reported that the antiandrogen compound Casodex inhibited the protective effects of androstenedione on ovariectomy-induced bone loss, whereas administration of an aromatase inhibitor was ineffective. Furthermore, in female rats, nonaromatizable androgens have been shown to prevent or reverse bone loss induced by ovariectomy, these effects being mediated by a reduction in bone turnover in trabecular bone and increased periosteal and endosteal bone formation.[23,24]

Circulating androgens in women

The ovaries and the adrenal glands are responsible for production of testosterone, androstenedione and DHEA. However, only the adrenals produce dehydroepiandrosterone sulfate (DHEAS). Approximately half of the testosterone is produced by peripheral conversion of circulating pre-androgens, with androstendione being the predominant precursor, the rest deriving from the ovaries.[25] Only 1–2% of total circulating testosterone is biologically available for tissue exposure; the remainder is bound by SHBG, cortisol binding globulin (CBG), and albumin.[11]

With age, the mean circulating levels of androgens in women decline, such that by the time women are 40 years of age, their levels are almost half of those in their twenties.[11] As levels of DHEA and DHEAS fall linearly with age, this is reflected in age-related decline of their metabolite, testosterone.[13,26] After menopause, direct ovarian production is responsible for as much as 50% of circulating testosterone with adrenals serving a less important role.[27] Data from research by Labrie et al.[28] show that most of the decrease in DHEAS levels occurs between the ages of 50 and 60, and thereafter decreases at a lesser rate.

Surgical removal of the ovaries is the most common cause of iatrogenic androgen insufficiency and results in sudden decline (~50%) of both testosterone and androstenedione.[15] Unlike natural menopause, surgical menopause is associated with dramatic decreases in estrogen, progesterone, and testosterone. Testosterone levels, in particular, may drop to ~5.0 ng/dL (~50% drop from the normal levels in healthy women) within the first 24–48 h after bilateral salpingo-oophorectomy with or without total abdominal hysterectomy.[16] Mean blood production rates of both androstenedione and testosterone are significantly lower than the respective values in the control group.

Implications of endogenous androgens for bone in humans

Several epidemiologic studies have investigated the association of endogenous androgens with bone mass or presence of osteoporotic fractures. In cross-sectional settings, women with android-type body fat distribution, which is characterized by high waist-to-hip ratio have higher BMD than those with a more gynoid-type body fat distribution.[29] This in part can be attributable to a lower SHBG concentration and thereby higher circulating concentration of sex steroids. Independently of age, body mass index, and other sex steroid confounders, bioavailable testosterone – but not DHEAS, DHEA, androstenedione, or SHBG – has been shown to be an independent predictor of BMD at the spine and hip.[30] In the study by Bagur et al.[31] both endogenous estradiol and testosterone levels were significant predictors of BMD at the spine. Moreover, testosterone was also significant independent predictor of BMD at the total hip and the total skeleton. In women under 65 years of age, estradiol levels exceeding 10 pg/mL were associated with increased BMD, which was however not applicable for the older group. Adding complexity to the relative importance of androgens to BMD, Tok et al.[32] not only confirmed the positive correlation of BMD with measures of serum testosterone and DHEAS, but also found that serum free testosterone had an apparent greater role for spine BMD, whereas DHEAS was more closely associated with hip BMD. Longcope

et al.[33] measured androgens and estradiol levels in postmenopausal women with or without vertebral crush fractures. Women with vertebral crush fractures were found to have significantly lower metabolic clearance rates of testosterone and estrone compared with the control group. In addition there was a significant decrease in androgen levels in the crush fracture group.

Other supporting evidence comes from studies undertaken in women with polycystic ovary syndrome (PCOS). In these women, a significant correlation of elevated testosterone and androstenedione with BMD is a common finding. A direct effect of hyperandrogenism on bone mass was illustrated by a study that observed that nonobese, young, hirsute oligomenorrheic and amenorrheic women had higher BMD than nonhirsute oligomenorrheic and amenorrheic controls.[34] In a subgroup of PCOS patients with amenorrhea, spine and femoral BMD values were comparable to control values but were lower than the BMD in women with idiopathic hirsutism and nonamenorrheic PCOS, despite comparable estradiol values.[34] The importance of endogenous androgens and BMD is further illustrated by a decrease in BMD after the use of androgen antagonists both in eumenorrheic women with hyperandrogenemia and in women with PCOS.[35]

The number of longitudinal observations assessing the relative importance of sex steroids for bone loss is sparse. In the Rancho Bernardo study, DHEA was positively associated with BMD at all skeletal sites measured 4 years later, whereas higher bioavailable testosterone was only associated with BMD at the ultra-distal radius.[36] The strongest correlate of BMD was bioavailable estradiol. In another analysis of the same cohort, bioavailable testosterone was an independent predictor of height loss (a surrogate marker of vertebral crush fracture), independent of age, BMI, smoking habits, alcohol intake, and the use of thiazides and HRT.[37] These latter observations provide strong support for the importance of testosterone effects for the maintenance of bone integrity in postmenopausal women.

Credits and limitations of hormone replacement therapy

The Women's Health Initiative study with more than 16 000 participants was the first large-scale randomized clinical trial to demonstrate a reduction in hip and vertebral fracture risk with HRT use.[38,39] Before this proof, support for estrogen use to prevent bone loss and fractures in post-menopausal women had come from three lines of evidence: (1) numerous randomized trials have consistently shown that estrogen prevents post-menopausal bone loss (e.g.[40,41]), (2) observational studies consistently suggested that post-menopausal HRT reduces the risk of hip and other types of fracture (e.g.[42,43]), and (3) risk-versus-benefit studies suggested that HRT would increase life expectancy for most menopausal women, since protection against hip fractures and coronary heart disease would outweigh the increase in the risk of breast cancer (e.g.[42,44]).

Although the skeletal benefits of HRT for pre-venting bone loss can hardly be challenged, one might be wary of published evidence that pro-longed HRT use unequivocally reduces the risk of fracture.[45] An evaluation of incident fracture rates in the Study of Osteoporotic Fractures population illustrates the limitations of HRT. In women who reported taking estrogen continuously since the menopause (an average of 25 years), the rate of bone loss was noted to accelerate with increasing age, and those on estrogen therapy continued to lose bone density, as did those without estrogen.[46] Furthermore, as reported very recently, almost 20% experienced a nontraumatic, nonvertebral fracture during a 10-year follow-up period.[47] This was fully two-thirds the number observed in women who had never taken estrogen. The extent to which estrogen was associated with lower rates of vertebral and hip fracture was similar. Thus, many women who take estrogen will ultimately suffer osteoporotic fractures.[48] Therefore, low bone mass and fractures remain serious threats in older postmenopausal women, even in the pres-ence of hormone replacement. This brings us to ask the question what factors might counter the efficacy of HRT over time and whether interven-tions outbalancing these effects can be defined.

Impact of ERT on the endogenous androgen milieu

Although the changes of menopause and aging are important with regard to the bioavailability of androgens, these changes are minor in compari-son to those induced by standard doses of HRT, particularly when it is administered by the oral route. Oral estrogens dominate the market with more than 85% of women choosing this form of estrogen replacement therapy (ERT). Because the pituitary–ovarian axis appears to remain intact after a natural menopause,[49] ERT at standard 'physiologic' or higher doses has a significant suppressive effect on gonadotropins (negative feedback), particularly luteinizing hormone (LH)[50] and, thereby, reduces the production of andro-gens from the early postmenopausal ovary. The changes in gonadotropin secretion occur about equally for both oral and parenteral estrogens when administered at equipotent doses.[50]

ERT and HRT also dramatically alter the circulat-ing levels of SHBG and CBG.[15] Testosterone and dihydrotestosterone are primarily bound to SHBG (66% and 78%, respectively).[51] In addition, testos-terone is bound to CBG and albumin.[51] Although small oral doses of ERT have a dramatic impact on SHBG concentrations, it requires larger doses of estradiol to significantly increase CBG. Judd et al.[15] demonstrated that doses of conjugated equine estrogens as low as 0.15 mg daily signi-ficantly increased SHBG, while standard doses (0.625 mg daily) increased SHBG by approx-imately 300% above baseline. Similarly, they showed that 0.625 mg of conjugated equine estro-gens could significantly increase CBG, although only to a small degree, while 1.25 mg of conju-gated equine estrogens was capable of increasing CBG concentrations by approximately 25% over baseline levels.[15]

Several studies demonstrate the clinical impor-tance of these binding globulin changes. Tazuke et al.[52] studied the plasma steroid hormone and SHBG levels in frozen plasma obtained from 977 women aged 50–79 years during the period 1972–1974. Almost all the 301 ERT users were taking oral conjugated equine estrogens; none reported use of any progestogen. After adjusting statistically for both age and obesity, DHEAS, androstenedione, and free testosterone were all significantly lower in the women currently taking estrogen than in the women not using estrogen. These differences were independent of cigarette smoking. Prospective observations in a random-ized clinical trial indicated no changes in total testosterone, but standard doses of esterified estrogens (0.625 mg, 1.25 mg) increased SHBG in a dose-dependent fashion, and thereby reduced bioavailable testosterone significantly. DHEAS and androstenedione were also reduced at the higher estrogen doses.

Effects of androgens on bone turnover and bone mass

The relative advantages of combining estrogen with androgen were recently demonstrated by an elegant double blind, randomized clinical trial.[53] Postmenopausal women received daily treatment with either a combination of 1.25 mg esterified estrogen and 2.5 mg methyltestosterone or of 1.25 mg conjugated equine estrogen only for 9 weeks. Similar decreases in the urinary excretion of the bone resorption markers (deoxypyridinoline, pyridinoline, and hydroxyproline) were noted in both groups. Women treated with conjugated equine estrogen showed decreased serum markers of bone formation (bone-specific alkaline phosphatase, osteocalcin, and C-terminal procollagen peptide), whereas the estrogen–androgen treatment evoked significant increases. Levels of SHBG increased with conjugated equine estrogen therapy, but significantly decreased during the estrogen–androgen therapy. These observations can be translated to a greater positive calcium balance accompanying estrogen–androgen treatment, which can be expected to elicit greater increases in BMD over time compared with the benefits of treatment with estrogen only.

Indeed, numerous studies have documented the positive effects of androgens on BMD in naturally and surgically postmenopausal women. Early studies used subcutaneous implants containing the sex steroids. A prospective, open-labeled study[54] included 20 naturally menopausal women, who had been receiving long-term oral estrogen therapy. Upon entering the study, they were treated either with estrogen–testosterone implants (group 1, subcutaneous implant containing 75 mg estradiol plus 100 mg testosterone) or oral estrogen only (group 2, 1.25 mg conjugated equine estrogen) for 1 year. At the end of the treatment, women who continued treatment with oral estrogen showed no considerable changes in BMD. In contrast, those treated with the pellets revealed significant increases in BMD at the spine (5.7%) and the femoral neck (5.2%). This study illustrates that androgens may elicit anabolic bone-building potentials even in those in whom the beneficial effects of estrogen is likely maximal.

Later, the long-term benefits of subcutaneous estrogen plus androgen administration on BMD was evaluated in a prospective, 2-year, single blind trial including 34 postmenopausal women.[55] Patients were randomly assigned to receive either estradiol (50 mg pellets) or estradiol/androgen (50 mg estradiol +50 mg testosterone pellet) once every 3 months. Cyclic oral progestins were given to women who had an intact uterus. Those women receiving androgen supplementation showed more rapidly emerging and greater increases in BMD (total body, lumbar vertebral, and hip) by the end of the treatment period compared with those who received ERT/HRT. In the study by Garnett et al.[56] 50 postmenopausal women were allocated randomly to receive estradiol (E_2) (75 mg) alone or with testosterone (100 mg) every 6 months for 1 year. Women with an intact uterus received cyclic norethindrone (5 mg) for 10 days of each calendar month. Twenty-five untreated women were recruited to act as a reference group. Both treatment regimens elicited significant gains in BMD at both the hip and spine, without considerable differences between the treatment groups.

The efficacy of the oral formulation of estrogen–androgen therapy on BMD has also been demonstrated by properly designed randomized clinical trials. In the study by Watts et al.,[57] 66 surgically menopausal women were treated with either 1.25 mg oral esterified estrogens or 1.25 mg esterified estrogens +2.5 mg methyltestosterone for 2 years. Although both treatments prevented bone loss at the spine and hip, only the combined therapy elicited significant increases in spine BMD (3.4%). In a 2-year, parallel group, double blind study including 311 surgical menopausal women were randomly assigned to receive daily treatment with the following regimens: 1) 0.625 mg conjugated estrogen, 2) 1.25 mg conjugated estrogen, 3) 1.25 mg esterified estrogens plus 1.25 mg methyltestosterone, 4) 1.25 mg esterified estrogens plus 2.5 mg methyltestosterone.[58] The gain in BMD at the spine and hip from baseline induced by the combination therapy was significantly greater than those elicited by estrogens only. Importantly, whereas the higher dose of conjugated estrogen induced a 1.3% change in hip BMD from baseline, the increase associated with the higher dose of the combination therapy was 3.5%.

The corresponding effects on spine BMD was also twofold higher (4.3% vs. 2.3%).

These initial results with estrogen–androgen therapy signal particularly impressive benefits in terms of increasing hip BMD, which represent one part of hip fracture prevention. However, the combination therapy offers additional benefits in this context. Studies by Dobs et al.[59] elegantly demonstrated that estrogen–androgen replacement can increase body lean mass and lower-body muscle strength, which might both exert beneficial effects on BMD and the risk of hip fracture in the elderly by lowering the risk of falls.

The efficacy of androgen only therapy was also tested in a small study by Labrie et al.[60] Elderly women 60–70 years old received treatment with 10% DHEA cream for 12 months. The treatment induced increases in BMD, which seemed most pronounced at the hip. The most interesting findings of the study was the revelation of a marked (>200%) increase in serum osteocalcin, a marker of bone formation accompanied with moderate decrease in bone resorption. DHEAS might be particularly useful when treating osteoporosis at the hip.

Androgenic progestogens

Progesterone or progestogens are prescribed for only one reason: to protect the endometrium in naturally menopausal women who are on estrogen therapy.[61] Progesterone is available in the micronized form or as synthetic progestogens. The latter are divided into derivatives that are structurally related to progesterone and have minimal or no androgenic activity, such as medroxyprogesterone acetate and megestrol acetate; and those that are related to testosterone and do have variable androgenic activity, such as norethindrone and norethindrone acetate. In clinical trials,[40] micronized progesterone and medroxyprogesterone acetate did not contribute significantly to the bone-protective effects of estrogen-alone therapy. In contrast, women receiving norethisterone acetate (NETA), in a dose of 1 mg daily, when additionally given either 5 μg or 10 μg of ethinyl E_2 daily, displayed a significant increase in their BMD when compared with matched controls or with estrogen-alone treated patients.[62] On the basis of the results of this and other studies, it may be concluded that

NETA – by changing the bone remodeling cycle in favor of bone formation – has an additive effect on BMD when combined with estrogen therapy.[63] Unopposed NETA, at doses higher than that needed for hormone therapy, has also been shown to increase BMD.[64]

Other androgen compounds

DHEA, the anabolic steroids (i.e., nandrolone decanoate), and a unique tissue-specific compound, tibolone, have all been demonstrated to have bone-building potential. Nandrolone decanoate, especially when used together with hormone therapy, significantly increases BMD.[65] It could be a useful option for elderly women, who may also benefit from its recognized anabolic effect on muscle. Tibolone is a unique product that has mild estrogenic (one-tenth the potency of ethinyl E_2), progestogenic (one-eighth the potency of norethindrone), and androgenic (one-fiftieth of 17-methyltestosterone) effects.[66] The biologic efficacy of tibolone is mediated through three of its metabolites that have weak affinity for the progesterone, estrogen, and androgen receptors and by tissue-specific stimulation of various enzyme systems. Clinical trials have shown that bone loss can be prevented in the spine and hip with doses ranging from 1.25 mg to 2.5 mg per day. In comparative studies, tibolone (2.5 mg) is as effective as traditional hormone replacement regimens.[66]

Safety

The various studies that have investigated the use of androgens in women have found that androgens are well tolerated and devoid of serious adverse effects. In addition to the dose of the androgen component, the relative dose of the added estrogen may also have an important role in the development of androgenic symptoms. Estrogen and androgen have reciprocal effect on circulating SHBG and thus the bioavailability of testosterone for tissue exposure. Low-dose androgen replacement therapy as used in women, 1.25 mg esterified estrogen + 2.5 mg methyltestosterone, or a half-strength preparation, 0.625 mg EE plus 1.25 mg methyltestosterone, is unlikely to produce commonly described side effects.[67]

Symptoms of virilization

Approximately 15–20% of women on testosterone implants develop a slight increase in downy facial hair after several years. The vast majority does not find this alarming, and it regresses on halving or omitting the testosterone from subsequent implants. Less than 1% develop hirsutism or acne, and virilism is an exceptionally rare finding.[68] These symptoms are more likely when supraphysiologic androgen levels are reached.

Endometrial histology

Endometrial protection is a critical aspect of HRT. Studies indicate that addition of testosterone neither facilitates nor antagonizes the stimulatory effect of estrogens on the endometrium.[69] These findings draw attention to the need to add a progestational agent to the regimen when treating postmenopausal women with intact uterus.

Lipid alterations

The influence of androgens on lipid profile may depend on the dose and the route of administration. Oral estrogen–androgen replacement – relative to estrogen only – may reduce high-density lipoprotein cholesterol (HDL-C) levels. However, total cholesterol, low-density lipoprotein cholesterol (LDL-C), and triglycerides also decreases during the combined therapy which is likely outbalancing the atherogenic risk posed by the HDL-lowering effect. Furthermore, the HDL-lowering effect is more likely in heavy smokers.[68]

Parenteral treatments have little to negligible effects on lipid profile. Subcutaneous pellets do not seem to cause changes in cholesterol, triglycerides, and HDL-C,[70] but testosterone may enhance the effects of estrogen on LDL-C.[71] During long-term treatment with intramuscular estrogen–androgen depot injections, no adverse effects on lipid profile were apparent compared with estrogen-treated or placebo-treated surgically menopausal women.[72]

Conclusions

Collectively, emerging evidence argue for a significant role of androgens in the pathogenesis of osteoporosis in postmenopausal women, especially in those who underwent surgical removal of the ovaries. While HRT continues to have an undeniable efficacy for the prevention and treatment of osteoporosis, it seems reasonable to believe that the clinical benefits (in terms of increasing BMD) could be further enhanced by proper supplementation with androgens. The considerable gain in BMD at the femoral neck during estrogen–androgen therapy is particularly a noteworthy finding and warrants further investigations. Also additional studies are required to determine whether androgen supplementation could enhance the efficacy of HRT in terms of reducing the risk for vertebral and nonvertebral fractures.

References

1. Melton LJ, 3rd. Epidemiology worldwide. Endocrinol Metab Clin North Am 2003; 32:1–13.
2. Papaioannou A, Watts NB, Kendler DL et al. Diagnosis and management of vertebral fractures in elderly adults. Am J Med 2002; 113:220–228.
3. Nelson HD, Helfand M, Woolf SH, & Allan JD. Screening for postmenopausal osteoporosis: a review of the evidence for the U.S. Preventive Services Task Force. Ann Intern Med 2002; 137:529–541.
4. McLellan AR. Identification and treatment of osteoporosis in fractures. Curr Rheumatol Rep 2003; 5:57–64.
5. Gourlay M, Richy F, & Reginster JY. Strategies for the prevention of hip fracture. Am J Med 2003; 115:309–317.
6. Cummings SR, Melton LJ. Epidemiology and outcomes of osteoporotic fractures. Lancet 2002; 359:1761–1767.
7. Lindsay R. Hormones and bone health in postmenopausal women. Endocrine 2004; 24:223–230.
8. Balasch J. Sex steroids and bone: current perspectives. Hum Reprod Update 2003; 9:207–222.
9. Manolagas SC, Kousteni S, & Jilka RL. Sex steroids and bone. Recent Prog Horm Res 2002; 57:385–409.

10. Compston JE. Sex steroids and bone. Physiol Rev 2001; 81:419–447.

11. Rannevik G, Carlstrom K, Jeppsson S et al. prospective long-term study in women from pre-menopause to post-menopause: changing profiles of gonadotrophins, oestrogens and androgens. Maturitas 1986; 8:297–307.

12. Rannevik G, Jeppsson S, Johnell O et al. A longitudinal study of the perimenopausal transition: altered profiles of steroid and pituitary hormones, SHBG and bone mineral density. Maturitas 1995; 21:103–113.

13. Meldrum DR. Changes in circulating steroids with aging in postenopausal women. Obstet Gynecol 1997; 57:624–628.

14. Overlie I, Moen MH, Morkrid L et al. The endocrine transition around menopause–a five years prospective study with profiles of gonadotropines, estrogens, androgens and SHBG among healthy women. Acta Obstet Gynecol Scand 1999; 78:642–647.

15. Judd HL. Hormonal dynamics associated with the menopause. Clin Obstet Gynecol 1976; 19:775–788.

16. Longcope C. Adrenal and gonadal androgen secretion in normal females. Clin Endocrinol Metab 1986; 15:213–228.

17. Yildiz A, Sahin I, Gol K et al. Bone loss rate in the lumbar spine: a comparison between natural and surgically induced menopause. Int J Gynaecol Obstet 1996; 55:153–159.

18. Simon JA. Estrogen replacement therapy: effects on the endogenous androgen milieu. Fertil Steril 2002; 77:S77–S82.

19. Komulainen M, Kroger H, Tuppurainen MT et al. Prevention of femoral and lumbar bone loss with hormone replacement therapy and vitamin D3 in early postmenopausal women: a population-based 5-year randomized trial. J Clin Endocrinol Metab 1999; 84:546–552.

20. Kasperk CH, Wakley GK, Hierl T, Ziegler R. Gonadal and adrenal androgens are potent regulators of human bone cell metabolism in vitro. J Bone Miner Res 1997; 12:464–471.

21. Goulding A, Gold E. Flutamide-mediated androgen blockade evokes osteopenia in the female rat. J Bone Miner Res 1993; 8:763–769.

22. Lea CK, Flanagan AM. Physiological plasma levels of androgens reduce bone loss in the ovariectomized rat. Am J Physiol 1998; 274:E328–E335.

23. Tobias JH, Compston JE. Does estrogen stimulate osteoblast function in postmenopausal women? Bone 1999; 24:121–124.

24. Turner RT, Wakley GK, Hannon KS. Differential effects of androgens on cortical bone histomorphometry in gonadectomized male and female rats. J Orthop Res 1990; 8:612–617.

25. Haning RV Jr, Chabot M, Flood CA et al. Metabolic clearance rate (MCR) of dehydroepiandrosterone sulfate (DS), its metabolism to dehydroepiandros-

terone, androstenedione, testosterone, and dihydrotestosterone, and the effect of increased plasma DS concentration on DS MCR in normal women. J Clin Endocrinol Metab 1989; 69:1047–1052.

26. Mushayandebvu T, Castracane VD, Gimpel T et al. Evidence for diminished midcycle ovarian androgen production in older reproductive aged women. Fertil Steril 1996; 65:721–723.

27. Judd HL, Lucas WE, Yen SS. Effect of oophorectomy on circulating testosterone and androstenedione levels in patients with endometrial cancer. Am J Obstet Gynecol 1974; 118:793–798.

28. Labrie F, Belanger A, Cusan L et al. Marked decline in serum concentrations of adrenal C19 sex steroid precursors and conjugated androgen metabolites during aging. J Clin Endocrinol Metab 1997; 82: 2396–2402.

29. Heiss CJ, Sanborn CF, Nichols DL et al. Associations of body fat distribution, circulating sex hormones, and bone density in postmenopausal women. J Clin Endocrinol Metab 1995; 80:1591–1596.

30. Zofkova I, Bahbouh R, Hill M. The pathophysiological implications of circulating androgens on bone mineral density in a normal female population. Steroids 2000; 65:857–861.

31. Bagur A, Oliveri B, Mautalen C et al. Low levels of endogenous estradiol protect bone mineral density in young postmenopausal women. Climacteric 2004; 7:181–188.

32. Tok EC, Ertunc D, Oz U et al. The effect of circulating androgens on bone mineral density in post-menopausal women. Maturitas 2004; 48:235–242.

33. Longcope C, Baker RS, Hui SL, Johnston CC Jr. Androgen and estrogen dynamics in women with vertebral crush fractures. Maturitas 1984; 6:309–318.

34. Dixon JE, Rodin A, Murby B et al. Bone mass in hirsuit women with androgen excess. Clin Endocrinol (Oxford) 1989; 30:271–277.

35. Di Carlo C, Shoham Z, MacDougall J et al. Polycystic ovaries as a relative protective factor for bone mineral loss in young women with amenorrhea. Fertil Steril 1992; 57:314–319.

36. Barrett-Connor E, Kritz-Silverstein D, Edelstein SL. A prospective study of dehydroepiandrosterone sulfate (DHEAS) and bone mineral density in older men and women. Am J Epidemiol 1993; 137:201–206.

37. Greendale GA, Edelstein S, Barrett-Connor E. Endogenous sex steroids and bone mineral density in older women and men: the Rancho Bernardo Study. J Bone Miner Res 1997; 12:1833–1843.

38. Rossouw JE, Anderson GL, Prentice RL et al. Writing Group for the Women's Health Initiative Investigators. Risks and benefits of estrogen plus progestin in healthy postmenopausal women: principal results from the Women's Health Initiative randomized controlled trial. JAMA 2002; 288:321–333.

39. Anderson GL, Limacher M, Assaf AR et al. Women's Health Initiative Steering Committee. Effects of

conjugated equine estrogen in postmenopausal women with hysterectomy: the Women's Health Initiative randomized controlled trial. JAMA 2004; 291:1701–1712.

40. Effects of hormone therapy on bone mineral density: results from the postmenopausal estrogen/progestin interventions (PEPI) trial. The Writing Group for the PEPI. JAMA 1996; 276:1389–1396.

41. NIH Consensus Development Panel on Osteoporosis Prevention, Diagnosis, and Therapy, March 7–29, 2000: highlights of the conference. South Med J 2001; 94:569–573.

42. Grady D, Rubin SM, Petitti DB et al. Hormone therapy to prevent disease and prolong life in postmenopausal women. Ann Intern Med 1992; 117:1016–1037.

43. Lindsay R. Estrogen deficiency. In: BL Riggs, LJ Melton III (Eds.). Osteoporosis: Etiology, Diagnosis, and Management, 2nd ed. 1995 Philadelphia: Lippincott-Raven Publishers, 133–160.

44. Burkman RT, Collins JA, Greene RA. Current perspectives on benefits and risks of hormone replacement therapy. Am J Obstet Gynecol 2001; 185:S13–S23.

45. Reginster JY, Bruyere O, Audran M et al. Do estrogens effectively prevent osteoporosis-related fractures? The Group for the Respect of Ethics and Excellence in Science. Calcif Tissue Int 2000; 67:191–194.

46. Ensrud KE, Palermo L, Black DM et al. Hip and calcaneal bone loss increase with advancing age: longitudinal results from the study of osteoporotic fractures. J Bone Miner Res 1995; 10:1778–1787.

47. Nelson HD, Rizzo J, Harris E et al. Study of Osteoporotic Fractures Research Group. Osteoporosis and fractures in postmenopausal women using estrogen. Arch Intern Med 2002; 162:2278–2284.

48. Orwoll ES, Nelson HD. Does estrogen adequately protect postmenopausal women against osteoporosis: an iconoclastic perspective. J Clin Endocrinol Metab 1999; 4:1872–1874.

49. Andreyko L, Monroe SE, Marshall LA et al. Concordant suppression of serum immunoreactive LH, FSH, alpha subunit, bioactive LH and testosterone in postmenopausal women by a potent gonadotropin-releasing hormone antagonist (detirelix). J Clin Endocrinol Metab 1992; 74: 399–405.

50. Chetkowski RJ, Meldrum DR, Steingold KA et al. Biological effects of transdermal estradiol. N Engl J Med 1986; 314:1615–1620.

51. Dunn JF, Nisula BC, Rodbard D. Transport of steroid hormones: binding of 21 endogenous steroids to both testosterone-binding globulin and corticosteroid-binding globulin in human plasma. J Clin Endocrinol Metab 1981; 53:58–68.

52. Tazuke S, Shaw KT, Barrett-Connor E. Exogenous estrogen and endogenous sex hormones. Medicine 1992; 71:44–51.

53. Raisz LG, Wiita B, Artis A et al. Comparison of the effects of estrogen alone and estrogen plus androgen on biochemical markers of bone formation and resorption in postmenopausal women. J Clin Endocrinol Metab 1996; 81:37–43.

54. Savvas M, Studd JW, Norman S et al. Increase in bone mass after one year of percutaneous oestradiol and testosterone implants in post-menopausal women who have previously received long-term oral oestrogens. Br J Obstet Gynaecol 1992; 99: 757–760.

55. Davis SR, McCloud P, Strauss BJ, Burger H. Testosterone enhances estradiol's effects on postmenopausal bone density and sexuality. Maturitas 1995; 21:227–236.

56. Garnett T, Studd J, Watson N et al. The effects of plasma estradiol levels on increases in vertebral and femoral bone density following therapy with estradiol and estradiol with testosterone implants. Obstet Gynecol 1992; 79:968–972.

57. Watts NB, Notelovitz M, Timmons MC et al. Comparison of oral estrogens and estrogens plus androgen on bone mineral density, menopausal symptoms, and lipid-lipoprotein profiles in surgical menopause. Obstet Gynecol 1995; 85:529–537.

58. Barrett-Connor E, Young R, Notelovitz M et al. A two-year, double-blind comparison of estrogen-androgen and conjugated estrogens in surgically menopausal women. Effects on bone mineral density, symptoms and lipid profiles. J Reprod Med 1999; 44:1012–1020.

59. Dobs AS, Nguyen T, Pace C, Roberts CP. Differential effects of oral estrogen versus oral estrogen-androgen replacement therapy on body composition in postmenopausal women. J Clin Endocrinol Metab 2002; 87:1509–1516.

60. Labrie F, Diamond P, Cusan L et al. Effect of 12-month dehydroepiandrosterone replacement therapy on bone, vagina, and endometrium in postmenopausal women. J Clin Endocrinol Metab 1997; 82:3498–3505.

61. Gambrell RD Jr, Bagnell CA, Greenblatt RB. Role of estrogens and progesterone in the etiology and prevention of endometrial cancer: review. Am J Obstet Gynecol 1983; 146:696–707.

62. Speroff L, Rowan J, Symons J et al. The comparative effect on bone density, endometrium, and lipids of continuous hormones as replacement therapy (CHART study). A randomized controlled trial. JAMA 1996; 276:1397–1403.

63. Christiansen C, Riis BJ, Nilas L et al. Uncoupling of bone formation and resorption by combined oestrogen and progestagen therapy in postmenopausal osteoporosis. Lancet 1985; 2:800–801.

64. Abdalla HI, Hart DM, Lindsay R et al. Prevention of bone mineral loss in postmenopausal women by norethisterone. Obstet Gynecol 1985; 66:789–792.

65. Erdtsieck RJ, Pols HA, van Kuijk C et al. Course of bone mass during and after hormonal replacement

therapy with and without addition of nandrolone decanoate. J Bone Miner Res 1994; 9:277–283.

66. Berning B, Bennink HJ, Fauser BC. Tibolone and its effects on bone: a review. Climacteric 2001; 4:120–136.

67. Simon JA. Safety of estrogen/androgen regimens. J Reprod Med. 2001; 46:281–290.

68. Sands R & Studd J. Exogenous androgens in post-menopausal women. Am J Med 1995; 98:76S–79S.

69. Gelfand MM, Ferenczy A, Bergeron C. Endometrial response to estrogen-androgen stimulation. Prog Clin Biol Res 1989; 320:29–40.

70. Teran AZ, Greenblatt RB, Chaddha JS. Changes in lipoproteins with various sex steroids. Obstet Gynecol Clin North Am 1987; 14:107–119.

71. Farish E, Fletcher CD, Hart DM et al. The effects of hormone implants on serum lipoproteins and steroid hormones in bilaterally oophorectomised women. Acta Endocrinol (Copenh) 1984; 106:116–120.

72. Sherwin BB, Gelfand MM, Schucher R, Gabor J. Postmenopausal estrogen and androgen replacement and lipoprotein lipid concentrations. Am J Obstet Gynecol 1987; 156:414–419.

Chapter 11

Practical aspects of estrogen–androgen hormone replacement therapy

Camille Sylvestre and Morrie M Gelfand

Summary

The decline in androgens and estrogens in the perimenopausal years produce symptoms that affect the quality of life of several women. One problem in particular is the loss of sexual desire. This chapter reviews this problem, the ways to approach it, the investigations, and the available treatments.

Introduction

With life expectancy extending well into the eighth decade, women are now living longer in the postmenopausal phase of their lives. This is particularly important for those who undergo a surgical menopause before their natural menopause. Bilateral removal of ovaries is still frequent for a variety of reasons, including ovarian tumors (including cancer), estrogen-sensitive breast cancer, endometriosis, and uterine fibroids. Hormonal changes after surgical menopause are more drastic than after natural menopause.

The three major hormones produced by the ovaries are estrogen, progesterone and androgens. The decline in estrogens and androgens typically produces hot flashes and night sweats, sleep disruption, vaginal dryness, and loss of sexual desire. It is our responsibility as health professionals to know how to manage these hormonal deficiencies and their symptoms, and to help women experiencing these problems to maintain a quality of life in the postmenopausal years. Minimal attention is generally paid to the sexual consequences of menopause because physicians and patients are uncomfortable discussing this issue; some physicians have also minimal training in this area, and there are few treatments available to address these effects. This chapter is a brief overview of sexual problems in menopause with an emphasis on low sexual desire, which is the most common dysfunction, of practical points on opening a discussion with the patient on sexual function, and of investigations and options of treatment available.

Sexual dysfunction in menopause

One of the major complaints in menopausal women is the lack of sexual desire. It is now called hypoactive sexual desire disorder (HSDD) and is characterized by a persistent or recurring lack of sexual fantasies, thoughts, and/or desire for or openness to sexual activity, resulting in personal distress.[1] There is strong indirect evidence from the recent trials of the testosterone patch that testosterone replacement is associated with increase in both sexual desire and response (arousability) in surgically menopausal women. With the loss of ovarian function, estrogen deficiency can also cause vaginal atrophy, decreased lubrication, and decreased clitoral blood flow and sensory perception, which often cause dyspareunia and reduced sexual responsivity. Chronic illnesses and medications can play a role in HSDD.

In addition to these physiologic factors, psychologic and relationship factors can contribute to sexual dysfunction. Changes in a woman's self-perception, self-confidence and self-worth following the loss of her reproductive organs can have a dramatic impact on sexual interest and responsiveness, and cause tensions in relationships. Studies show that HSDD may be detrimental to emotional wellbeing and quality of life, because it is associated with anxiety, depression, and marital difficulties.

Discussing sex with patients

Identification of sexual problems should be part of the routine gynecologic history. As mentioned before, this could be challenging for both the patient and the physician. Patients are more likely to report sexual problems and feel comfortable talking about them if their physician initiates and leads the discussion in a relaxed, nonthreatening manner. The suggestions in Table 11.1 may help to create a comfortable atmosphere.

Investigations

Complete assessment of suspected HSDD requires a detailed sexual, medical, psychologic, and psychosocial history. To establish patient's sexual history, ask about childhood/adolescent development, past experience, nature and duration of problems, and current functioning and practices. To distinguish between organic and psychologic factors, it is important to determine if the low sexual desire is lifelong or acquired, and situational or generalized.

Chronic illnesses and medications that can affect sexual desire and function should be identified. Common medical conditions such as cardiovascular disease, hyperlipidemia, diabetes, thyroid disorders and anemia may contribute to sexual problems. Sexual dysfunction in women receiving

Table 11.1 Recommendations for discussing sex with patients

- Request the patient's permission to discuss sexual issues
- Reassure patient about confidentiality
- Consider optimal timing of discussion during office visit (e.g. before patient has disrobed)
- Convey concern about sexual wellness
- Be relaxed, confident, and comfortable
- Be understanding and a sympathetic listener
- Offer encouragement and positive feedback
- Start discussion with 'easy', less sensitive questions to build confidence and trust
- Use sexual and nonsexual terminology familiar to the patient; avoid technical language and medical jargon
- Avoid bias and refrain from being judgmental
- Consider the patient's individual ethnic, cultural, religious, and personal background, and sexual orientation
- Speak to both partners whenever possible

Adapted from Utian.[1]

treatments that suppress adrenal function is usually due to hormonal deficiency. Medications that may influence sexual desire include cardiovascular and antihypertensive medications, hormonal agents and psychoactive medications, for example antipsychotics, benzodiazepines, and selective serotonin reuptake inhibitors. Psychologic disorders such as depression and anxiety need to be investigated. In women being treated with antidepressants, it may be difficult to differentiate sexual adverse effects from mood disorder or the effects of medications.

A complete psychosocial evaluation is critical in the assessment of HSDD. History may focus on recent life changes such as the departure of the children from home, retirement, stress, financial problems; historical events such as abuse or trauma; and intrapersonal conflicts such as religious/moral beliefs and social limitations. Physician should inquire about relationship distress or conflict, differences in needs, functions, and practices between the patient and her partner, and problems with communication or technique. Finally it is important to evaluate the impact of the patient's sexual dysfunction on her psychologic and emotional wellbeing, interpersonal relationships, and occupational performance.

On physical examination, look for signs of abuse, and on pelvic examination, focus on signs of vaginal atrophy or infection, vulvodynia, deep

Table 11.2 Investigations undertaken before estrogen–androgen replacement therapy

- Follicle-stimulating hormone
- Thyroid-stimulating hormone
- Estradiol
- Androgen profile
  — Total testosterone
  — Sex hormone binding globulin
  — Free testosterone
  — Bioavailable testosterone

- Lipid profile
- Complete blood count

tenderness, or complications of surgery. General laboratory testing is recommended including lipid profile, complete blood count, and hormonal profile (see Table 11.2). Analysis of testosterone level is included in the baseline investigation and should be used as a follow-up measure every 6–12 months when the patient is undergoing therapy.

Management of HSDD

Patients with HSDD will benefit from a multidisciplinary approach. This should involve a nurse practitioner, a psychologist/psychiatrist, a dietician, and a gynecologist. The patient needs to be reassured that there is help available for her problem, and that it could be psychologic support and/or hormonal replacement. The physician has to explain to her the need to eliminate all other physiologic or psychologic causes of decreased desire. However, if hormonal deficiency seems to be the only cause, she needs to be told that it is probably the decrease in androgens and estrogens that causes her decrease in libido. She should expect to be evaluated by all the other professionals before treatment is instituted.

In absence of any contraindication, estrogen replacement therapy is recommended in a symptomatic menopausal woman who has undergone hysterectomy and bilateral oophorectomy or hysterectomy and natural menopause. If her uterus is present, progestin should be added to prevent endometrial hyperplasia. Estrogen therapy, in addition to relieve hot flashes and night sweats, can preserve sexual function by improving vaginal health. Alternative therapies may be suggested for women who do not wish to take estrogens,

including dietary supplements, lubricants, and stress management strategies. Vaginal estrogens (such as Vagifem®) that do not increase the serum estradiol levels may be tried. Vagifem® is used in women with breast cancer.

Since the 1950s, several small studies have shown that androgens combined with estrogens might help in the treatment of menopausal symptoms. In the mid eighties, Sherwin and Gelfand[2–7] did extensive research in estrogen–androgen hormone replacement therapy (EA-HRT) and demonstrated that the treatment increased sexual desire and quality of life. In women with uterus in situ, progestins need to be added to the EA-HRT.

In the USA, EA therapy is available in the form of methyltestosterone with estrogen orally (Estratest) (Table 11.3). It decreases the triglyceride levels. Andriol (an oral androgen, testosterone undecanoate) is available in Canada. Another EA combination is injectable testosterone enanthate and estradiol (Climacteron). It is injected every 5–8 weeks depending on the response. Subcutaneous pellets of estradiol combined with testosterone are also available. It is administered subcutaneously in the lower abdomen every 3 months. These various treatments have been proved to increase energy, libido, sexuality, and wellbeing, and decrease breast tenderness. The lipid profile was not changed in the different studies. Testosterone therapy in males has been associated with possible positive effects on Alzheimer disease. This could be an advantage for women as well. The negative side effects of androgen treatment are mild hirsutism, increase in sexuality, and rarely voice changes that are reversible. If the uterus is present, the addition of progestins can cause bleeding episodes and a possible negative effect on lipids.

A testosterone patch has been recently developed. It provides bioidentical testosterone at a sex-appropriate androgen dose level. It is undergoing phase II and III trials and has been shown to improve sexual function, such as sexual desire and activity and decrease in personal distress.[8,9] It is a good choice for patients with low high density lipoprotein (HDL). Pure testosterone has no effect on lipids.[10]

Follow-up

Regardless of the treatment option, good follow-up care will ensure the best possible outcome.

Table 11.3 Testosterone preparations available for women

Component (trade name)	Method of administration	Dose	Frequency
Testosterone undecanoate (Andriol)	Oral	40 mg	Every 2 days
Methyltestosterone (MT) and conjugated estrogens (E) (Estratest)	Oral	2.5 mg MT + 1.25 mg E	Every day
Testosterone enanthate (T) and estradiol benzoate (EB) and estradiol dienanthate (ED) (Climacteron)	Intramuscular	150 mg T + 1 mg EB + 7.5 mg ED	Every 5 to 8 weeks
Testosterone cream 1–2%	Transdermal on the thigh	10 mg	Every day
Testosterone (T) and estradiol (E) implants	Subcutaneous inserted in lower abdomen	50 mg T + 40 mg E	Every 3 months
Testosterone patch (Intrinsa)	Transdermal	300 µg daily	Once a week

Patients should be reviewed after 3 months and the need for professional counseling possibly by a psychologist or sex therapist should be reassessed. Lipid profile should be every 6–12 months as well as side effects and response monitored. It is important to note that there is no available long-term safety and efficacy data on the use of testosterone therapy in female sexual dysfunction, but there is ongoing research to determine the long-term effects of EA-HRT.

Conclusion

The effects of menopause on sexual health and general wellbeing have to be carefully evaluated. The most common sexual dysfunction is HSDD, which is multifactorial in origin. The possible causes of HSDD should be examined and ideally a multidisciplinary team should manage the patient. Depletion of testosterone may be a common contributor to loss of desire and EA-HRT can be offered as a treatment option. Careful follow-up of these patients will ensure a successful outcome.

References

1. Utian W. Problems with desire and arousal in surgically menopausal women: advances in assessment, diagnosis and treatment. Menopause Management 2005; 14:10–22.

2. Gelfand MM. Estrogen-androgen hormone replacement therapy. In: R. Paoletti et al. (Eds.). Women's Health and Menopause 1999:189–194. Massachucetts: Kluwer Academic Publishers and Fondazione Giovanni Lorenzini.

3. Sherwin BB, Gelfand MM. Effects of parenteral administration of estrogen and androgen on plasma hormone levels and hot flashes in the surgical menopause. Am J Obstet Gynecol 1984; 148:552–557.

4. Sherwin BB, Gelfand MM. Differential symptom response to parenteral estrogen and/or androgen administration in the surgical menopause. Am J Obstet Gynecol 1985; 151:153–160.

5. Sherwin BB, Gelfand MM, Brender W. Androgen enhances sexual motivation in females: a crossover study of sex steroid administration in the surgical menopause. Psychosom Med 1985; 47:339–351.

6. Sherwin BB, Gelfand MM. Sex steroids and effect in the surgical menopause: A double blind, crossover study. Psychoneuroendocrinology 1985; 10:325–335.

7. Sherwin BB, Gelfand MM. The role of androgen in the maintenance of sexual functioning in oophorectomized women. Psychosom Med 1987; 49:397–409.

8. Shifren JL, Braunstein GD, Simon JA et al. Transdermal testosterone treatment in women with impaired sexual function after oophorectomy. N Engl J Med 2000; 343:682–688.

9. Simon JA, Nachtigal LE, Davis SR et al. Transdermal testosterone patch improves sexual activity and desire in surgically menopausal women. Obstet Gynecol 2004; 103(Suppl):64S.

10. Notelovitz M. Hot flashes and androgens: a biological rationale for clinical practice. Mayo Clin Proc 2004; 79(Suppl):S8–S13.

Chapter 12

Androgens, DHEA and breast cancer

*Fernand Labrie, Richard Poulin, Jacques Simard,
Van Luu-The, Claude Labrie, and Alain Bélanger*

Summary

Androgens exert underestimated but important physiologic functions in women. The mammary gland possesses all the enzymatic machinery required to transform dehydroepiandrosterone into both androgens and estrogens although it predominantly synthesizes androgens. Testosterone and anabolic steroids have beneficial effects on breast cancer comparable with those of other hormonal therapies; however, masculinizing effects are a limiting factor. In vitro and in vivo preclinical studies show that androgens exert a direct inhibitory effect on normal epithelial as well as breast cancer cell proliferation. In addition to other modulatory influences, proliferation of both the normal mammary gland and breast cancer results from the balance between the stimulatory effect of estrogens and the inhibitory effect of androgens. By taking advantage of the inhibitory effect of androgens on breast cancer proliferation, the efficacy of currently used and well tolerated estrogen-deprivation therapies could potentially be improved.

Introduction

The recent observation that women synthesize at least two-thirds as much androgens as men do suggests that androgens exert important, but so far underestimated, physiologic roles in women.[1,2] In fact, the excretion of androgenic compounds in the urine of adult women was demonstrated more than 50 years ago.[3]

Estrogens and breast cancer

Breast cancer is the most frequent (212 930 new cases predicted in the USA in 2005) and the second cause of cancer deaths (40 870 deaths predicted in the USA in 2005).[4] In fact, because of its frequent diagnosis at an early age, its occurrence in otherwise healthy individuals, and its frequent fatal outcome, breast cancer is probably the most feared disease in women.

Among all risk factors, it is well recognized that estrogens play the predominant role in breast cancer development and growth.[5–7] However, existing surgical or medical ablative procedures do not result in complete elimination of estrogens in women[8] due to the contribution of the adrenal glands that secrete high levels of dehydroepiandrosterone (DHEA) and DHEA sulfate (DHEAS) which are converted into estrogens in peripheral target tissues.[9–11] Considerable attention has thus focused on the development of blockers of estrogen biosynthesis and action[12–19] for the treatment of breast cancer.

In fact, a most important characteristic of the endocrine physiology of the mammary gland is that the normal mammary gland, as well as early breast cancer, absolutely require estrogens for proliferation and growth. Proof of the predominant role of estrogens in early breast cancer is well illustrated by the observation that treatment with the selective estrogen receptor modulator (SERM) raloxifene (Evista) caused a dramatic 76% decrease in breast cancer incidence following 3 years of its administration in osteoporotic postmenopausal women.[20]

In agreement with the important role of estrogens, inhibitors of estrogen formation and action have shown positive results in breast cancer, these benefits being accompanied by an exceptionally good tolerance compared with chemotherapy. In fact, in addition to the well recognized benefits of the antiestrogens tamoxifen and fulvestrant, these data pertain to the inhibitors of estrogen formation (the aromatase inhibitors anastrozole, letrozole, and exemestane),[21–24] as well as medical castration with luteinizing hormone releasing hormone (LHRH) agonists (Zoladex (goserelin), Lupron (leuprolide), Decapeptyl (triptorelin), and buserelin). While being much better tolerated, these compounds used alone or in combination show results that are usually superior to chemotherapy, especially in early disease, the most frequent stage of breast cancer at diagnosis.

Potential role of androgens in breast cancer

The 70–95% reduction in the formation of DHEA and DHEAS by the adrenals during aging[1] results in a dramatic reduction in the formation of androgens and estrogens in peripheral target tissues. Such a decrease in DHEA availability could well be involved in the pathogenesis of age-related diseases including the metabolic syndrome illustrated by insulin resistance and diabetes[25,26] as well as obesity.[27,28] Low circulating levels of DHEAS and DHEA have also been found in patients with breast cancer[29] and DHEA has been found to exert antioncogenic activity in a series of animal models.[30–32] DHEA has also been shown to have immunomodulatory effects in vitro[33] and in vivo in fungal and viral diseases,[34] including infection with human immunodeficiency virus (HIV).[35] On the other hand, a stimulatory effect of DHEA on the immune system has been described in postmenopausal women.[36]

Physiology of sex steroid formation in women: intracrinology

Double source of androgens and estrogens

Humans, along with the other primates, are unique among animal species in having adrenals that secrete large amounts of the inactive precursor steroids DHEA and, especially, DHEAS, which are converted into potent androgens and/or estrogens in peripheral tissues[9,10,37–41] (Figure 12.1). In fact, plasma DHEAS levels in adult women are 10 000 times higher than those of testosterone and 3000–30 000 times higher than those of estradiol (E_2), thus providing a large reservoir of substrates for conversion into androgens and/or estrogens in the peripheral intracrine tissues which possess the enzymatic machinery necessary to transform DHEA into active sex steroids.

The secretion of DHEA and DHEAS by the adrenals increases during adrenarche in children at the age of 6–8 years. Maximal values of circulating DHEAS are reached between the ages of 20 and 30 years. Thereafter, serum DHEA and DHEAS levels decrease markedly (Figure 12.2).[1] In fact, at 70 years of age, serum DHEAS levels are decreased by 80% of their peak values, while they can be decreased by 95% by the age of 85–90 years. On the other hand, much attention has been given to the benefits of DHEA administered to postmenopausal women, especially on the bone, skin, vaginum, and wellbeing after oral[42,43] and percutaneous[44,45] administration.

It is thus remarkable that humans, in addition to possessing sophisticated endocrine and paracrine systems, have largely vested in sex steroid formation in peripheral tissues.[29,46–47] Transformation of the adrenal precursor steroids DHEAS and DHEA into androgens and/or estrogens in peripheral target tissues depends upon the level of expression of the various steroidogenic and metabolizing enzymes in each cell of these tissues.[9] This branch of endocrinology, which focuses on the intracellular formation and action of hormones, has been called intracrinology[9,46] (Figures 12.3 and 12.4). As mentioned above, this situation of a high secretion rate of adrenal precursor sex steroids in men and women is thus completely different from all animal models used in the laboratory, namely rats, mice, guinea pigs, and all others (except monkeys), where the secretion of sex steroids takes place exclusively in the gonads.[48] One explanation for the delayed progress in our understanding of the formation of sex steroids in peripheral target tissues or intracrinology is the fact that the adrenals of the animal models usually used do not secrete significant amounts of DHEA or DHEAS, thus focusing all attention on the testes and ovaries as the exclusive sources of androgens and estrogens. The term intracrinology was thus coined[46] to describe the synthesis of active steroids in peripheral target

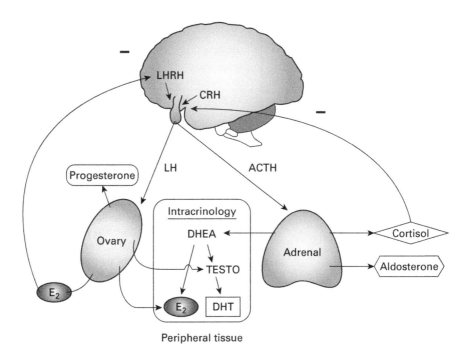

Figure 12.1

Schematic representation of the role of ovarian and adrenal sources of sex steroids in premenopausal women. After menopause, the secretion of estradiol by the ovaries ceases and then 100% of estrogens and close to 100% of androgens are made locally in peripheral target intracrine tissues. LHRH, luteinizing hormone releasing hormone; CRH, corticotropin releasing hormone; LH, luteinizing hormone; ACTH, adrenocorticotropic hormone; DHEA, dehydroepiandrosterone; DHT, dihydrotestosterone.

tissues where the action is exerted in the same cells where synthesis takes place without release in significant amounts of the active steroids in the extracellular space and general circulation.[9]

In women, the role of the adrenal precursors DHEA and DHEAS in the peripheral formation of sex steroids is even more important than in men. In fact, in men, androgen secretion by the testes continues at a high level throughout life while, in women, estrogen secretion by the ovaries completely ceases at menopause, thus leaving the adrenals as the only source of sex steroids. In fact, the best estimate is that the intracrine formation of estrogens in peripheral tissues in women accounts for 75% of all estrogens before menopause, and close to 100% after menopause.[9-11] In addition to E_2, another important but still largely unrecognized estrogen is androst-5-ene-3β, 17β-diol (5-diol). This steroid of adrenal origin has in fact been shown to exert direct estrogenic effects in both normal and malignant estrogen-sensitive tissues at concentrations found in the circulation of normal adult women.[48-50]

Since ovarian estrogen secretion ceases at menopause, the major role of peripheral estrogen formation in postmenopausal women is clearly demonstrated, as mentioned above, by the major benefits of aromatase inhibitors in breast cancer[21-24,51] as well as by the findings of a 76% decrease in breast cancer incidence in postmenopausal osteoporotic women who received the SERM raloxifene for 3 years.[20] These important benefits on breast cancer are entirely due to the blockade of estrogens normally made in peripheral tissues by normal intracrine mechanisms.

It should be added that mammary cells not only synthesize estrogens but also possess complex regulatory mechanisms that allow for the strict control of the intracellular levels of both stimulatory and inhibitory sex steroids. For instance, our data show that the androgen dihydrotestosterone (DHT) favors the degradation of estradiol (E_2) into estrone (E_1), thus suggesting that the potent antiproliferative activity of DHT in E_2-stimulated ZR-75-1 human breast cancer cells is, at least partially,

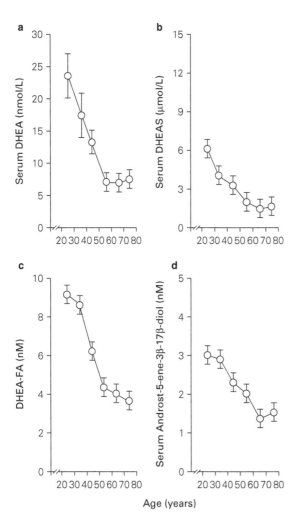

Figure 12.2

Effect of age (20–30 to 70–80 years old) on serum concentration of DHEA (A), DHEAS (B), DHEA-fatty acid esters (DHEA-FA) (C), and androst-5-ene-3β, 17β-diol (5-diol) (D) in women.[1] DHEA(S), dehydroepiandrosterone (sulfate).

exerted on 17β-HSD activity.[52–54] Conversely, we have found that estrogens cause a marked increase in the production of the glucuronidated androgen metabolites androstane-3α, 17β-diol glucuronide (3α-diol-G), androstane-3β, 17β-diol-G (3β-diol-G) and androsterone-G (ADT-G) in MCF-7 cells, thus decreasing the inhibitory androgenic activity.[55] In fact, since glucuronidation is the predominant route of androgen inactivation, androgen-inactivating enzymes constitute an important site of regulation of breast cancer growth.

Androgen steroidogenic and steroid-inactivating enzymes

Steroidogenic enzymes

As mentioned above, transformation of the adrenal precursor steroids DHEA and DHEAS into androgens and/or estrogens in peripheral target tissues depends upon the level of expression of the various steroidogenic and metabolizing enzymes in each cell of these tissues. Knowledge in this area has recently made rapid progress with the elucidation of the structure of most of the tissue-specific genes that encode the steroidogenic enzymes responsible for the transformation of DHEA and DHEAS into androgens and/or estrogens in peripheral intracrine tissues[9,11,39,56–59] (see Figure 12.4).

Because the molecular structure of most of the key non–P-450 dependent enzymes required for sex steroid formation has not been elucidated and knowing that local formation of sex steroids is most likely to play a major role in the control of activity of both normal and tumoral hormone-sensitive tissues, a major portion of our research program and that of other groups has been devoted to this exciting and therapeutically promising area.[12,37,39–41,57–60] Since the main emphasis of this review is on androgens, we will limit the discussion to the type 5 17β-HSD, an androgen-synthesizing enzyme in peripheral tissues.

Type 5 17β-HSD

Type 3 17β-HSD synthesizes testosterone from 4-dione in the Leydig cells of the testes,[61] thus providing approximately 50% of the total amount of androgens in men. However, in the peripheral target tissues of both men and women, as well as in the ovary, the same enzymatic reaction is catalyzed by a different enzyme, namely type 5 17β-HSD.[62] This enzyme is highly homologous with types 1 and 3 3α-HSDs as well as 20α-HSD and thus belongs to the aldo-keto reductase family.

In the postmenopausal ovary, hypertrophied stromal cells are localized mainly at the periphery and hilus.[63] These stromal cells contain both 3β-HSD and type 5 17β-HSD, thus permitting the transformation of DHEA into 4-dione and then into testosterone. In fact, the amount of stromal hyperplasia in postmenopausal ovaries is correlated with the ovarian vein levels of 4-dione and testosterone.[64] These hyperplastic stromal cells

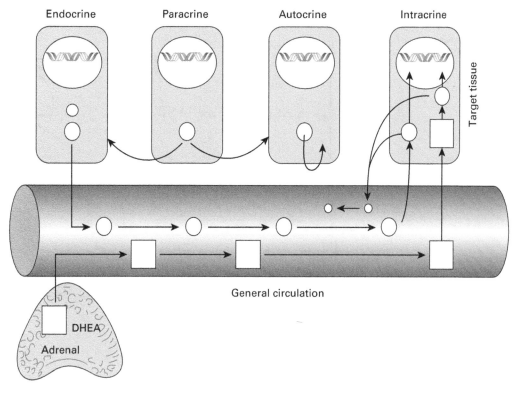

Figure 12.3

Schematic representation of endocrine, paracrine, autocrine, and intracrine secretion. Classically, endocrine activity refers to the specialized glands which synthesize in large quantities hormones that are released into the general circulation and thus transported to distant target cells which possess the specific receptors required to mediate their action. On the other hand, hormones released from one cell can influence neighboring cells (paracrine activity) or can exert a positive or negative action on the cell of origin (autocrine activity). Intracrine activity, on the other hand, refers to the formation of active hormones which exert their action in the same cells where synthesis takes place with no or minimal release into the pericellular compartment and the general circulation.[9] This mechanism explains why serum levels of active sex steroids do not adequately reflect the intracellular concentration and activity of sex steroids.

are thus responsible for the synthesis of 4-dione and testosterone in the postmenopausal ovary.

Type 5 17β-HSD is not only expressed in the ovary but is also present in a large series of peripheral tissues including the mammary gland. The epithelium lining the acini and ducts of the mammary gland is composed of two layers, an inner epithelial layer and an outer discontinuous layer of myoepithelial cells. By immunocytochemistry, 3β-HSD is seen in the epithelial cells of acini and ducts as well as in stromal fibroblasts.[65] Immunostaining is also observed in the walls of blood vessels, including the endothelial cells. On the other hand, the labeling is mainly cytoplasmic. No significant labeling was detected in the myoepithelial cells. On the other hand,

immunostaining for type 5 17β-HSD gave results almost superimposable to those obtained for 3β-HSD, the cytoplasmic labeling being observed in both epithelial and stromal cells as well as in blood vessel walls.[65] Studies performed at the electron microscopic level revealed that in sections stained for 3β-HSD or type 5 17β-HSD, labeling was not associated with any specific membrane-bound organelles in the different reactive cell types.[66]

Steroid-inactivating enzymes

The androgen DHT formed in peripheral tissues is essentially metabolized locally before its appearance in the circulation.[2] The metabolites of DHT include ADT, 3α-diol and 3β-diol, which are formed

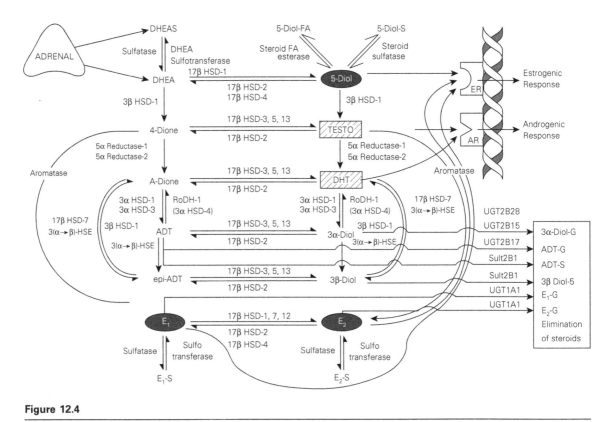

Figure 12.4

Human steroidogenic and steroid-inactivating enzymes in peripheral intracrine tissues. DHEA, dehydroepiandrosterone; 5-diol, androst-5-ene-3β, 17β-diol; DHT, dihydrotestosterone; HSD, 17β-hydroxysteroid dehydrogenase; ADT, androsterone; UGT, UDP-glucuronosyl transferase.

by the action of a series of 3α/β-HSDs and 17β-HSD isoforms (see Figure 12.4).[41,67,68] However, most if not all of the androgen-target tissues express HSD isoforms that are capable of back converting these metabolites into DHT, thus suggesting that a fine regulation of these enzymes is extremely important for controlling the concentration of DHT in andro-gen-target tissues. Another important aspect of the control of intracellular DHT is the inactivation of DHT by the UDP-glucuronosyl transferases (UGTs).

In fact, the serum levels of the glucuronide derivatives of androgens are increased after oral or topical administration of DHEA in the presence of no change or minimal change in the blood levels of nonconjugated androgen metabolites.[2] These observations further support the concept that 5α-reduced androgen glucuronides found in the cir-culation are produced in situ in peripheral tissues after conversion of the adrenal and/or gonadal steroid precursors into DHT first and, subsequently,

into androgen metabolites without release of these intermediate steroid precursors and metabolites into the circulation.[2,9,11] Consequently, the glu-curonidation of androgen metabolites by the UGT enzymes in androgen-sensitive tissues should be considered as the end of the androgenic signal. In the circulation, two major androgen metabolites, namely ADT-G and 3α-diol-G have been identified, but low amounts of testo-G, DHT-G and 3β-diol-G have also been detected.

DHEA is mainly transformed into androgens, thus leading to large amounts of androgens synthesized in women

The rapid fall in circulating estradiol at menopause, coupled with the demonstrated beneficial effects of exogeneous estrogens on menopausal symptoms[69,70] and bone resorption[71-73] have focused most of the efforts of hormone replacement therapy on various forms of estrogens as well as to combinations of estrogen and progestin to avoid the risk of endometrial cancer induced by estrogens administered alone.

In fact, the almost exclusive focus on the role of ovarian estrogens in women's reproductive physiology has removed the attention from the dramatic fall in circulating DHEA which already starts at the ages of 20–30 years to reach 70% at menopause[2] (see Figure 12.2). In fact, since DHEA is transformed to both androgens and/or estrogens in peripheral tissues, such a fall in serum DHEA and DHEAS explains why women at menopause are not only lacking estrogens but have also been deprived from androgens for quite a few years.

Using the serum concentrations of ADT-G and 3α-diol-G as estimates of total androgens, the average sum of the serum concentrations of these conjugated metabolites of DHT are 37.5 nM and 8.47 nM, respectively, in men compared to 32.5 nM and 4.28 nM, respectively, in women.[2] In fact, the average serum concentrations of ADT-G and 3α-diol-G measured in women between the ages 20 and 80 years are thus 86.6% (ADT-G) and 50.5% (3α-diol-G), compared to those found in men of the same age (20–80 years).[2] Although the metabolic clearance rates of the three main androgen metabolites are likely to show differences between men and women, an estimate of the relative amount of total androgens in women and men calculated on the basis of the sum of the serum concentrations of these two metabolites suggests that total androgen production in women is more than two-thirds of that observed in men.[1,2]

Such data are based upon the knowledge that the active androgens are inactivated to glucuronide derivatives before their diffusion from the intracellular compartment into the circulation where they can be measured as ADT-G and 3α-diol-G. Such data showing the presence of relatively high levels of androgens in normal women strongly suggest that the androgens play a major but so far underestimated physiologic role in women. Moreover, since the testicular secretion of androgens, which accounts for 50% of androgens in men, shows little decline with age while women rely almost exclusively on adrenal DHEA for their production of androgens, the 70–95% fall in serum DHEA after menopause leads to a major androgen deficiency in postmenopausal women.

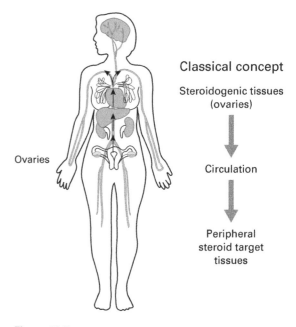

Classical concept

Steroidogenic tissues (ovaries)

↓

Circulation

↓

Peripheral steroid target tissues

Ovaries

Figure 12.5

Schematical representation of the classical concept of sex steroid physiology whereby all steroids were assumed to be made by the endocrine glands.

Serum testosterone is not a reliable parameter of the androgen pool in women

As illustrated schematically in Figure 12.5, the classical concept of androgen and estrogen secretion assumed that all androgens and estrogens were secreted into the circulation by the classical endocrine glands (ovaries) and circulated in the blood stream before reaching the target tissues. According to this classical concept, it was erroneously believed that measurement of the active steroids in the circulation was providing a reliable measure of the general exposure of the organism to sex steroids. In fact, this concept is not valid when applied to humans, especially in postmenopausal women, where all estrogens and almost all androgens are made in peripheral tissues in the same cells where they exert their action without release of significant amounts in the circulation.[9] In fact, the active sex steroids produced locally in peripheral tissues act locally and are inactivated locally before being released

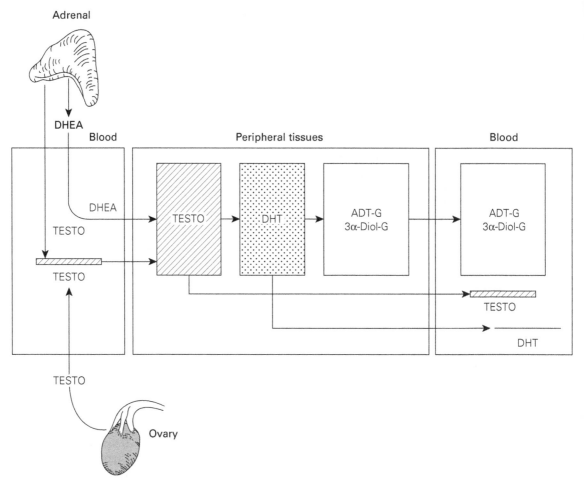

Figure 12.6

Distribution in adult women of the active androgens testosterone and DHT, the sex steroid precursor DHEA, and the main metabolites of androgens (ADT-G and 3α-diol-G) in the circulation and in peripheral intracrine tissues. The height of the bars is proportional to the concentration of each steroid or its derivatives in individual compartments.[75] See Figure 12.4 legend for abbreviations.

as glucuronide derivatives that can be measured in the circulation (Figures 12.6 and 12.7).

As mentioned above, the active androgens and estrogens synthesized in peripheral target tissues exert their action in the cells of origin and very little extracellular diffusion of the active sex steroids occurs, thus resulting in very low levels of active sex steroids in the circulation.[2] In fact, as we have observed in postmenopausal women, the most striking effects of DHEA administration are seen on the circulating levels of the glucuronide derivatives of the metabolites of DHT, namely

ADT-G and 3α-diol-G, these metabolites being produced locally in the peripheral intracrine tissues which possess the appropriate steroidogenic enzymes to synthesize testosterone and DHT from the adrenal precursors DHEA and DHEAS. These peripheral target tissues also contain the steroid-inactivating enzymes required to metabolize androgens into inactive and more water soluble conjugates, namely glucuronide derivatives[9,11] (see Figure 12.7). Such local biosynthesis and action of androgens in target tissues eliminates the exposure of other tissues to androgens

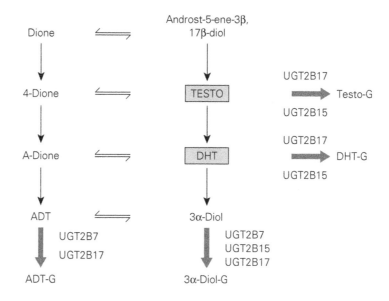

Figure 12.7

Enzymes involved in the peripheral metabolism or inactivation of testosterone and DHT in humans. See Figure 12.4 legend for abbreviations.

and thus minimizes the risks of undesirable masculinizing or other androgen-related side effects. The same applies to estrogens, although we feel that a reliable parameter of total estrogen secretion (comparable to the glucuronides for androgens) has not yet been identified.

The serum concentrations of the conjugated metabolites of DHT, namely ADT-G and 3α-diol-G, are thus the most reliable parameters of the total androgen pool in women while serum testosterone is almost exclusively a measure of direct secretion of testosterone by the ovaries and/or adrenals. In fact, while the vast majority of testosterone and DHT is synthesized in the peripheral tissues in women, only a small proportion – estimated at 10–15% of the intracellular content of these androgens – diffuses out of the intracellular compartment without prior metabolism and can be measured as active androgen in the circulation (see Figure 12.6). This is due to the fact that testosterone and DHT, instead of being released as intact molecules into the circulation, are rapidly metabolized and glucuronidated into ADT-G and 3α-diol-G (see Figure 12.7). Since the individual glucuronosyltransferases responsible for the inactivation of androgens in the human mammary gland have not yet been identified, the human prostate can be used as an example of the types

of glucuronosyltransferases involved.[75,76] The glucuronidated metabolites are much more water soluble than DHT and can thus easily diffuse into the general circulation where they can be measured en route for their elimination mainly by the kidneys (see Figure 12.6). As mentioned above, the serum concentration of the above-indicated conjugated androgen metabolites decreases by 47.5–72.7% between the 20–30 and 70–80 age groups in women, thus suggesting a parallel decrease in the total androgen pool with age.[1]

Proof that changes of the intracellular concentration of sex steroids cannot be estimated by the measurement of serum testosterone and E_2 in the circulation has been obtained in a study performed in postmenopausal women.[2] This study analyzed in detail the serum concentrations of the active androgens and estrogens, as well as a series of free and conjugated forms of their precursors and metabolites, after daily application for 2 weeks of a 10 mL 20% DHEA solution on the skin to avoid first passage of DHEA through the liver.

The data from that study show that elevations in serum DHEA within the physiologic range found in young adult women lead to only small or even no significant changes in serum testosterone, DHT, or E_2, whereas, in contrast, the concentrations of the conjugated metabolites of DHT were markedly elevated, in parallel with the changes in serum DHEA, DHEAS, and 5-diol. Such data obtained in normal postmenopausal women offer unique proof that the serum levels of androgens and estrogens are not valid indicators of total androgenic and estrogenic activities in women. In fact, as mentioned earlier, serum testosterone and E_2 reflect almost exclusively the contribution of the small amount of sex steroids secreted by the ovaries and/or adrenals.

Measurement of the conjugated metabolites of androgens is thus the only valid approach that permits an accurate estimate of the total androgen pool in women. It is likely that a similar situation exists for estrogens, although as mentioned above, a precise evaluation of the pharmacokinetics of estrogen metabolism and identification of the multiple metabolites remains to be achieved.

Androgens inhibit breast cancer

Androgens have been suspected for many decades of being estrogen antagonists and have been used to treat or prevent breast cancer.[77,78]

Clinical data

As mentioned above, estrogens have long been known to play a predominant role in the development and growth of human breast cancer.[5,6] On the other hand, well recognized observations have shown that androgens such as testosterone,[77,79–81] fluoxymesterone,[82–84] calusterone,[85] and anabolic steroids[86,87] used in the adjuvant therapy of breast cancer in women have an efficacy comparable to that achieved with other types of endocrine manipulation. Most importantly, a higher response rate and a longer time to disease progression were observed when androgens were combined with an antiestrogen compared with an antiestrogen alone.[83,84] The benefits of combined treatment with fluoxymesterone and tamoxifen versus tamoxifen alone were observed in postmenopausal women with metastatic breast cancer,[84] both in terms of response rate and time to progression of disease.

Interestingly, the observation that an increased response rate can be obtained by combining

androgens and an antiestrogen therapy in breast cancer[83,84] is in agreement with our observations summarized later in the chapter, which show that the mechanisms of the inhibition exerted by the two types of agent are different, while their effects, at least in part, are additive. It should also be mentioned that androgens have been shown to induce an objective remission after failure of antiestrogen therapy and hypophysectomy. Such clinical observations indicate that the benefits obtained with androgen therapy in breast cancer cannot solely be due to a suppression of pituitary gonadotropin secretion but must result, at least in part, from a direct effect on tumor growth, a mechanism which is supported by a series of experimental data described later.

The above-mentioned clinical data are also well supported by the observation of a synergistic effect of DHEA and of the pure antiestrogen EM-800 on prevention of the development of dimethylbenz(a)anthracene (DMBA)-induced mammary tumors in the rat.[88] Moreover, the almost exclusive androgenic component of the action of DHEA on the histomorphology and structure of the rat mammary gland has recently been shown,[89,90] thus suggesting that the inhibitory effect of DHEA is due to its transformation into androgens. Moreover, the effect of androgens as direct inhibitors of breast cancer growth is well supported by the presence of androgen receptors (AR) in a large proportion of human breast cancers.[90–93] There is also genetic evidence in agreement with a protective role of androgens against breast cancer.[94,95]

The overwhelming clinical evidence for tumor regression observed in 20–50% of premenopausal and postmenopausal breast cancer patients treated with various androgens[86] favors the view that naturally occurring androgens might constitute an as yet overlooked direct inhibitory control of mammary cancer cell growth. It is thus reasonable to suggest, as strongly supported by a series of preclinical data to be summarized later, that the balance between androgenic and estrogenic stimuli controls the proliferation of breast tumors (Figure 12.8).

In this context, it has been found that Western women having a low excretion of adrenal androgenic metabolites respond more poorly to endocrine therapy and have a shorter survival time.[96–98] However, the association in case–control studies between serum androgen levels and breast cancer risk has led to contradictory data.

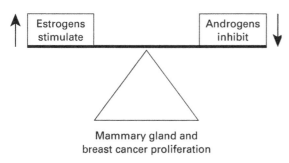

Figure 12.8

Schematic representation of the balance between the stimulatory action of estrogens and the inhibitory effect of androgens on mammary gland and breast cancer proliferation.

Accordingly, subnormal levels of serum androgens have been reported in women with increased risk of breast cancer[29,99–101] while opposite findings have also been reported.[102–105] In fact, most (if not all) of the epidemiologic studies reported have one or more serious limitations which compromise the possibility of reaching valid conclusions. These limitations include lack of reliability of serum steroid levels always measured by radioimmunoassays, comparison of normal control subjects with patients already having breast cancer and, frequently, small number of patients.

In fact, it is now recognized that all steroid measurements performed by radioimmunoassays lack the required precision and will have to be repeated by mass spectrometry. In fact, much more convincing and scientifically rigorous data are provided by the clinical studies mentioned above where androgens or anabolic steroids have shown inhibition of breast cancer in a manner comparable to other endocrine therapies.[77,79–87]

Despite these limitations, epidemiological studies have generally observed a protective effect of DHEA on breast cancer, especially in Western women.[29,99,101,106] In fact, low serum DHEA levels have been associated with breast cancer in women[29] while women with breast cancer were found to have low urinary levels of androsterone and etiocholanolone, two metabolites of DHEA.[107,108] Moreover, women with primary operable breast cancer had urinary levels of 11-deoxy-17-ketosteroids (derived mainly from DHEAS and DHEA) lower than normal, thus suggesting that a low secretion rate of DHEA and DHEAS could precede the development of breast cancer.

Preclinical data

The evidence from preclinical studies demonstrating the inhibitory effect of androgens on breast cancer is extremely strong.

Inhibitory effect of androgens

Lacassagne in 1936 first observed[109] that treatment of mice with testosterone propionate delayed the occurrence of estrone-stimulated mammary tumors. On the other hand, in DMBA-induced tumors, high doses of DHT (0.5–4.0 mg/day) for several weeks caused the regression of 60% of established tumors.[78] Similar effects have been observed with testosterone propionate[110] and dromostanolone propionate.[111,112]

In support of the clinical data mentioned above, our studies have clearly demonstrated that androgens exert a potent and direct inhibitory effect, at physiologic concentrations, on the proliferation of human breast cancer cells.[53,54,113–116] In fact, the first demonstration of a potent and direct inhibitory effect of androgens on human breast cancer growth was obtained in the estrogen-sensitive human breast cancer cell line ZR-75-1.[53] In that study, as shown in Figure 12.9A, DHT not only completely blocked the stimulatory effect of E_2 on cell proliferation but it also reduced cell growth in the absence of estrogens. At low cell density, it can be seen in Figure 12.9B that DHT completely prevented breast cancer cell growth.

DHT has been shown to be formed from testosterone and 4-dione in human breast cancer tissue both in vitro in tissue pieces and in vivo.[117] Such data indicate the presence of 5α-reductase in breast cancer tissue, an enzyme originally thought to be specific for classic androgen-dependent tissues such as the prostate. In ZR-75-1 cells, concentrations of DHT in the incubation medium similar to the plasma levels found in normal women[118–120] and breast cancer patients[121] (0.3–0.7 nM) are potent inhibitors of the mitogenic effect of E_2 and even inhibit growth in the absence of estrogens.[53] Furthermore, testosterone, at concentrations observed in adult women (1–2 nM), is also a potent inhibitor of cell growth. 4-Dione also led to significant growth inhibition in ZR-75-1 cells, although the active concentrations (IC_{50} 15 nM) are in the upper range of the plasma concentrations (1–10 nM) found in women.[118–121]

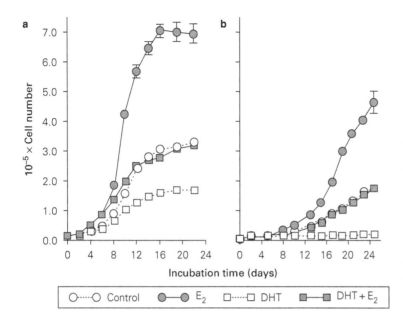

Figure 12.9

Time course of the effect of dihydro-testosterone (DHT) and/or 17β-estradiol (E_2) on the proliferation of ZR-75-1 cells. (A) Cells were plated at 1×10^4 cells/ 2.0 cm² well and 48 h later (zero time), 1 nM E_2 (●), 10 nM DHT (□), or both steroids (■) were added and cell numbers determined at the indicated time intervals. Control cells received the ethanol vehicle only. (B) Same as in (A) except that the initial density was 5.0×10^3 cells/2.0 cm² well.[53]

Following our demonstration of the inhibitory effect of DHT and antiestrogens on ZR-75-1 cell proliferation in vitro,[52,53,113–115,122] we extended our study to the in vivo situation using ovariectomized athymic mice bearing tumors with the same human breast cancer cells to more closely mimic the situation found in women. We thus examined the effect of DHT on tumor growth stimulated by 'physiologic' doses of E_2 administered by silastic implants.

As illustrated in Figure 12.10, E_2 caused a progressive increase in total tumor area from 100% (which corresponds to an average of 0.23 ± 0.08 cm²) at start of the experiment to $226 \pm 31\%$ after 100 days of treatment. The addition of DHT, on the other hand, not only completely reversed the stimulatory effect of E_2 on tumor growth but it decreased total tumor area to $48 \pm 10\%$ of its original size. The androgen DHT is thus a potent inhibitor of the stimulatory effect of E_2 on ZR-75-1 human breast carcinoma growth in vivo in athymic mice. Since ovariectomized animals supplemented by exogenous estrogen were used in these studies, such data provide further support for a direct inhibitory action of androgens at the tumor cell level under in vivo conditions, thus adding to the well known inhibitory effect of androgens exerted on the pituitary–gonadal axis in intact women.[123]

Considering the potential importance of androgens in breast cancer therapy, and to better understand the molecular mechanisms responsible for the antagonism between androgens and estrogens, we studied the effect of androgens on estrogen receptor (ER) expression in the ZR-75-1 human carcinoma cell line. The specific uptake of [³H]E_2 in intact ZR-75-1 cell monolayers was decreased by as much as 88% after 10-day preincubation with increasing concentrations of DHT (Figure 12.11). A half-maximal effect of DHT on [³H]E_2 uptake was observed at 70 pM.[113] The addition of hydroxyflutamide, a nonsteroidal antiandrogen devoid of agonistic activity and having no significant affinity for receptors other than the AR[124,125] competitively reversed inhibition of [³H]E_2-specific uptake by DHT. The inhibition constant (K_i) value for the reversal of DHT action by hydroxyflutamide was estimated at 39 nM, in agreement with the affinity of the antagonist for the AR.[125] Similar results were observed on PR levels, thus showing a direct inhibitory effect of DHT in human breast cancer cells.[114]

This study showed for the first time that androgens strongly suppress ER content in the human breast cancer cell line ZR-75-1, as measured by radioligand binding and anti-ER monoclonal antibodies. Similar inhibitory effects were observed on the levels of ER messenger RNA (mRNA)

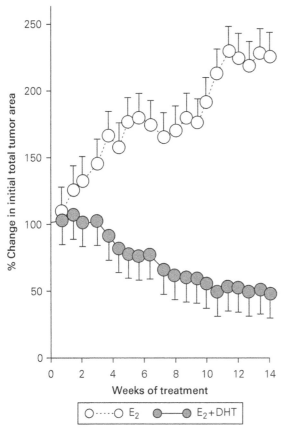

Figure 12.10

Effect of 100-day treatment of ovariectomized (OVX) athymic mice with silastic implants of 17β-estradiol (E_2) (1/3000, E_2/cholesterol, w/w) alone or in combination with silastic implants of dihydrotestosterone (DHT) (1/5, DHT/cholesterol, w/w) on average total ZR-75-1 tumor area in nude mice. Results are expressed as percentage of pretreatment values (means±SEM of 11 tumors in the E_2 group and nine tumors in the E_2+DHT group).[13]

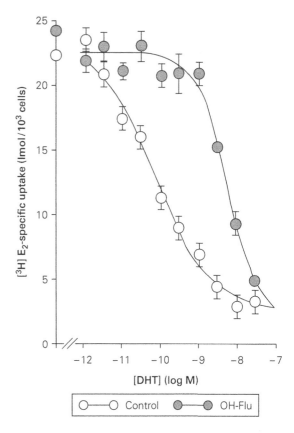

Figure 12.11

Effect of preincubation with increasing concentrations of dihydroxytestosterone (DHT) on [^{3}H]E_2-specific binding in ZR-75-1 human breast cancer cells in a hydroxylapatite exchange assay of [^{3}H]E_2-specific binding of cytosol and nuclear (cytosol+nuclear=total) extracts obtained from ZR-75-1 cells preincubated for 11 days with the indicated concentrations of DHT. E_2-specific uptake of [^{3}H]E_2 in intact ZR-75-1 cells preincubated for 10 days with the indicated concentrations of DHT alone (o, control) or in the presence of 3 μM antiandrogen hydroxyflutamide (●, OH-FLU). Values are given as means ±SE from triplicate determinations.[114]

measured by ribonuclease protection assay.[113] The androgenic effect was observed at sub-nanomolar concentrations of the nonaromatizable androgen DHT, regardless of the presence of estrogens, and was competitively reversed by the antiandrogen hydroxyflutamide. Such data on ER expression provide an explanation for at least part of the antiestrogenic effects of androgens on breast cancer cell growth and provide an explanation for the observations showing that the specific inhibitory effects of androgen therapy are additive to the standard treatment limited to blockade of estrogens by antiestrogens.[122] Another possible clue to the mechanism of action of DHT in breast cancer cells is provided by the observation that androgens and estrogens exert opposite effects on PR levels.[126]

The effect of androgens on ZR-75-1 cell proliferation, however, cannot be solely explained by the suppression of ER expression. This is because androgens still exert potent inhibitory effects on

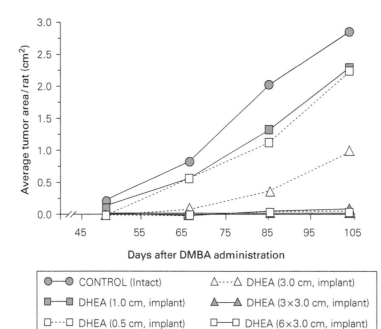

Figure 12.12

Effect of increasing doses of dehydroepiandrosterone (DHEA) constantly released from silastic implants and administered 7 days before the intragastric administration of 20 mg of DMBA in intact 50–52-day-old female rats on average tumor area (cm²) per rat at the indicated time intervals.[32]

growth in the absence of estrogens, even after prolonged periods of estrogen deprivation before exposure to androgens.[55,114] Moreover, the antiproliferative activity of androgens in estrogen-deprived ZR-75-1 cells is more pronounced and is additive to that exerted by antiestrogens.[53,127]

Downregulation of ER expression by androgens is likely to be of crucial importance in their physiologic mode of action, i.e. when estrogens are simultaneously present in normal as well as cancerous mammary gland tissue. In the specific case of human breast cancer, endogenous androgens may reduce the tumor cell sensitivity to estrogens by decreasing ER levels. Thus, in normal breast tissue, endogenous as well as locally produced androgens are likely to contribute to the regulation of the level of ER, thus modulating the sensitivity to estrogens (see Figure 12.8).

In agreement with the in vitro data, Dauvois et al.[129] have shown that constant release of the androgen DHT in ovariectomized rats bearing DMBA-induced mammary carcinoma caused a marked inhibition of tumor growth induced by E_2. That DHT acts through interaction with the androgen receptor in DMBA-induced mammary carcinoma is well supported by the finding that simultaneous treatment with the antiandrogen

flutamide completely prevented DHT action. Such data demonstrated, for the first time, that androgens are potent inhibitors of DMBA-induced mammary carcinoma growth by an action independent from inhibition of gonadotropin secretion. The data suggested an action exerted directly at the tumor level, thus further supporting in vitro data obtained with the human ZR-75-1 breast cancer cell line.[53,113]

Inhibitory effect of DHEA on breast cancer

Prevention of mammary tumor development by DHEA

As described above, the human adrenals secrete large amounts of the precursor steroids DHEA and DHEAS, which are converted into androgens in target intracrine tissues.[9,10,37,38,46,129,130] To investigate the possibility that DHEA and its metabolites could have a preventive effect on the development of mammary carcinoma, we studied the effect of increasing circulating levels of DHEA constantly released from silastic implants on the development of mammary carcinoma induced by DMBA in the rat. The DMBA-induced mammary carcinoma in the rat has been widely used as a model of hormone-sensitive breast cancer in women.[7,128,131]

Treatment with increasing doses of DHEA delivered constantly by silastic implants of increasing length and number caused a progressive inhibition of tumor development[32] (Figure 12.12). It is of interest to see that tumor size in the group of animals treated with the highest dose (6×3.0 cm long implants) of DHEA was similar to that found in ovariectomized animals, thus showing a complete blockade of estrogen action by DHEA. Such data clearly demonstrate that circulating levels of the precursor adrenal steroid DHEA, comparable to those observed in normal adult premenopausal women, exert a potent inhibitory effect on the development of mammary carcinoma induced by DMBA in the rat.

Inhibitory effects of DHEA on the growth of human breast cancer xenografts

As mentioned above, androgens have been clearly demonstrated to inhibit the growth of human breast cancer in women with breast cancer[77,79–87] as well as in laboratory studies in vitro[12,13,52,53,113–116,128,132,133] while DHEA is predominantly transformed into androgens in the mammary gland.[89] Hence we studied the possibility that DHEA could inhibit the growth of the human ZR-75-1 breast cancer cells in vivo in nude mice. To avoid the inhibitory effects of DHEA-derived steroids on gonadotropin secretion, we used ovariectomized animals supplemented with E_1.

As illustrated in Figure 12.13, the size of the ZR-75-1 tumors increased by 9.4-fold over a 291-day period (9.5 months) in ovariectomized nude mice supplemented with E_1; in contrast, in control ovariectomized mice that received the vehicle alone, tumor size decreased to 36.9% of the initial value during the course of the study.[134] Treatment with increasing doses of percutaneous DHEA caused a progressive inhibition of estrogen-stimulated ZR-75-1 tumor growth. In fact, inhibitions of 50.4%, 76.8%, and 80.0% were achieved at 9.5 months of treatment with the daily doses of DHEA of 0.3 mg, 1.0 mg, and 3.0 mg per animal, respectively (see Figure 12.13). In agreement with the decrease in total tumor load, treatment with DHEA led to a marked decrease in the average weight of the tumors remaining at the end of the experiment. To our knowledge, these data provided the first demonstration of the inhibitory effect of DHEA on the growth of human breast cancer xenografts in nude mice.

Most likely, the inhibition of tumor growth seen after DHEA treatment in ovariectomized animals results from its intracrine in situ conversion into androgens in the mammary gland.[9,10,37,38,46] In agreement with these data, we have shown that DHEA exerts an almost exclusively androgenic effect in the rat mammary gland.[89] Taken together, these data strongly suggest that DHEA exerts its inhibition of breast cancer development and growth through its conversion to androgens and activation of the androgen receptor.

A group of researchers have reported that DHEA is inhibitory on breast cancer growth in the presence of estrogens while it can be stimulatory on experimental models where estrogens are absent.[105,135] It should be mentioned, however, that an absence of estrogens does not exist in women where comparable levels of E_2 are found in breast cancer tissue in premenopausal and postmenopausal women.[137] In fact, such an hypothetical situation of an absence of estrogens does not exist in normal women, even after menopause.

While DHT exerts a potent inhibitory effect on the proliferation of ZR-75-1 human breast cancer cells,[52,53] DHT has not always been found to inhibit the growth of MCF-7 cells. The lack of inhibitory action of DHT in some MCF-7 cell lines is most likely due to the presence of a high level of 3α-HSD activity in these cells, thus preventing DHT from exerting its inhibitory effect before its transformation into 3β-diol, a compound having intrinsic estrogenic activity (Labrie et al. unpublished data; reference 137). That the inhibitory effect of DHEA on breast cancer MCF-7 cell growth is due to interaction with AR is supported by the finding that the antiandrogen flutamide reversed the inhibitory effect of DHEA on MCF-7 human breast cancer cell proliferation while the antiestrogen tamoxifen had no effect.[138]

Additive inhibitory effects of DHEA and the antiestrogen EM-800 (acolbifene) on the growth of DMBA-induced mammary tumors

Antiestrogens[13,15,139–141] as well as DHEA[32] can independently inhibit the development of DMBA-induced mammary carcinoma. Hence we studied

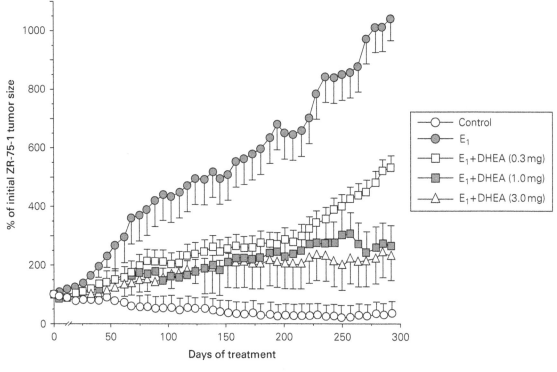

Figure 12.13

Effect of increasing doses of dehydroepiandrosterone (DHEA) (a total dose of 0.3 mg, 1.0 mg or 3.0 mg) administered percutaneously in two doses daily on average ZR-75-1 tumor size in ovariectomized nude mice supplemented with 0.5 μg estrone (E_1) daily. Ovariectomized mice receiving the vehicle alone were used as additional controls. The initial tumor size was taken as 100%. DHEA (0.3 mg, 1.0 mg, or 3.0 mg per animal per day) was administered percutaneously on the dorsal skin in a 0.02 mL solution of 50% ethanol–50% propylene glycol.[135]

the potential benefits of combining the new antiestrogen EM-800 (prodrug of EM-652 or acolbifene) with DHEA on the development of mammary carcinoma induced by DMBA in the rat. As illustrated in Figure 12.14, 95% of control animals developed palpable mammary tumors by 279 days after DMBA administration. Treatment with DHEA or EM-800 alone partially prevented the development of DMBA-induced mammary carcinoma, the incidence being thus reduced to 57% ($P < 0.01$) and 38% ($P < 0.01$), respectively. Interestingly, a combination of the two compounds led to a significantly greater inhibitory effect than that achieved by each compound administered alone ($P < 0.01$ versus DHEA or EM-800 alone). In fact, the only two tumors that developed in the group of animals treated with both compounds disappeared before the end of the experiment.

Such data obtained in vivo support our previous findings that the inhibitory effects of androgens and antiestrogens on mammary carcinoma are exerted at least in part by different mechanisms and that the combination of an androgenic compound with a pure antiestrogen could well have improved efficacy compared to each compound used alone in the prevention and treatment of breast cancer in women. In agreement with Figure 12.8, such an antagonism between androgens and estrogens on breast cancer proliferation is illustrated schematically in Figure 12.15. It can be seen in Figure 12.15 that DHEA, secondary to its predominant transformation into androgens in the mammary gland tissue,[89] exerts inhibitory effects on mammary carcinoma development and growth. This action counteracts and can even completely neutralize the stimulatory effect of

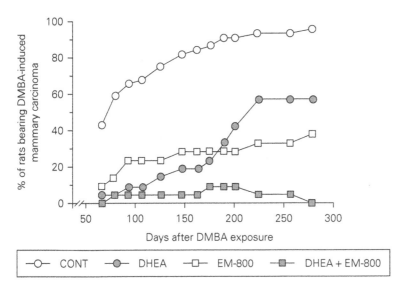

Figure 12.14

Effect of treatment with dehydroepiandrosterone (DHEA) (10 mg, percutaneously, once daily) or EM-800 (75 µg, orally, once daily) alone or in combination for 9 months on the incidence of dimethybenz(a)anthracene (DMBA)-induced mammary carcinoma in the rat throughout the 279-day observation period. Data are expressed as percentage of the total number of animals in each group.[143]

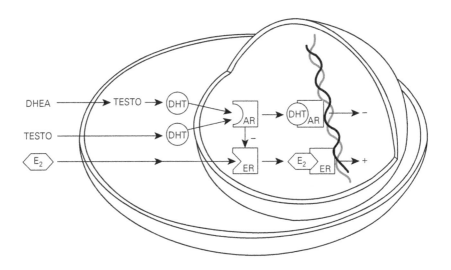

Figure 12.15

Antagonism between the inhibitory effects of androgens or dehydroepiandrosterone (DHEA) and the stimulatory effects of estrogens on breast cancer proliferation. E_2, 17β-estradiol; DHT, dihydrotestosterone; AR, androgen receptor; ER, estrogen receptor.

estrogens (see Figure 12.8). It might be relevant to mention that treatment with DHEA markedly delayed the appearance of breast tumors in C3H mice which were genetically bred to develop breast cancer.[143]

It should be added that treatment of ovariectomized monkeys with testosterone decreased by about 40% the stimulation of mammary epithelial proliferation induced by estradiol.[144] Moreover, it is possible that part of the increased risk of breast cancer in *BRCA-1* mutant patients is associated with the decreased efficiency of the mutated *BRCA-1* gene to interact with the androgen receptor.[145] It is also pertinent to mention that female athletes and transsexuals taking androgens show atrophy of mammary gland epithelial tissue.[146,147]

The data summarized above demonstrate the direct inhibitory effects of androgens and DHEA on breast cancer proliferation. However, it is likely that endogenous androgens and DHEA play an important physiologic and functional role. In addition, it is likely that this antagonism between androgens and estrogens is operative in both the normal mammary gland and breast cancer (see Figures 12.8 and 12.15).

References

1. Labrie F, Bélanger A, Cusan L et al. Marked decline in serum concentrations of adrenal C19 sex steroid precursors and conjugated androgen metabolites during aging. J Clin Endocrinol Metab 1997; 82: 2396–2402.

2. Labrie F, Bélanger A, Cusan L, Candas B. Physiological changes in dehydroepiandrosterone are not reflected by serum levels of active androgens and estrogens but of their metabolites: intracrinology. J Clin Endocrinol Metab 1997; 82:2403–2409.

3. Geist SH. Androgen therapy in the human female. J Clin Endocrinol 1941; 1:154–161.

4. Jemal A, Murray T, Ward E et al. Cancer statistics, 2005. CA Cancer J Clin 2005; 55:10–30.

5. McGuire WL, Carbone PP, Sears ME, Escher GC. Estrogen receptors in human breast cancer: an overview. In: WL McGuire, PP Carbone & EP Vollmer, (Eds.). Estrogen Receptors in Human Breast Cancer. 1975:1–7. New York: Raven Press.

6. Davidson NE, Lippman ME. The role of estrogens in growth regulation of breast cancer. Crit Rev Oncol 1989; 1:89–111.

7. Asselin J, Labrie F. Effects of estradiol and prolactin on steroid receptor levels in 7,12-dimethylbenz(a)anthracene-induced mammary tumors and uterus in the rat. J Steroid Biochem 1978; 9: 1079–1082.

8. Miller WR. Fundamental research leading to improved endocrine therapy for breast cancer. J Steroid Biochem 1987; 27:477–485.

9. Labrie F. Intracrinology. Mol Cell Endocrinol 1991; 78:C113–C118.

10. Labrie F, Bélanger A, Simard J et al. DHEA and peripheral androgen and estrogen formation: Intracrinology. Ann NY Acad Sci 1995; 774:16–28.

11. Labrie F, Luu-The V, Labrie C et al. Endocrine and intracrine sources of androgens in women: inhibition of breast cancer and other roles of androgens and their precursor dehydroepiandrosterone. Endocr Rev 2003; 24:152–182.

12. de Launoit Y, Dauvois S, Dufour M et al. Inhibition of cell cycle kinetics and proliferation by the androgen 5α-dihydrotestosterone and antiestrogen N, n-butyl-N-methyl-11-(16'α-chloro-3',17β-dihydroxy-estra-1',3',5'-(10')triene-7'α-yl)undecanamide in human breast cancer ZR-75-1 cells. Cancer Res 1991; 51: 2797–2802.

13. Dauvois S, Geng CS, Lévesque C et al. Additive inhibitory effects of an androgen and the antiestrogen EM-170 on estradiol-stimulated growth of human ZR-75-1 breast tumors in athymic mice. Cancer Res 1991; 51:3131–3135.

14. Lévesque C, Mérand Y, Dufour JM et al. Synthesis and biological activity of new halo-steroidal antiestrogens. J Med Chem 1991; 34:1624–1630.

15. Labrie F, Li S, Labrie C et al. Inhibitory effect of a steroidal antiestrogen (EM-170) on estrone-stimulated growth of 7,12 dimethylbenz(a)anthracene (DMBA)-induced mammary carcinoma in the rat. Breast Cancer Res Treat 1995; 33:237–244.

16. Wakeling AE, Bowler J. Biology and mode of action of pure antiestrogens. J Steroid Biochem 1988; 30: 141–147.

17. Labrie C, Martel C, Dufour JM et al. Novel compounds inhibit estrogen formation and action. Cancer Res 1992; 52:610–615.

18. Gronemeyer H, Benhamou B, Berry M et al. Mechanisms of antihormone action. J Steroid Biochem Mol Biol 1992; 41:217–221.

19. Gauthier S, Caron B, Cloutier J et al. (S)-(+)-4-[7-(2,2-dimethyl-1-oxopropoxy)-4-methyl-2-[4-[2-(1-piperidinyl)-ethoxy]phenyl]-2H-1-benzopyran-3-yl]-phenyl 2,2-dimethylpropanoate (EM-800): a highly potent, specific, and orally active nonsteroidal antiestrogen. J Med Chem 1997; 40: 2117–2122.

20. Cummings SR, Eckert S, Krueger KA et al. The effect of raloxifene on risk of breast cancer in postmenopausal women: results from the MORE randomized trial. Multiple Outcomes of Raloxifene Evaluation. JAMA 1999; 281:2189–2197.

21. Bonneterre J, Thurlimann B, Robertson JF et al. Anastrozole versus tamoxifen as first-line therapy for advanced breast cancer in 668 postmenopausal women: results of the Tamoxifen or Arimidex Randomized Group Efficacy and Tolerability study. J Clin Oncol 2000; 18:3748–3757.

22. Mouridsen H, Gershanovich M, Sun Y et al. Superior efficacy of letrozole versus tamoxifen as first-line therapy for postmenopausal women with advanced breast cancer: results of a phase III study of the international letrozole breast cancer group. J Clin Oncol 2001; 19:2596–2606.

23. Goss P. Anti-aromatase agents in the treatment and prevention of breast cancer. Cancer Control 2002; 9(2 Suppl):2–8.

24. Goss PE, Ingle JN, Martino S et al. A randomized trial of letrozole in postmenopausal women after

five years of tamoxifen therapy for early-stage breast cancer. N Engl J Med 2003; 19:1793–1802

25. Schriock ED, Buffington CK, Hubert GD et al. Divergent correlations of circulating dehydroepiandrosterone sulfate and testosterone with insulin levels and insulin receptor binding. J Clin Endocrinol Metab 1988; 66:1329–1331.

26. Coleman DL, Schwizer RW, Leiter EH. Effect of genetic background on the therapeutic effects of dehydroepiandrosterone (DHEA) in diabetes-obesity mutants and in aged normal mice. Diabetes 1984; 33:26–32.

27. MacEwen EG, Kurzman ID. Obesity in the dog: role of the adrenal steroid dehydroepiandrosterone (DHEA). J Nutr 1991; 121:S51–S55.

28. Tchernof A, Després JP, Bélanger A et al. Reduced testosterone and adrenal C19 steroid levels in obese men. Metabolism 1995; 44:513–519.

29. Zumoff B, Levin J, Rosenfeld RS et al. Abnormal 24-hr mean plasma concentrations of dehydroepiandrosterone and dehydroisoandrosterone sulfate in women with primary operable breast cancer. Cancer Res 1981; 41:3360–3363.

30. Schwartz AG, Pashko L, Whitcomb JM. Inhibition of tumor development by dehydroepiandrosterone and related steroids. Toxicol Pathol 1986; 14:357–362.

31. Gordon GB, Shantz LM, Talalay P. Modulation of growth, differentiation and carcinogenesis by dehydroepiandrosterone. Adv Enzyme Regul 1987; 26:355–382.

32. Li S, Yan X, Bélanger A, Labrie F. Prevention by dehydroepiandrosterone of the development of mammary carcinoma induced by 7,12-dimethylbenz(a)anthracene (DMBA) in the rat. Breast Cancer Res Treat 1993; 29:203–217.

33. Suzuki T, Suzuki N, Daynes RA, Engleman EG. Dehydroepiandrosterone enhances IL2 production and cytotoxic effector function of human T cells. Clin Immunol Immunopathol 1991; 61:202–211.

34. Rasmussen KR, Arrowood MJ, Healey MC. Effectiveness of dehydroepiandrosterone in reduction of cryptosporidial activity in immunosuppressed rats. Antimicrob Agents Chemother 1992; 36:220–222.

35. Henderson E, Yang JY, Schwartz A. Dehydroepiandrosterone (DHEA) and synthetic DHEA analogs are modest inhibitors of HIV-1 IIIB replication. Aids Res Hum Retroviruses 1992; 8:625–631.

36. Casson PR, Andersen RN, Herrod HG et al. Oral dehydroepiandrosterone in physiologic doses modulates immune function in postmenopausal women. Am J Obstet Gynecol 1993; 169:1536–1539.

37. Labrie F, Luu-The V, Lin SX et al. The key role of 17β-HSDs in sex steroid biology. Steroids 1997; 62:148–158.

38. Labrie F, Simard J, Luu-The V et al. The 3β-hydroxysteroid dehydrogenase/isomerase gene family:

lessons from type II 3β-HSD congenital deficiency. In: V Hansson, FO Levy, K Taskén (Eds.). Signal Transduction in Testicular Cells. Ernst Schering Research Foundation Workshop. 1996:185–218. Berlin: Springer-Verlag.

39. Labrie F, Luu-The V, Lin S-X et al. Intracrinology: role of the family of 17β-hydroxysteroid dehydrogenases in human physiology and disease. J Mol Endocrinol 2000; 25:1–16.

40. Labrie F, Luu-The V, Labrie C, Simard J. DHEA and its transformation into androgens and estrogens in peripheral target tissues: intracrinology. Front Neuroendocrinol 2001; 22:185–212.

41. Luu-The V. Analysis and characteristics of multiple types of human 17beta-hydroxysteroid dehydrogenase. J Steroid Biochem Mol Biol 2001; 76: 143–151.

42. Baulieu EE, Thomas G, Legrain S et al. Dehydroepiandrosterone (DHEA), DHEA sulfate, and aging: contribution of the DHE Age Study to a sociobiomedical issue. Proc Natl Acad Sci USA 2000; 97: 4279–4284.

43. Morales AJ, Nolan JJ, Nelson JC, Yen SS. Effects of replacement dose of dehydroepiandrosterone in men and women of advancing age. J Clin Endocrinol Metab 1994; 78:1360–1367.

44. Diamond P, Cusan L, Gomez JL et al. Metabolic effects of 12-month percutaneous DHEA replacement therapy in postmenopausal women. J Endocrinol 1996; 150:S43–S50.

45. Labrie F, Diamond P, Cusan L et al. Effect of 12-month DHEA replacement therapy on bone, vagina, and endometrium in postmenopausal women. J Clin Endocrinol Metab 1997; 82:3498–3505.

46. Labrie C, Bélanger A, Labrie F. Androgenic activity of dehydroepiandrosterone and androstenedione in the rat ventral prostate. Endocrinology 1988; 123: 1412–1417.

47. Bélanger B, Bélanger A, Labrie F et al. Comparison of residual C-19 steroids in plasma and prostatic tissue of human, rat and guinea pig after castration: unique importance of extratesticular androgens in men. J Steroid Biochem 1989; 32:695–698.

48. Adams JB. Control of secretion and the function of C19-Δ5 steroids of the human adrenal gland. Mol Cell Endocrinol 1985; 41:1–17.

49. Poulin R, Labrie F. Stimulation of cell proliferation and estrogenic response by adrenal C19-Δ5-steroids in the ZR-75-1 human breast cancer cell line. Cancer Res 1986; 46:4933–4937.

50. Simard J, Vincent A, Duchesne R, Labrie F. Full oestrogenic activity of C19-Δ5-adrenal steroids in rat pituitary lactotrophs and somatotrophs. Mol Cell Endocrinol 1988; 55:233–242.

51. Mouridsen H, Gershanovich M, Sun Y et al. Phase III study of letrozole versus tamoxifen as first-line therapy of advanced breast cancer in postmenopausal women: analysis of survival and update of

efficacy from the International Letrozole Breast Cancer Group. J Clin Oncol 2003; 21:2101–2109.

52. Poulin R, Simard J, Labrie C et al. Down-regulation of estrogen receptors by androgens in the ZR-75-1 human breast cancer cell line. Endocrinology 1989; 125:392–399.

53. Poulin R, Baker D, Labrie F. Androgens inhibit basal and estrogen-induced cell proliferation in the ZR 75-1 human breast cancer cell line. Breast Cancer Res Treat 1988; 12:213–225.

54. Couture P, Thériault C, Simard J, Labrie F. Androgen receptor-mediated stimulation of 17β-hydroxysteroid dehydrogenase activity by dihydrotestosterone and medroxyprogesterone acetate in ZR-75-1 human breast cancer cells. Endocrinology 1993; 132:179–185.

55. Roy R, Dauvois S, Labrie F, Bélanger A. Estrogen-stimulated glucuronidation of dihydrotestosterone in MCF-7 human breast cancer cells. J Steroid Biochem Mol Biol 1992; 41:579–582.

56. Labrie F, Sugimoto Y, Luu-The V et al. Structure of human type II 5α-reductase. Endocrinology 1992; 131:1571–1573.

57. Labrie F, Simard J, Luu-The V et al. Structure, function and tissue-specific gene expression of 3β-hydroxysteroid dehydrogenase/5-ene-4-ene isomerase enzymes in classical and peripheral intracrine steroidogenic tissues. J Steroid Biochem Mol Biol 1992; 43:805–826.

58. Luu-The V, Zhang Y, Poirier D, Labrie F. Characteristics of human types 1, 2 and 3 17β-hydroxysteroid dehydrogenase activities: oxidation-reduction and inhibition. J Steroid Biochem Mol Biol 1995; 55: 581–587.

59. Labrie Y, Durocher F, Lachance Y et al. The human type II 17β-hydroxysteroid dehydrogenase gene encodes two alternatively-spliced messenger RNA species. DNA Cell Biol 1995; 14:849–861.

60. Labrie F, Sugimoto Y, Luu-The V et al. Structure of human type II 5 alpha-reductase gene. Endocrinology 1992; 131:1571–1573.

61. Geissler WM, Davis DL, Wu L et al. Male pseudohermaphroditism caused by mutations of testicular 17β-hydroxysteroid dehydrogenase 3. Nat Genet 1994; 7:34–39.

62. Dufort I, Rheault P, Huang XF et al. Characteristics of a highly labile human type 5 17beta-hydroxysteroid dehydrogenase. Endocrinology 1999; 140:568–574.

63. Russell P, Bannatyne P. Surgical pathology of the ovaries. 1989. Churchill Livingstone, New York: Edinburgh.

64. Sluijmer AV, Heineman MJ, Koudstaal J et al. Relationship between ovarian production of estrone, estradiol, testosterone, and androstenedione and the ovarian degree of stromal hyperplasia in postmenopausal women. Menopause 1998; 5:207–210.

65. Pelletier G, Luu-The V, Tetu B, Labrie F. Immunocytochemical localization of type 5 17β-hydroxysteroid dehydrogenase in human reproductive tissues. J Histochem Cytochem 1999; 47:731–737.

66. Pelletier G, Luu-The V, El-Alfy M et al. Immunoelectron microscopic localization of 3β-hydroxysteroid dehydrogenase and type 5 17β-hydroxysteroid dehydrogenase in the human prostate and mammary gland. J Mol Endocrinol 2001; 26:11–19.

67. Dufort I, Labrie F, Luu-The V. Human types 1 and 3 3 alpha-hydroxysteroid dehydrogenases: differential lability and tissue distribution. J Clin Endocrinol Metab 2001; 86:841–846.

68. Labrie F, Luu-The V, Lin S-X et al. Role of 17β-hydroxysteroid dehydrogenases in sex steroid formation in peripheral intracrine tissues. Trends Endocrinol Metab 2000; 11:421–427.

69. Lomax P & Schonbaum E. Postmenopausal hot flushes and their management. Pharmacol Ther 1993; 57:347–358.

70. Archer DF, Furst K, Tipping D et al. A randomized comparison of continuous combined transdermal delivery of estradiol-norethindrone acetate and estradiol alone for menopause. CombiPatch Study Group. Obstet Gynecol 1999; 94:498–503.

71. Weiss NS, Ure CL, Ballard JH et al. Decreased risk of fractures of the hip and lower forearm with postmenopausal use of estrogen. N Engl J Med 1980; 303:1195–1198.

72. Christiansen C, Christensen MS, Larsen NE, Transbol IB. Pathophysiological mechanisms of estrogen effect on bone metabolism. Dose-response relationships in early postmenopausal women. J Clin Endocrinol Metab 1982; 55:1124–1130.

73. Women's Health Initiative. Risks and benefits of estrogen plus progestin in healthy postmenopausal women. JAMA 2002; 288:321–333.

74. Munnuz-Torres M, Jodar E, Quesada M, Escobar-Jimenez F. Bone mass in androgen-insensitivity syndrome: response to hormonal replacement therapy. Calcif Tissue Int 1995; 57:94–96.

75. Barbier O, Girard C, Lapointe H et al. Cellular localization of uridine diphosphoglucuronosyltransferase 2B enzymes in the human prostate by in situ hybridization and immunohistochemistry. J Clin Endocrinol Metab 2000; 85:4819–4826.

76. Turgeon D, Carrier JS, Levesque E et al. Relative enzymatic activity, protein stability, and tissue distribution of human steroid-metabolizing UGT2B subfamily members. Endocrinology 2001; 142:778–787.

77. Ulrich P. Testosterone (hormone mâle) et son role possible dans le traitement de certains cancers du sein. Acta Unio Internationalis Contra Cancrum 1939:377–379.

78. Huggins C, Briziarelli G, Sutton HJ. Rapid induction of mammary carcinoma in the rat and the influence of hormone on the tumors. J Exp Med 1959; 109:25–42.

79. Fels E. Treatment of breast cancer with testosterone propionate. A preliminary report. J Clin Endocrinol 1944; 4:121–125.

80. Segaloff A, Gordon D, Horwitt BN et al. Hormonal therapy in cancer of the breast. 1. The effect of testosterone propionate therapy on clinical course and hormonal excretion. Cancer 1951; 4:319–323.

81. Cooperative Breast Cancer Group. Testosterone propionate therapy of breast cancer. JAMA 1964; 188:1069–1072.

82. Kennedy BJ. Fluxymesterone therapy in treatment of advanced breast cancer. N Engl J Med 1958; 259: 673–675.

83. Tormey DC, Lippman ME, Edwards BK, Cassidy JG. Evaluation of tamoxifen doses with and without fluoxymesterone in advanced breast cancer. Ann Intern Med 1983; 98:139–144.

84. Ingle JN, Twito DI, Schaid DJ et al. Combination hormonal therapy with tamoxifen plus fluoxymesterone versus tamoxifen alone in postmenopausal women with metastatic breast cancer. A phase II study. Cancer 1991; 67:886–891.

85. Gordan GS, Halden A, Horn Y et al. Calusterone (7β,17α-dimethyltestosterone) as primary and secondary therapy of advanced breast cancer. Oncology 1973; 28:138–146.

86. Gordan GS. Anabolic-androgenic steroids. 1976: 499–513. In: Arimasa N, Kochakian CD (Eds). Handbook of Experimental Pharmacology. New York: Springer Verlag.

87. Segaloff A. The use of androgens in the treatment of neoplastic disease. Pharm Ther 1977; C2:33–37.

88. Luo S, Sourla A, Labrie C et al. Combined effects of dehydroepiandrosterone and EM-800 on bone mass, serum lipids, and the development of dimethylbenz(a)anthracene (DMBA)-induced mammary carcinoma in the rat. Endocrinology 1997; 138:4435–4444.

89. Sourla A, Martel C, Labrie C, Labrie F. Almost exclusive androgenic action of dehydroepiandrosterone in the rat mammary gland. Endocrinology 1998; 139:753–764.

90. Trams G & Maass H. Specific binding of estradiol and dihydrotestosterone in human mammary cancers. Cancer Res 1977; 37:258–261.

91. Allegra JC, Lippman ME, Thompson EB et al. Distribution, frequency and quantitative analysis of estrogen, progesterone, androgen and glucocorticoid receptors in human breast cancer. Cancer Res 1979; 39:1447–1454.

92. Miller WR, Telford J, Dixon JM, Hawkins RA. Androgen receptor activity in human breast cancer and its relationship with estrogen and progesterone receptor activity. Eur J Cancer Clin Oncol 1985; 21:539–542.

93. Bryan RM, Mercer RJ, Bennett RC et al. Androgen receptors in breast cancer. Cancer 1984; 54: 2436–2440.

94. Wooster R, Mangion J, Eeles R et al. A germline mutation in the androgen receptor in two brothers with breast cancer and Reifenstein syndrome. Nat Genet 1992; 2:132–134.

95. Lobaccaro JM, Lumbroso S, Belon C et al. Androgen receptor gene mutation in male breast cancer. Hum Mol Genet 1993; 2:1799–1802.

96. Bulbrook RD, Herian M, Tong D et al. Effect of steroidal contraceptives on levels of plasma androgen sulphates and cortisol. Lancet 1973; 1: 628–631.

97. Juret P, Hayem M. New biological evidence on the hormone dependence of breast cancer (preliminary note). Rev Fr Etud Clin Biol 1968; 13:884–887.

98. Masnyk IJ, Silverrman DT, Hankey BF. Prediction of response to adrenalectomy in the treatment of advanced breast cancer. J Natl Cancer Inst 1978; 60: 271–278.

99. Bulbrook RD, Hayward JL, Spicer CC. Relation between urinary androgen and corticoid excretion and subsequent breast cancer. Lancet 1971; 2: 395–398.

100. Brennan MJ, Wang DY, Hayward JL et al. Urinary and plasma androgens in benign breast disease. Possible relation to breast cancer. Lancet 1973; 1:1076–1079.

101. Wang DY, Bulbrook RD, Hayward JL. Urinary and plasma androgens and their relation to familial risk of breast cancer. Eur J Cancer 1975; 11:873–877.

102. Dorgan JF, Longcope C, Stephenson HE, Jr et al. Relation of prediagnostic serum estrogen and androgen levels to breast cancer risk. Cancer Epidemiol Biomarkers Prev 1996; 5:533–539.

103. Berrino F, Muti P, Micheli A et al. Serum sex hormone levels after menopause and subsequent breast cancer. J Natl Cancer Inst 1996; 88:291–296.

104. Secreto G, Toniolo P, Berrino F et al. Increased androgenic activity and breast cancer risk in premenopausal women. Cancer Res 1984; 44(12 Pt. 1): 5902–5905.

105. Secreto G, Toniolo P, Berrino F et al. Serum and urinary androgens and risk of breast cancer in potmenopausal women. Cancer Res 1991; 51: 2572–2576.

106. Segaloff A, Hayward BF, Carter AC et al. Identification of breast cancer patients with high risk of early recurrence after radical mastectomy. III. Steroid hormones meausred in urine. Cancer 1980; 46:1087–1092.

107. Bulbrook RD, Hayward JL, Spicer CC, Thomas BS. Abnormal excretion of urinary steroids by women with early breast cancer. Lancet 1962; 2:1238–1240.

108. Cameron EHD, Griffiths K, Gleave EN et al. Benign and malignant breast disease in south Wales: a study of urinary steroids. Br Med J 1970; 4:768–771.

109. Lacassagne A. Hormonal pathogenesis of adenocarcinoma of the breast. Am J Cancer 1936; 27: 217–228.

110. Costlow ME, Buschow RA, McGuire WL. Prolactin receptors and androgen-induced regression of 7,12-dimethylbenz(a)anthracene-induced mammary carcinoma. Cancer Res 1976; 36(9 pt.1):3324–3329.

111. Quadri SK, Kledzik GS, Meites J. Counteraction by prolactin of androgen-induced inhibition of mammary tumor growth in rats. J Natl Cancer Inst 1974; 52:875–878.

112. Teller MN, Budinger JM, Zvilichovsky G et al. Oncogenicity of purine 3-oxide and unsubstituted purine in rats. Cancer Res 1978; 38:2229–2232.

113. Poulin R, Baker D, Poirier D, Labrie F. Androgen and glucocorticoid receptor-mediated inhibition of cell proliferation by medroxyprogesterone acetate in ZR-75-1 human breast cancer cells. Breast Cancer Res Treat 1989; 13:161–172.

114. Simard J, Hatton AC, Labrie C et al. Inhibitory effects of estrogens on GCDFP-15 mRNA levels and secretion in ZR-75-1 human breast cancer cells. Mol Endocrinol 1989; 3:694–702.

115. Dumont M, Dauvois S, Simard J. Antagonism between estrogens and androgens on GCDFP-15 gene expression in ZR-75-1 cells and correlation between GCDFP-15 and estrogen as well as progesterone receptor expression in human breast cancer. J Steroid Biochem 1989; 34:397–402.

116. Simard J, Dauvois S, Haagensen DE et al. Regulation of progesterone-binding breast cyst protein GCDFP-24 secretion by estrogens and androgens in human breast cancer cells: a new marker of steroid action in breast cancer. Endocrinology 1990; 126:3223–3231.

117. Thériault C, Labrie F. Hormonal regulation of estradiol 17β-hydroxysteroid dehydrogenase activity in the ZR-75-1 human breast cancer cell line. Ann NY Acad Sci 1990; 595:419–421.

118. Rochefort H, Garcia M. The estrogenic and antiestrogenic activities of androgens in female target tissues. Pharmacol Ther 1983; 23:193–216.

119. Abraham GE. Ovarian and adrenal contribution to peripheral androgens during the menstrual cycle. J Clin Endocrinol Metab 1974; 39:340–346.

120. Vermeulen A, Verdonck L. Factors affecting sex hormone levels in postmenopausal women. J Steroid Biochem 1979; 11:899–904.

121. Mistry P, Griffiths K, Maynard PV. Endogenous C19-steroids and estradiol levels in human primary breast tumor tissues and their correlation with androgen and estrogen receptors. J Steroid Biochem 1986; 24:1117–1125.

122. de Launoit Y, Veilleux R, Dufour M et al. Characteristics of the biphasic action of androgens and of the potent antiproliferative effects of the new pure antiestrogen EM-139 on cell cycle kinetic parameters in LNCaP human prostatic cancer cells. Cancer Res 1991; 51:5165–5170.

123. Cusan L, Dupont A, Cossette M, Labrie F. Flutamide in the treatment of female androgenic alopecia. Can J Dermatol 1993; 5:421–427.

124. Neri R, Peets E, Watnick A. Anti-androgenicity of flutamide and its metabolite Sch 16423. Biochem Soc Trans 1979; 7:565.

125. Simard J, Luthy I, Guay J et al. Characteristics of interaction of the antiandrogen Flutamide with the androgen receptor in various target tissues. Mol Cell Endocrinol 1986; 44:261–270.

126. MacIndoe JH, Etre LA. An antiestrogenic action of androgens in human breast cancer cells. J Clin Endocrinol Metab 1981; 53:836–842.

127. Poulin R, Mérand Y, Poirier D. Antiestrogenic properties of keoxifene, trans-4-hydroxytamoxifen and ICI164384, a new steroidal antiestrogen, in ZR-75-1 human breast cancer cells. Breast Cancer Res Treat 1989; 14:65–76.

128. Dauvois S, Li S, Martel C, Labrie F. Inhibitory effect of androgens on DMBA-induced mammary carcinoma in the rat. Breast Cancer Res Treat 1989; 14:299–306.

129. Labrie C, Simard J, Zhao HF et al. Stimulation of androgen-dependent gene expression by the adrenal precursors dehydroepiandrosterone and androstenedione in the rat ventral prostate. Endocrinology 1989; 124:2745–2754.

130. Labrie C, Flamand M, Bélanger A, Labrie F. High bioavailability of DHEA administered percutaneously in the rat. J Endocrinol 1996; 150: S107–S118.

131. Asselin J, Kelly PA, Caron MG, Labrie F. Control of hormone receptor levels and growth of 7,12-dimethylbenz(a)anthracene-induced mammary tumors by estrogens, progesterone and prolactin. Endocrinology 1977; 101:666–671.

132. Hackenberg R, Luttchens S, Hofmann J et al. Androgen sensitivity of the new human breast cancer cell line MFM-223. Cancer Res 1991; 51:5722–5727.

133. Dauvois S, Spinola PG, Labrie F. Additive inhibitory effects of bromocriptine (CB-154) and medroxyprogesterone acetate (MPA) on dimethylbenz(a)anthracene (DMBA)-induced mammary tumors in the rat. Eur J Cancer Clin Oncol 1989; 25:891–897.

134. Couillard S, Labrie C, Bélanger A. Effect of dehydroepiandrosterone and the antiestrogen EM-800 on the growth of human ZR-75-1 breast cancer xenografts. J Natl Cancer Inst 1998; 90:772–778.

135. Boccuzzi G, Aragno M, Brignardello E et al. Opposite effects of dehydroepiandrosterone on the growth of 7,12-dimethylbenz(a)anthracene-induced rat mammary carcinomas. Anticancer Res 1992; 12:1479–1484.

136. Poortman J, Thijssen JH, von Landeghem AA et al. Subcellular distribution of androgens and oestrogens in target tissue. J Steroid Biochem 1983; 19(1C):939–945.

137. Najid A, Ratinaud MH. Comparative studies of steroidogenesis inhibitors (econazole, ketoconazole) on human breast cancer MCF-7 cell proliferation by growth experiments, thymidine incorporation and flow cytometric DNA analysis. Tumori 1991; 77:385–390.

138. Boccuzzi G, Di Monaco M, Brignardello E et al. Dehydroepoandrosterone antiestrogenic action through androgen receptor in MCF-7 human breast cancer cell line. Anticancer Res 1993; 13:2267–2272.

139. Jordan VC. Effect of tamoxifen (ICI 46,474) on initiation and growth of DMBA-induced rat mammary carcinoma. Eur J Cancer 1976; 12:419–424.

140. Jordan VC. Use of the DMBA-induced rat mammary carcinoma system for the evaluation of Tamoxifen as a potential adjuvant therapy. Rev Endocr Relat Cancer Suppl 1978:49–55.

141. Kawamura I, Mizota T, Kondo N et al. Antitumor effects of droloxifene, a new antiestrogen drug, against 7,12-dimethylbenz(a)anthracene-induced mammary tumors in rats. Jpn J Pharmacol 1991; 57:215–224.

142. Luo S, Labrie C, Bélanger A, Labrie F. Effect of dehydroepiandrosterone on bone mass, serum lipids, and dimethylbenz(a)anthracene-induced mammary carcinoma in the rat. Endocrinology 1997; 138:3387–3394.

143. Schwartz AG. Inhibition of spontaneous breast cancer formation in female C3H (Avy/a) mice by long-term treatment with dehydroepiandrosterone. Cancer Res 1979; 39:1129–1132.

144. Zhou J, Ng S, Adesanya-Famuiya O et al. Testosterone inhibits estrogen-induced mammary epithelial proliferation and suppresses estrogen receptor expression. FASEB J 2000; 14: 1725–1730.

145. Park JJ, Irvine RA, Buchanan G et al. Breast cancer susceptibility gene 1 (BRCAI) is a coactivator of the androgen receptor. Cancer Res 2000; 60: 5946–5949.

146. Korkia P & Stimson GV. Indications of prevalence, practice and effects of anabolic steroid use in Great Britain. Int J Sports Med 1997; 18:557–562.

147. Burgess HE, Shousha S. An immunohistochemical study of the long-term effects of androgen administration on female-to-male transsexual breast: a comparison with normal female breast and male breast showing gynaecomastia. J Pathol 1993; 170:37–43.

Chapter 13
Side effects of androgen treatment

Orhan Bukulmez and Bruce R Carr

Summary

Currently there is no FDA-approved androgen therapy for postmenopausal women presenting with signs and symptoms of androgen insufficiency. Off-label use of androgens in women should therefore incorporate in-depth discussion of their potential adverse effects. Based on the current limited information, these are generally mild. Transdermal testosterone provides the best balance between achieving physiologic testosterone concentrations and most favorable safety profile in terms of lipid profile, cardiovascular and liver effects. Full-strength oral methyltestosterone–esterified estrogen combination may cause acne and hirsutism. Because there are no large studies of over 2 years' duration, any conclusions regarding the potential effects of androgen therapy on the risks of cardiovascular disease and malignancies should be treated with caution.

Introduction

The concept of androgen therapy in women with or without estrogen to enhance general wellbeing dates back to 1940s. The studies in which methyltestosterone was used, the treatment was considered beneficial for menopausal symptoms and general wellbeing and for libido.[1,2] In 1960s methyltestosterone was incorporated to the esterified estrogens and approved by the US Food and Drug Administration (FDA) only for menopausal symptoms that did not respond adequately to estrogens alone.

There has been a recent surge of interest in the use of androgen replacement therapy for postmenopausal women for the symptoms and signs consistent with female androgen insufficiency syndrome which include sexual dysfunction.[3] In fact, there are no FDA-approved androgen therapies for the latter indication. Products in use for this purpose are oral methyltestosterone, micronized testosterone, and dehydroepiandrosterone (DHEA), compounded topical 2% testosterone ointment, intramuscular testosterone injections, and testosterone implants. This off-label use of androgens in the USA must be communicated to the patient along with their potential side effects. In addition, patients should be well-informed regarding the most recent safety data of androgen therapy alone or in combination with estrogens.

General overview of the androgen preparations

The studies from the 1980s concentrated on the effect of injected testosterone versus the effect of estrogen alone in oophorectomized women.[4–6] The potential effects of testosterone has been attempted to be predicted from serum levels of testosterone. Injected testosterone provided a rapid pharmacologic peak effect of the steroid with testosterone values often above 150 ng/dL and even higher levels with repeated dosing.

These studies were followed by trials on the use of estrogen with methyltestosterone. In these regimens, 1.25–2.5 mg/day of methyltestosterone is added to esterified estrogens. The circulating levels of methyltestosterone remains low in the range of 20–30 ng/dL. Nevertheless, since methyltestosterone is at least as potent as testosterone, some androgenic effects do occur. In addition, there is increase in biologically active, unbound testosterone associated with methyltestosterone use due to the reduction in sex hormone binding globulin (SHBG) levels. Despite concomitant oral estrogen use, SHBG levels may be suppressed by approximately 45%.[7] In this way the testosterone-SHBG ratio increases by 25–50% resulting in upper-normal range unbound testosterone levels.

The synthesis of SHBG is influenced by the type and route of estrogen treatment. After 3 months of treatment, conjugated equine estrogen (CEE) 0.625 mg/day orally, increases SHBG levels by 100% over baseline values. After 1 mg of 17β-estradiol orally and 50 μg of transdermal estrogen, SHBG levels increase by 42% and 12%, respectively.[8] The addition of androgen to estrogen treatment changes this response. Again, methyltestosterone 2.5 mg combined with 1.25 mg of esterified estrogen daily decreases SHBG levels by more than 40%, whereas esterified estrogen alone at 1.25 mg/day increases plasma SHBG levels by 95% after 3 months of treatment.[9] These findings have implications for androgen-related side effects.

There are various androgen preparations as detailed elsewhere in this book. Generally, women treated with injectable testosterone achieve pharmacologic levels of testosterone with associated peaks and valleys and the risk of steroid accumulation. Currently available oral micronized testosterone is absorbed poorly. Regarding oral DHEA, in a double blind, prospective, placebo controlled, randomized cross-over study, oral DHEA (50 mg/day) has been shown to increase circulating androgen levels to the physiologic range in women with adrenal dysfunction.[10] The DHEA products, however, are available as an over the counter supplement and regulated minimally. The packages of DHEA have been shown to contain no DHEA to 150% of the labeled claim.[11] Hence the effects of the commercially available preparations of DHEA may be highly unpredictable.

Methyltestosterone or fluorinated testosterone in large doses as used in males, are not recommended for females. In lower does, methyltestosterone (1.25–2.5 mg/day) with esterified estrogens has been shown to be beneficial for menopausal symptoms, bone mass and the quality of life. In fact most frequently used product available in the USA for women with androgen insufficiency is esterified estrogen in combination with 1.25–2.5 mg/day of methyltestosterone. Some data suggest safety and the efficacy with this regimen,[12,13] although it will be reviewed in more detail.

At this point, it would be appropriate to review the effects of androgens and androgen-containing preparations on various organ systems in relevance to their safety.

Effects on cardiovascular system

Overview

The belief that testosterone is a risk factor for cardiac disease is based on the observation that men have higher incidence of cardiovascular disease than women. However, the data supporting a causal relationship between higher testosterone levels and heart disease are far from being conclusive.[14–16] Several studies suggest higher testosterone levels may actually have a favorable effect on the risk of cardiovascular disease in men.[17–20] Furthermore, studies of testosterone therapy in men have not demonstrated any increased incidence of cardiovascular disease or any acute events such as myocardial infarction, stroke, or angina.[21] In fact, there is almost no evidence that parenteral testosterone administration is likely to have adverse cardiovascular consequences, and in fact it has been suggested it may be beneficial.[22]

It has been suggested that relative androgen excess may predict an increased risk of cardiovascular disease in women over the age of 50. Hyperandrogenicity in combination with obesity, hirsutism, namely the polycystic ovary syndrome (PCOS), has been reported to be associated with increased risk of coronary heart disease.[23] Longitudinal results from the Massachusetts Women's Health Study suggested that the higher levels of DHEA and DHEAS (DHEA sulfate) in middle-aged women may indicate a higher cardiovascular disease risk.[24] On the other hand, it has been demonstrated that postmenopausal women who were in the highest tertiles of free testosterone and androstenedione levels had significantly lower carotid intimal–medial thickness and plaque.[25]

There are no long-term studies with adequate power to determine the potential effects of androgens on cardiovascular system. Some extrapolations can be attempted by reviewing the current literature on androgen effects on various tested surrogate parameters related with cardiovascular disease risk. These parameters include serum lipid profile, effects on blood vessel tone, blood viscosity, and insulin resistance.

Lipid profile changes

Most of the trials of androgen therapy for women have also studied the changes in lipid profile (Table 13.1). The duration of these trials ranged from 1 month to 2 years. The trials have utilized various androgens with different forms of administration.

The aromatizable androgen preparations such as transdermal testosterone are generally neutral to the lipid profile. Oral androgens like methyltestosterone, however, significantly decrease total cholesterol, triglyceride (TG) and high-density lipoprotein cholesterol (HDL-C) levels. The effect of methyltestosterone on low-density lipoprotein cholesterol (LDL-C) levels is mostly neutral (see Table 13.1)

In a recent double blind, randomized trial, 118 postmenopausal women experiencing hypoactive sexual desire received either esterified estrogens 0.625 mg/day or esterified estrogens plus methyltestosterone (1.25 mg/day) for 4 months.[32] Estrogen–methyltestosterone treatment resulted in a significant decrease in HDL-C levels (−12.4 mg/dL) in contrast with a significant increase with estrogen alone (+3.2 mg/dL). Also, the estrogen–methyltestosterone combination caused a significant decrease in TG levels (−31.1 mg/dL).

Increased TG levels is a risk factor for cardiovascular disease in women.[41] Low HDL-C levels in elderly postmenopausal women are considered as stronger risk factor for coronary artery disease than the elevated LDL-C levels.[40] Hence it is difficult to predict the influence of lipid profile changes induced by methyltestosterone–estrogen combination on future cardiovascular risk. The most unfavorable lipid profile is seen in women taking oral anabolic androgens such as nandrolone decanoate which increases total cholesterol and LDL-C levels and decreases HDL-C levels (see Table 13.1).

Most of the data available on the association between DHEA concentrations and cardiovascular disease have been reported in men. Twelve such studies suggested a mild potential relationship or

no relationship after controlling for confounding variables.[42] Oral micronized dehydroepiandrosterone (DHEA) also has been used in clinical trials.[43,44] Clinical trials of DHEA in women suggested the possibility of a mild decrease in HDL-C which is of unknown clinical significance.[44,45]

In a double blind, prospective, placebo controlled, randomized cross-over study, oral DHEA (50 mg/day) was shown to increase circulating androgen levels to the physiologic range in women with adrenal dysfunction.[10] In this study, serum concentrations of SHBG, total cholesterol, and HDL-C were found to be decreased significantly by 4 months of DHEA therapy. In addition to DHEA lowering HDL-C levels, it may potentially affect hepatic function. For these reasons if to be used, vaginal or transdermal administration of DHEA have been recommended.

In summary, the clinical implications of the changes in the lipid profile in women receiving androgen therapy is not known due to lack of long-term trials. It may only be concluded that the transdermal testosterone preparations are least likely to change the lipid profile. In contrast, methyltestosterone decreases total cholesterol, triglyceride and HDL-C levels. Nonaromatizable anabolic agents seem to induce atherogenic effects on the lipid profile. Methyltestosterone with its triglyceride-lowering effect could be chosen in women with hypertriglyceridemia. Testosterone is a lipid neutral drug and can be preferred if the patient's HDL-C level is low.[46]

Vascular tone

It is known that testosterone in men acts as a coronary vasodilator.[18] The vascular effects of testosterone implants (50 mg) have been evaluated in 33 postmenopausal women who were also receiving estrogen replacement. Six weeks of cotreatment with testosterone improved both endothelial-dependent (flow-mediated) and endothelium-independent brachial artery vasodilation as compared with control women.[22]

In another study, 20 postmenopausal women who were on estrogen replacement for at least a year were randomized either to esterified estrogens at 1.25 mg/day or esterified estrogens at the same dose plus methyltestosterone at 2.5 mg/day for 8 weeks.[47] Blood flow to the fingertip and the vagina was determined by laser Doppler velocimetry at

Table 13.1 Effect of androgen treatment on lipid profiles of women involved in prospective studies*

Author	Study design	No. of subjects	Androgen	Estrogen	Duration	Androgen effects
Burger et al.[26]	Pre/Post	17	T 100 mg s.c. implant	Estradiol 40 mg s.c. implant	6 months	None
Sherwin et al.[27]	Prospective, controlled	11 controls 20 E/T 11 Estrogen	T enanthate 150 mg) + estradiol (diananthate 7.5 mg, benzoate 1.0 mg) i.m.	Estradiol valerate 10 mg i.m.	30 days	None
Hickok et al.[7]	Prospective, randomized, double blind	26 (13/13)	MT 1.25 mg/d + esterified estrogen (0.625 mg/d) p.o.	Esterified estrogen 0.625 mg/d	6 months	T Chol ↓, LDL↓, HDL↓, ApoA-I ↓ TG ↔
Watts et al.[38]	Prospective, randomized, double blind, surgical menopause	66 (33/33)	MT 2.5 mg/d + esterified estrogen (1.25 mg/d) p.o.	Esterified estrogen 1.25 mg/d	2 years	T Chol ↓, TG ↓, HDL ↓ LDL ↔
Raisz et al.[28]	Prospective, randomized	28 (13MT+E/15CEE)	MT 2.5 mg/d + esterified estrogen (1.25 mg/d) p.o.	Conjugated equine estrogen 1.25 mg/d	9 weeks	ApoA-I ↓, T Chol ↓, TG ↓. HDL ↓ LDL ↔
Lovejoy et al.[35]	Prospective, randomized	30 10NDC/10Sp/ 10 placebo	Nandrolone decanoate 30 mg every 2 weeks vs Spironolactone (Sp) vs placebo	None	9 months	T Chol ↑, LDL ↑, TG ↔ HDL ↓
Buckler et al.[37]	Prospective, randomized, women with premenstrual syndrome	44 (22/22)	T SQ implants 100 mg every 6 months vs controls	None	2 years	HDL ↓, ApoA-I ↓ LDL ↔, TG ↔, T Chol ↔
Gruber et al.[29]	Prospective, randomized	39 (20/19)	Dihydrotestosterone topical 100 mg twice daily vs placebo	None	6 months	None
Miller et al.[33]	Prospective, randomized premenopausal women with AIDS wasting	53 (18/18/17)	Transdermal T, 150 μg or 300 μg twice weekly or placebo	None	12 weeks	None
Barrett-Connor et al.[39]	Prospective, double blind randomized, surgical menopause	311 (81 low-dose MT, 73 low-dose MT, 79 low-dose E, 78 high-dose E)	MT 1.25 mg + esterified estrogens 0.625 mg/d or MT 2.5 mg + esterified estrogens 1.25 mg/d	CEE 0.625 mg daily or CEE 1.25 mg daily	2 years	T Chol ↓, LDL ↓, HDL ↓, TG ↓
Davis et al.[30]	Prospective, single blind, randomized	32 (17 ET/15 E)	Estradiol 50 mg + T 50 mg implants every 3 months	Estradiol 50 mg implants every 3 months	2 years	T Chol ↓ LDL ↓ HDL ↔
Shifren et al.[34]	Prospective, randomized	75 (25 low-dose T, 25 high-dose T, 25 placebo)	Transdermal T 150 μg/d or 300 μg/d or placebo	CEE 0.625 mg daily to all patients	12 weeks	None
Basaria et al.[36]	Prospective, randomized	40 (20 EA, 20 E)	MT 2.5 mg/d + esterified estrogen 1.25 mg/d	Esterified estrogen 1.25 mg/d	16 weeks	T Chol ↓, HDL ↓, TG ↓ LDL ↔
Lobo et al.[32]	Prospective, randomized	218 (107 E/MT, 111 E)	MT 2.5 mg/d + esterified estrogen 0.625 mg/d	Esterified estrogen 0.625 mg/d	16 weeks	T Chol ↓, HDL ↓, TG ↓ LDL ↔
Floter et al.[31]	Prospective, randomized, cross-over surgical menopause	50	Estradiol valerate 2 mg plus T undecenoate 40 mg/d	Estradiol valerate 2 mg/d plus placebo	24 weeks	↑LDL ↓ HDL ↓ ↑T Chol ↔, TG↔, ↑Lipoprotein (a) ↔

*Modified from Basaria & Dobs[40] with permission. †Decreased as compared to the baseline state.
ApoA-I, apolipoprotein A-I; CEE, conjugated equine estrogen; E, estrogen; HDL, high-density lipoprotein; i.m., intramuscularly; LDL, low-density lipoprotein; MT, methyltestosterone;

baseline and then every 4 weeks. The women assigned to estrogen-methyltestosterone arm showed a statistically nonsignificant increase in the blood flow in those regions. It has been concluded that estrogen–androgen treatment does not diminish the vasodilator effects of estrogen treatment in postmenopausal women. Once again, since the studies of long duration and adequate power are lacking, this issue is far from conclusive. Nevertheless, these studies on androgen therapy are reassuring in terms of the lack of short-term adverse effects on peripheral vascular tone.

Clotting parameters

There is paucity of data on the effect of androgen treatment on the coagulation factors. In a study of 32 men treated for 52 weeks, the effects of supraphysiologic doses of testosterone (200 mg of intramuscular testosterone enanthate weekly) on factors involved in hemostasis and thrombosis were investigated.[48] Initial decreases in plasminogen activator inhibitor, protein C, and free protein S levels appeared to be counterbalanced by increases in levels of antithrombin III. All these factors returned to pretreatment levels with continued treatment. There was a sustained fall in plasma fibrinogen levels. There was no effect on platelet activation as measured by β-thromboglobulin concentration.

In a prospective, randomized 16 week study, fibrinogen levels were significantly increased in women who had received esterified estrogen (1.25 mg/day) plus methyltestosterone 2.5 mg/day as compared with women who had been on esterified estrogen 1.25 mg/day.[36] Another study compared the clotting factors of 22 premenopausal women who had been on testosterone implants for 2 years with 22 age-matched controls.[37] At the end of two years, all clotting factors were within the reference range in women who were on testosterone. These levels were not different from the control group as well. Testosterone appears to be more neutral on clotting parameters.

Polycythemia

Higher testosterone levels appear to act as a stimulus for erythropoiesis. Adult men have higher hemoglobin levels than adult women. Although an increase in the hematocrit is beneficial for patients with anemia, elevation above the normal range may have adverse effects particularly in the elderly, since an attendant increase in blood viscosity could aggravate vascular events in the coronary, cerebrovascular or peripheral vascular system. Hence polycythemia is a risk factor for cardiovascular disease. The risk of hemoconcentration is greater if the patient also has a condition that is associated with an increase in the hematocrit, such as chronic obstructive pulmonary disease.[49,50]

It has been shown that polycythemia may develop in elderly men undergoing testosterone replacement therapy.[51] Polycythemia can also occur in female-to-male transsexuals.[52] Injections appear to be associated with a greater risk of erythrocytosis than topical preparations.[50,53,54] However, no case of polycythemia has been demonstrated in studies of androgen replacement in women. A study including premenopausal women with acquired immune deficiency syndrome related wasting showed a slight increase in hematocrit levels with transdermal testosterone.[33] Nevertheless, it has been recommended that polycythemia at baseline should be an absolute contraindication for androgen therapy.[40]

Insulin resistance

In a 12-week study utilizing transdermal testosterone patches, no changes have been detected in fasting plasma insulin or glucose levels.[34] In another study, obese postmenopausal women were randomized to nandrolone decanoate (NDC) (an anabolic steroid with weak androgenic activity), spironolactone, or placebo for 9 months.[35] All women also received simultaneous calorie restriction for weight loss. Women in all three groups lost comparable amounts of weight, but the NDC-treated women gained lean mass relative to the other two groups and lost more body fat than women in the spironolactone group. Nandrolone decanoate treatment produced a gain in visceral fat, as determined by computed tomography scan, and a relatively greater loss of subcutaneous abdominal fat. In women taking nandrolone decanoate there were no significant changes in fasting glucose, fasting insulin or insulin sensitivity.[35] The results from these limited studies appear to be reassuring although none of them utilized any valid techniques to determine insulin sensitivity precisely.

Effects on signs and symptoms of hyperandrogenism

Potential risks of androgen therapy include hirsutism, acne, irreversible deepening of the voice, and virilization. Virilization of the female fetus is a potential risk of androgen therapy in women of reproductive age.

Acne, hirsutism, and virilization are commonly seen in female-to-male transsexuals receiving supraphysiologic doses of androgens.[52] The appearance of virilizing effects depends on both the dose and the duration of androgen therapy. Doses of methyltestosterone above 10 mg/day may produce masculinization in women if given for longer than six months.[55] These effects have been rare in women undergoing low-dose androgens. Approximately 15–20% of women may experience mild hirsutism during such therapies.[40] This condition usually resolves with discontinuation of treatment. Hirsutism is mostly related with the decrease in the SHBG levels resulting in an increased free testosterone levels.

In studies using transdermal testosterone patches,[33,34] testosterone implants,[37] and intramuscular injections[5] there were no worsening of acne or hirsutism scores in the groups receiving androgens. Some studies utilizing methyltestosterone however, have demonstrated higher hirsutism and acne scores in the androgen treatment arms.[7,32,38] In one study, women taking nandrolone decanoate had higher hirsutism and acne scores when compared with women receiving placebo.[35]

Watts et al. reported that of the 33 women treated with methyltestosterone 2.5 mg with esterified estrogens 1.25 mg daily for 2 years, 36% experienced hirsutism and 30% experienced facial acne.[38] However, in another 2-year study of women taking either 2.5 mg daily or 1.25 mg daily methyltestosterone in combination with estrogens, no differences have been demonstrated in hirsutism scores as compared with estrogen-only arm.[39] The different effects seen in dose studies may be explained by variable sensitivity of hair follicle as an end-organ.

High-dose injectable androgens can cause virilization. Nine postmenopausal women with symptoms and signs of androgen excess due to long-term use of an injectable androgen-estrogen combination which contained testosterone enanthate 150 mg, estradiol dienanthate 7.5 mg, estradiol benzoate 1.0 mg, were studied retrospectively.[56] Cosmetically disturbing hirsutism was the major complaint in eight subjects. Other symptoms included hot flushes, decreased libido, mood changes, depression, temporal balding and postmenopausal bleeding in one patient with an intact uterus. Seven women had clitoromegaly. The androgen–estrogen combination was discontinued and oral or transdermal estrogen replacement was instituted. In five women followed serially for 16–24 months, elevated testosterone levels required 12–20 months to return to the normal premenopausal range. Apparently testosterone levels achieved with this preparation were 10 times the normal production rate.[56] In a case report, the antiandrogen flutamide proved to be an effective therapy for clitoromegaly and hirsutism in a young woman who had self-injected testosterone and nandrolone to gain muscle mass for weight lifting.[57]

In a prospective, placebo controlled study, 75 healthy women who had undergone bilateral salpingo-oophorectomy and hysterectomy before natural menopause and who had been on conjugated equine estrogens at a daily dose of at least 0.625 mg orally for at least 2 months were randomized to two different transdermal testosterone regimens.[34] These women began three consecutive 12-week treatment periods during which they received in random order transdermal testosterone patches of either 150 µg/day or 300 µg/day twice weekly or placebo patches twice weekly. All women continued to use oral conjugated equine estrogens. The hirsutism and acne scores did not change significantly during treatment. However, the mean facial-depilation rate (the number of times in the previous month that hair was removed from the chin or upper lip) increased with 300 µg of testosterone per day.[34]

In a double blind, randomized trial, 118 postmenopausal women experiencing hypoactive sexual desire received either esterified estrogens 0.625 mg/day or esterified estrogens plus methyltestosterone (1.25 mg/day) for 4 months.[32] The women receiving the estrogen–methyltestosterone combination were twice as likely to report acne compared with estrogen-treated women (5.6% vs 2.7%, respectively).

The human voice is quite sensitive to hormonal changes. Professional female singers may note a number of adverse vocal changes upon reaching age 50.[58] The postmenopausal women may have trouble reaching their highest registers and may experience impaired vocal control.[59] It has been shown that postmenopausal estrogen replacement with or without progestin counters the reductions occur in fundamental frequency and sound pressure level of sustained phonation and speaking voice samples.[60] In one study, adding nandrolone acetate 50 mg every 4 weeks to an estrogen/progestin therapy for 1 year resulted in altered voice in the form of a lower fundamental frequency during speech, a loss of high frequencies and an increase in voice instability and creakiness.[61] There have been no reports regarding the adverse voice effects of low-dose androgen–estrogen replacement in women.

Generally, in studies in which individual responses to treatment were presented in detail, the virilizing effects associated with oral androgen treatment were usually reported to be abated with either dose reduction or discontinuation of treatment.[62] Methyltestosterone use may be associated with mild reversible acne and hirsutism. Although transdermal testosterone patches have not been associated with worsening of acne or hirsutism, high-dose parenteral testosterone may result in virilization.

Liver toxicity

It has been reported that alkylated androgens at high doses may result in hepatotoxicity and hepatic adenomas.[51] The effect of oral androgens in liver dysfunction depends on the dose and duration of treatment. Such adverse effects are rare and confined to patients receiving androgen therapy alone. The clinical studies conducted on synthetic androgens, such as stanozolol, fluoxymesterone, and oxymetholone demonstrated reversible increase in liver enzymes.[62,63]

Long-term, high-dose methyltestosterone therapy can be associated with hepatotoxicity. Of 60 patients (42 female transsexuals and 18 impotent males) receiving long-term therapy with methyltestosterone 50 mg three times a day, 19 had abnormal findings on liver function tests and 33 out of 52 had abnormal findings on liver scans,

particularly those who had been treated for more than a year.[64] Historically, cases of hepatotoxicity have been associated with oral administration of methyltestosterone in men treated with dosages of 10–100 mg/day.[65]

In the pharmacy-based computer database 3641 women were identified who had filled one or more prescriptions for low-dose esterified estrogens combined with methyltestosterone between 1992 and 1996 which included 3016 person years of exposure.[65] There were no records of toxic hepatitis or liver necrosis. It should be kept in mind that both of these entities are in fact, rare occurrences in general population receiving prescription medications.

The studies on androgen therapy for women have not demonstrated any significant disturbance in liver function tests.[32–34,38,39,66] The changes seen in liver function tests associated with estrogen-androgen preparations have been compared with those of estrogen-alone preparation used in postmenopausal women in a meta-analysis.[67] It has been concluded that combined esterified estrogen–methyltestosterone therapy in daily doses of 0.625 mg of esterified estrogen plus 1.25 mg methyltestosterone or 1.25 mg esterified estrogen plus 2.5 mg methyltestosterone was safe regarding liver function in postmenopausal women during the course of 24 months in eight controlled clinical trials.

According to a review of DHEA use in menopause,[42] there is one report of transient jaundice and hepatic dysfunction occurring 1 week after a single dose of 150 mg of DHEA. Hepatic dysfunction and failure have been reported in patients receiving 17-alkylated androgens such as fluoxymesterone 150 mg/day, stanozolol 6 mg/day, and methyltestosterone 10–100 mg/day.[55] These dosages are significantly higher than the dose of methyltestosterone (1.25 mg/day or 2.5 mg/day) prescribed for androgen replacement therapy for women. There have been no documented serious adverse effects linked to low-dose androgen replacement therapy.

Although the reports of liver toxicity are almost nonexistent in the context of low dose estrogen–androgen replacement therapy, individual sensitivity to the potential hepatotoxic effect may vary considerably. It is prudent to manage all patients receiving oral methyltestosterone therapy individually since the rare liver effects may happen regardless of dose or duration of treatment.[68]

Effects on endometrium

Supraphysiologic doses of androgens used in female-to-male transsexuals have been associated with polycystic ovarian morphology and endometrial hyperplasia.[69] However, most of the studies did not report any increased risk of endometrial cancer or hyperplasia in postmenopausal women receiving low-dose androgen replacement therapy.

Methyltestosterone–estrogen combination was not associated with any significant changes in the endometrium.[7] In a 4-month study, endometrial hyperplasia was detected in 1 of 107 women receiving estrogen plus methyltestosterone as compared with 1 of 111 women receiving unopposed estrogen.[32] In only one earlier study in which postmenopausal women had received estradiol–testosterone implants combined with oral norethindrone, 6% incidence of cystic endometrial hyperplasia was reported.[70]

Briefly, low-dose androgens do not seem to be associated with endometrial hyperplasia or cancer although the studies of longer duration are still needed.

Breast cancer and androgens

Androgen receptor expression is abundant in normal mammary epithelium and in the majority of breast cancer lines.[71,72] Interestingly, the breast cancer antigen 1 (BRCA-1) gene product has recently been identified as an androgen receptor coactivator.[73] The BRCA-1 protein binds to the androgen receptor and potentiates androgen receptor mediated effects. Hence *BRCA-1* mutations may blunt androgen effects on breast. Germline mutations in the androgen receptor gene resulting in variable degrees of androgen insensitivity have been associated with the occurrence of breast cancer in men.[74]

There is a considerable amount of evidence that androgens may protect against estrogen's mitogenic and cancer-promoting effects on breast tissue.[75] Studies of the effects of androgens in various breast cancer cell lines predominantly support apoptotic and antiproliferative effects of androgens on the mitotic effects of estrogens. These antiproliferative effects depend on the estrogen status, type of androgen used, androgen concentration, and the type of breast cancer line studied.[76] It has been shown that DHEAS and androstenediol stimulated the growth of estrogen receptor positive MCF-7 breast cancer cell line in the absence of estradiol, but reduced its proliferation in the presence of estradiol.[77] Testosterone and dehydrotestosterone (DHT) at supraphysiologic concentrations inhibited the proliferation of MCF-7 cell line independently of the presence of estradiol. Furthermore prolonged DHT exposure increased androgen receptor content and overexpression of androgen receptor decreased estradiol-induced signaling. It has also been suggested that the therapeutic action of medroxyprogesterone acetate in advanced breast cancer may be partially mediated by the androgen receptor.[78]

There are also conflicting reports in cell-line studies. The two other breast cancer cell lines that had no hormone receptors were found to be stimulated by DHT.[79] In the ER-negative cell lines testosterone was a more potent inhibitor of cell proliferation than DHT whereas in ER-positive cell lines stronger inhibition was achieved with DHT.[80] It was thought that the partial transformation of testosterone to estrogen in ER-positive cells might be an explanation for this effect.

In terms of animal studies, it has been demonstrated in ovariectomized rhesus monkeys that the addition of testosterone to estrogen therapy significantly inhibits estradiol-induced mammary epithelial proliferation.[71] Testosterone treatment also reduced the mammary epithelial estrogen receptor expression. It has also been demonstrated in a rat model that testosterone may oppose the mitogenic action of estrogen in the breast by promoting apoptosis.[81]

Prostate-specific antigen (PSA) is a new favorable prognostic indicator for breast cancer which has been reported to be found in 30% of breast cancers and has been associated with an earlier stage and a longer relapse-free survival.[82] The genes encoding PSA are regulated by androgens.[83] Differential androgen induction of PSA was reported in different breast cancer cell lines with different coactivators and corepressors.[83]

A number of studies have analyzed the correlation between circulating androgens such as testosterone and the risk of breast cancer (Table 13.2). The results of these studies vary greatly possibly due to the presence of many potential sources of bias. The androgen assays used in studies for serum or urine are different and may

Table 13.2   Serum androgen levels and the risk of breast cancer*

Risk of breast cancer	Author	Comments
Increased	Dorgan et al.[86]	Serum testosterone was positively associated with postmenopausal breast cancer (71 with breast cancer, 2 controls for each case)
	Berrino et al.[87]	24 postmenopausal women with breast cancer and 88 controls. Mean total and free testosterone were significantly higher in case subjects than controls
	Secreto et al.[84]	75 women with postmenopausal breast cancer and 15 controls. Increased risk with higher serum and urine androgen levels
	Secreto et al.[88]	27 premenopausal breast cancer patients and 62 controls. Elevated luteal phase serum and urine testosterone levels were found in breast cancer patients
Decreased	Lee et al.[89]	Urinary androgens were lower in 34 premenopausal women with breast cancer as compared with 25 control women
	Thomas et al.[90]	Lower urinary androgens were associated with higher recurrence rates in 241 premenopausal women with early breast cancer
	Thomas et al.[91]	Telephone interview with men with history of breast cancer. Androgen deficiency states associated with testicular failure might be associated with increased breast cancer in men
No association	Lipworth et al.[92]	Serum androgens were measured postoperatively in 122 postmenopausal women with breast cancer and 122 controls
	Helzlsouer et al.[93]	Serum androstenedione levels of 51 women who developed breast cancer compared with controls
	Garland et al.[94]	Serum androgen levels of 442 postmenopausal women were determined; 42 women were diagnosed with breast cancer during the following years
	Wysowski et al.[85]	A female population studied for serum androgens; 17 premenopausal and 39 post menopausal breast cancers detected during the following years. No differences in endogenous hormones were found as compared with controls

*Modified from Dimitrakakis et al.[95] with permission.

not be sensitive enough for the low range of values commonly found in women. Most of these studies report findings from a single blood measurement of androgens, although normally those levels show variability within the day and from day to day in the same woman. Since the unbound free testosterone is more important for the biologic effects, measuring total testosterone may not reflect the biologic effects. Since most androgenic activity in women is due to the peripheral conversion of precursors such as DHEA into testosterone within the target cells, the peripheral levels may not predict the tissue effects. In addition, it is not possible to dissociate the risk associated with elevated estradiol levels from the androgen component since the androgens are precursors for estradiol synthesis.

In a study of 97 postmenopausal women with breast cancer it has been shown that the serum levels of estradiol and testosterone were higher in cancer cases.[96] There was also an association between serum free testosterone levels and breast cancer relative risk which was statistically independent of the estradiol associated risk. However, in another similar study, higher serum testosterone levels lost its significance when the analysis was adjusted for free estradiol levels.[97] Hence it is very difficult to separate potential direct effects of serum testosterone from its potential to be aromatized into estradiol.

In some studies, high plasma levels of testosterone have been implicated in breast cancer. Japanese women who develop breast cancer have been reported to have a higher blood testosterone levels.[98] It has been suggested that high urinary testosterone is a prognostic indicator of early breast cancer recurrence in node-positive patients.[99] In a case–control study, serum levels of testosterone, DHT, androstenedione, DHEAS, and SHBG, and urinary levels of testosterone and androstanediol were compared in 75 postmenopausal women with breast carcinoma and 150 age-matched healthy controls.[85] Risk of breast cancer was positively associated with levels of all androgens in serum and urine. A potential role for increased androgenic activity in premenopausal breast cancer has been suggested as well.[100] High concentrations of androgens have been reported to be found in the postmenopausal breast cancer tissues.[101]

It has been thought that since androgen receptors are found in most of the breast tumors, androgens may directly stimulate breast tissue.[102] The androgen effects on breast may also be carried out via estrogen receptors after aromatization of androgens to estrogens. In contrary to the above, the most recent cross-sectional study which included 171 premenopausal women with breast cancer and 170 age-matched controls found no significant difference in testosterone levels among groups.[103] In two other earlier prospective case–control studies, there were no association between total testosterone levels and breast cancer.[85,104]

Polycystic ovarian syndrome is characterized by anovulation and hyperandrogenism. Despite long-term exposure to unopposed estrogen and hyperandrogenism the risk of breast cancer is not increased in women with PCOS.[105–107]

The findings from case–control studies of the relation between endogenous testosterone levels and breast cancer risk may not translate to women treated with exogenous testosterone. Total testosterone level does not provide information about actual tissue androgen exposure. As mentioned above, variation in SHBG levels, stress level of the patients, sensitivity of the assay method use are all confounders of the evaluation of testosterone levels. In addition, most of the studies did not control for estradiol in their calculations. Currently, the evidence from clinical studies that the free fraction of testosterone is an independent risk factor for breast cancer is lacking.[76]

There is currently no report of increased breast cancer risk in women receiving low-dose androgen replacement therapy although long-term studies with adequate power are lacking. In a 2-year trial comparing methyltestosterone plus estrogen replacement with estrogen replacement in which mammograms were obtained at baseline, 12 months, and 24 months, there were no significant changes in women receiving androgen–estrogen combination.[39] A recent retrospective analysis of 511 Australian women treated with conventional estrogen therapy plus 50–150 mg testosterone implants with a mean follow-up of 5.7 ± 2.5 years but no control group, reported a breast cancer incidence of 240 per 1 000 000 women years.[108] This incidence was equivalent to the incidence in the general population as determined by the state cancer registry. Although the few clinical data are reassuring, studies on the use of exogenous androgen and breast cancer risk are limited and caution and appropriate follow-up is recommended in women receiving androgen therapy.

Mood and behavior

In terms of central nervous system effects, androgens have been shown to protect neurons directly. These effects may be via androgen receptor-independent mechanisms and via brain 5α-reductase mediated formation of dehydrotestosterone.[109] It has been suggested that combining esterified estrogen with methyltestosterone increases both free bioavailable estrogen and androgen and enhance the movement of both steroids across the blood–brain barrier into the central nervous system.[46] However, the neuroprotective effects of androgens is observed with lower doses of testosterone and higher concentrations of testosterone may be toxic to neurons.[110]

In relevance to short-term central nervous system effects, androgens influence mood and behavior. Intramuscular testosterone treatment at 200 mg weekly for 20 weeks in men have been associated with anger.[111] In a study involving surgically menopausal women taking 200 mg of intramuscular testosterone enanthate every month, increased hostility scores have been reported as compared with women receiving placebo or estrogen replacement therapy and as compared with women with intact ovaries.[112] These behavioral effects seem to be associated with high doses of injectable androgens. None of the studies using low-dose androgens showed such adverse effects.

Immune system

It has long been recognized that testosterone has an immune-modulating action. The greater incidence of immune-mediated disease in women and androgen-deficient men has been attributed to the immunosuppressive effects of androgens as compared with estrogens.[113] There are several reports of testosterone therapy in rheumatoid arthritis and systemic lupus erythematosus in which improvements of clinical condition and inflammatory markers have been demonstrated.[114,115]

Testosterone incubated in cell-culture attenuates the production of inflammatory cytokines in human cells such as macrophages,[116] monocytes,[117] osteoblasts,[118] and endothelial cells.[119] In a study involving 27 men with androgen deficiency, depot testosterone 100 mg intramuscular injection every 10 days resulted in reductions in inflammatory cytokines tumor necrosis factor-α and interleukin-1β (IL-1β), and an increase in IL-10, which is an anti-inflammatory cytokine.[120] Testosterone treatment was also associated with decreased total cholesterol levels. Although these immune suppressant effects may be beneficial in autoimmune conditions and even may be implicated favorably in the pathogenesis of coronary artery disease with regard to plaque biology and stability, the long-term effects are still not known.

Miscellaneous effects

Transdermal testosterone therapy in men is associated with a variety of skin reactions mainly erythema or pruritus which are more common with patches which can be seen in up to 66% of the users.[121] Intramuscular injections of testosterone can cause local pain, soreness, bruising, erythema, swelling, nodules, or furuncles.

It has been reported in a case report that transdermal estradiol combined with 6-monthly testosterone implants use may be associated with the development of endometriosis in postmenopausal hysterectomized women.[122] Testosterone replacement therapy has been associated with

exacerbation of sleep apnea or with the development of sleep apnea generally in men treated with higher doses of parenteral testosterone who have other risk factors for sleep apnea.[123,124] In studies, upper-airway dimensions were not unaffected by testosterone-replacement therapy. Therefore it has been suggested that testosterone may contribute to sleep-disordered breathing by central mechanisms rather than by means of anatomic changes in the airway. Hence any history or suspicion of sleep apnea may preclude androgen replacement therapy.

Fluid retention is uncommon but may occur. In one study comparing esterified estrogen 1.25 mg daily with esterified estrogen plus methyltestosterone 2.5 mg daily in a total of 40 postmenopausal patients treated for 16 weeks, two patients in estrogen–androgen arm withdrew due to adverse effects. One developed bloating and weight gain and the other had migraine.[125]

Monitoring androgen therapy in women

Before starting androgen therapy, the women should be evaluated to assure the absence of any contraindications which include pregnancy, lactation, androgen-dependent neoplasia, severe acne and/or hirsutism, androgenic alopecia, sleep apnea, conditions associated with polycythemia, situations where increased anger and hostility is a problem.[126]

Monitoring women using androgens includes the subjective assessment of general satisfaction with the therapy and also evaluation for the potential adverse effects.

In any patient who is a candidate for androgen therapy, careful clinical assessment for the presence of acne and hirsutism should be performed. The modified Ferriman–Gallwey Hirsutism Rating Scale is useful for assessing the degree of hair growth in the androgen-sensitive regions of the body.[127] In addition, careful monitoring of acne, temporal balding and/or deepening of the voice is mandatory. Determination of lipid profile, hemoglobin and liver enzymes should be done before and possibly 1–2 months following the initiation of therapy.[128] Then intermittent monitoring of these parameters is justified at the physician's discretion.

Conclusion

Androgen therapy in women is a relatively new area. Postmenopausal androgen replacement is becoming increasingly widespread. This is despite the lack of clear guidelines regarding the diagnosis of androgen insufficiency, optimal therapeutic doses, and long-term safety data. Furthermore, the medical community is still debating on what recommendations to make about hormone replacement therapy in general after the publication of Heart and Estrogen Replacement Study[129] and the Women's Health Initiative Study.[130–133] Therefore, any counseling about the androgen therapy should consider the fact that there are no long-term studies with adequate power to determine the potential effects of androgens on cardiovascular system, central nervous system and breast and endometrial cancer risks.

With regard to studies of short duration, the adverse effects of androgen replacement therapy are generally mild and the safety profile of transdermal testosterone seems to be more favorable than the other modes of androgen therapy. Transdermal testosterone therapy appears to give the best balance between achieving physiologic testosterone concentrations and most favorable safety profile in terms of lipid profile, cardiovascular and liver effects.[34,134]

Providing that circulating androgen concentrations are kept within, or close to, the upper limit of the normal physiologic range, masculinizing effects are extremely unlikely. Methyltestosterone 1.25 mg/day or 2.5 mg/day is absorbed well orally and is available in combination with esterified estrogens (0.625 mg/day or 1.25 mg/day). Full-strength formulation may cause acne and hirsutism in some patients.

In conclusion, given the paucity of long-term controlled trials of androgen therapy in women, patients should be fully informed of potential risks and carefully monitored for adverse reactions.

References

1. Lobo RA. Androgens in postmenopausal women: production, possible role, and replacement options. Obstet Gynecol Surv 2001; 56:361–376.
2. Chu MC, Lobo RA. Formulations and use of androgens in women. Mayo Clin Proc 2004; 79(4 Suppl):S3–S7.
3. Bachmann G, Bancroft J, Braunstein G et al. Female androgen insufficiency: the Princeton consensus statement on definition, classification, and assessment. Fertil Steril 2002; 77:660–665.
4. Sherwin BB, Gelfand MM, Brender W. Androgen enhances sexual motivation in females: a prospective, crossover study of sex steroid administration in the surgical menopause. Psychosom Med 1985; 47:339–351.
5. Sherwin BB, Gelfand MM. Differential symptom response to parenteral estrogen and/or androgen administration in the surgical menopause. Am J Obstet Gynecol 1985; 151:153–160.
6. Sherwin BB, Gelfand MM. The role of androgen in the maintenance of sexual functioning in oophorectomized women. Psychosom Med 1987; 49:397–409.
7. Hickok LR, Toomey C, Speroff L. A comparison of esterified estrogens with and without methyltestosterone: effects on endometrial histology and serum lipoproteins in postmenopausal women. Obstet Gynecol 1993; 82:919–924.
8. Nachtigall LE, Raju U, Banerjee S et al. Serum estradiol-binding profiles in postmenopausal women undergoing three common estrogen replacement therapies: associations with sex hormone-binding globulin, estradiol, and estrone levels. Menopause 2000; 7:243–250.
9. Simon J, Klaiber E, Wiita B et al. Differential effects of estrogen-androgen and estrogen-only therapy on vasomotor symptoms, gonadotropin secretion, and endogenous androgen bioavailability in postmenopausal women. Menopause 1999; 6:138–146.
10. Arlt W, Callies F, van Vlijmen JC et al. Dehydroepiandrosterone replacement in women with adrenal insufficiency. N Engl J Med 1999; 341: 1013–1020.
11. Parasrampuria J, Schwartz K, Petesch R. Quality control of dehydroepiandrosterone dietary supplement products. JAMA 1998; 280:1565.
12. Phillips E, Bauman C. Safety surveillance of esterified estrogens-methyltestosterone (Estratest and Estratest HS) replacement therapy in the United States. Clin Ther 1997; 19:1070–1084.
13. Phillips EH, Ryan S, Ferrari R, Green C. Estratest and Estratest HS (esterified estrogens and methyltestosterone) therapy: a summary of safety surveillance data, January 1989 to August 2002. Clin Ther 2003; 25:3027–3043.
14. Zmuda JM, Cauley JA, Kriska A et al. Longitudinal relation between endogenous testosterone and cardiovascular disease risk factors in middle-aged men. A 13–year follow-up of former Multiple Risk Factor Intervention Trial participants. Am J Epidemiol 1997; 146:609–617.
15. Kabakci G, Yildirir A, Can I et al. Relationship between endogenous sex hormone levels, lipoproteins and coronary atherosclerosis in men

undergoing coronary angiography. Cardiology 1999; 92:221–225.

16. Gyllenborg J, Rasmussen SL, Borch-Johnsen K et al. Cardiovascular risk factors in men: The role of gonadal steroids and sex hormone-binding globulin. Metabolism 2001; 50:882–888.

17. English KM, Steeds RP, Jones TH et al. Low-dose transdermal testosterone therapy improves angina threshold in men with chronic stable angina: a randomized, double-blind, placebo-controlled study. Circulation 2000; 102:1906–1911.

18. Webb CM, McNeill JG, Hayward CS et al. Effects of testosterone on coronary vasomotor regulation in men with coronary heart disease. Circulation 1999; 100:1690–1696.

19. English KM, Mandour O, Steeds RP et al. Men with coronary artery disease have lower levels of androgens than men with normal coronary angiograms. Eur Heart J 2000; 21:890–894.

20. Hak AE, Witteman JC, de Jong FH et al. Low levels of endogenous androgens increase the risk of atherosclerosis in elderly men: the Rotterdam study. J Clin Endocrinol Metab 2002; 87:3632–3639.

21. Hajjar RR, Kaiser FE, Morley JE. Outcomes of long-term testosterone replacement in older hypogonadal males: a retrospective analysis. J Clin Endocrinol Metab 1997; 82:3793–3796.

22. Worboys S, Kotsopoulos D, Teede H et al. Evidence that parenteral testosterone therapy may improve endothelium-dependent and independent vaso-dilation in postmenopausal women already receiving estrogen. J Clin Endocrinol Metab 2001; 86: 158–161.

23. Taylor AE. Polycystic ovary syndrome. Endocrinol Metab Clin North Am 1998; 27:877–902, ix.

24. Johannes CB, Stellato RK, Feldman HA et al. Relation of dehydroepiandrosterone and dehydro-epiandrosterone sulfate with cardiovascular disease risk factors in women: longitudinal results from the Massachusetts Women's Health Study. J Clin Epidemiol 1999; 52:95–103.

25. Bernini GP, Moretti A, Sgro M et al. Influence of endogenous androgens on carotid wall in post-menopausal women. Menopause 2001; 8:43–50.

26. Burger HG, Hailes J, Menelaus M et al. The management of persistent menopausal symptoms with oestradiol-testosterone implants: clinical, lipid and hormonal results. Maturitas 1984; 6:351–358.

27. Sherwin BB, Gelfand MM, Schucher R, Gabor J. Postmenopausal estrogen and androgen replacement and lipoprotein lipid concentrations. Am J Obstet Gynecol 1987; 156:414–419.

28. Raisz LG, Wiita B, Artis A et al. Comparison of the effects of estrogen alone and estrogen plus androgen on biochemical markers of bone formation and resorption in postmenopausal women. J Clin Endocrinol Metab 1996; 81:37–43.

29. Gruber DM, Sator MO, Kirchengast S et al. Effect of percutaneous androgen replacement therapy on body composition and body weight in post-menopausal women. Maturitas 1998; 29:253–259.

30. Davis SR, Walker KZ, Strauss BJ. Effects of estradiol with and without testosterone on body composition and relationships with lipids in postmenopausal women. Menopause 2000; 7:395–401.

31. Floter A, Nathorst-Boos J, Carlstrom K, von Schoultz B. Serum lipids in oophorectomized women during estrogen and testosterone replacement therapy. Maturitas 2004; 47:123–129.

32. Lobo RA, Rosen RC, Yang HM et al. Comparative effects of oral esterified estrogens with and without methyltestosterone on endocrine profiles and dimensions of sexual function in postmenopausal women with hypoactive sexual desire. Fertil Steril 2003; 79:1341–1352.

33. Miller K, Corcoran C, Armstrong C et al. Transdermal testosterone administration in women with acquired immunodeficiency syndrome wasting: a pilot study. J Clin Endocrinol Metab 1998; 83: 2717–2725.

34. Shifren JL, Braunstein GD, Simon JA et al. Trans-dermal testosterone treatment in women with impaired sexual function after oophorectomy. N Engl J Med 2000; 343:682–688.

35. Lovejoy JC, Bray GA, Bourgeois MO et al. Exogenous androgens influence body composition and regional body fat distribution in obese post-menopausal women – a clinical research center study. J Clin Endocrinol Metab 1996; 81:2198–2203.

36. Basaria S, Nguyen T, Rosenson RS, Dobs AS. Effect of methyl testosterone administration on plasma viscosity in postmenopausal women. Clin Endocrinol (Oxford) 2002; 57:209–214.

37. Buckler HM, McElhone K, Durrington PN et al. The effects of low-dose testosterone treatment on lipid metabolism, clotting factors and ultrasonographic ovarian morphology in women. Clin Endocrinol (Oxford) 1998; 49:173–178.

38. Watts NB, Notelovitz M, Timmons MC et al. Comparison of oral estrogens and estrogens plus androgen on bone mineral density, menopausal symptoms, and lipid-lipoprotein profiles in surgical menopause. Obstet Gynecol 1995; 85:529–537.

39. Barrett-Connor E, Young R, Notelovitz M et al. A two-year, double-blind comparison of estrogen-androgen and conjugated estrogens in surgically menopausal women. Effects on bone mineral density, symptoms and lipid profiles. J Reprod Med 1999; 44:1012–1020.

40. Basaria S, Dobs AS. Safety and adverse effects of androgens: how to counsel patients. Mayo Clin Proc 2004; 79(4 Suppl):S25–S32.

41. Gotto AM, Jr. Triglyceride as a risk factor for coronary artery disease. Am J Cardiol 1998; 82:22Q–25Q.

42. Katz S, Morales AJ. Dehydroepiandrosterone (DHEA) and DHEA-sulfate (DS) as therapeutic options in menopause. Semin Reprod Endocrinol 1998; 16:161–170.

43. Morales AJ, Nolan JJ, Nelson JC, Yen SS. Effects of replacement dose of dehydroepiandrosterone in men and women of advancing age. J Clin Endocrinol Metab 1994; 78:1360–1367.

44. Barnhart KT, Freeman E, Grisso JA et al. The effect of dehydroepiandrosterone supplementation to symptomatic perimenopausal women on serum endocrine profiles, lipid parameters, and health-related quality of life. J Clin Endocrinol Metab 1999; 84:3896–3902.

45. Diamond P, Cusan L, Gomez JL et al. Metabolic effects of 12-month percutaneous dehydroepiandrosterone replacement therapy in postmenopausal women. J Endocrinol 1996; 150(Suppl):S43–S50.

46. Notelovitz M. Hot flashes and androgens: a biological rationale for clinical practice. Mayo Clin Proc 2004; 79(4 Suppl):S8–S13.

47. Sarrel PM, Wiita B. Vasodilator effects of estrogen are not diminished by androgen in postmenopausal women. Fertil Steril 1997; 68:1125–1127.

48. Anderson RA, Ludlam CA, Wu FC. Haemostatic effects of supraphysiological levels of testosterone in normal men. Thromb Haemost 1995; 74:693–697.

49. Kim YC. Testosterone supplementation in the aging male. Int J Impot Res 1999; 11:343–352.

50. Viallard JF, Marit G, Mercie P et al. Polycythaemia as a complication of transdermal testosterone therapy. Br J Haematol 2000; 110:237–238.

51. Basaria S, Dobs AS. Hypogonadism and androgen replacement therapy in elderly men. Am J Med 2001; 110:563–572.

52. Moore E, Wisniewski A, Dobs A. Endocrine treatment of transsexual people: a review of treatment regimens, outcomes, and adverse effects. J Clin Endocrinol Metab 2003; 88:3467–3473.

53. Dobs AS, Meikle AW, Arver S et al. Pharmacokinetics, efficacy, and safety of a permeation-enhanced testosterone transdermal system in comparison with bi-weekly injections of testosterone enanthate for the treatment of hypogonadal men. J Clin Endocrinol Metab 1999; 84:3469–3478.

54. Singh AB, Hsia S, Alaupovic P et al. The effects of varying doses of T on insulin sensitivity, plasma lipids, apolipoproteins, and C-reactive protein in healthy young men. J Clin Endocrinol Metab 2002; 87:136–143.

55. Simon JA. Safety of estrogen/androgen regimens. J Reprod Med 2001; 46(3 Suppl):281–290.

56. Urman B, Pride SM, Yuen BH. Elevated serum testosterone, hirsutism, and virilism associated with combined androgen-estrogen hormone replacement therapy. Obstet Gynecol 1991; 77:595–598.

57. Howe RS, Chow RP, Stevens CL. Use of flutamide for self-induced androgen excess. A case report. J Reprod Med 1994; 39:838–840.

58. Boulet MJ, Oddens BJ. Female voice changes around and after the menopause – an initial investigation. Maturitas 1996; 23:15–21.

59. Abitbol J, Abitbol P, Abitbol B. Sex hormones and the female voice. J Voice 1999; 13:424–446.

60. Lindholm P, Vilkman E, Raudaskoski T et al. The effect of postmenopause and postmenopausal HRT on measured voice values and vocal symptoms. Maturitas 1997; 28:47–53.

61. Gerritsma EJ, Brocaar MP, Hakkesteegt MM, Birkenhager JC. Virilization of the voice in post-menopausal women due to the anabolic steroid nandrolone decanoate (Decadurabolin). The effects of medication for one year. Clin Otolaryngol 1994; 19:79–84.

62. Gelfand MM, Wiita B. Androgen and estrogen-androgen hormone replacement therapy: a review of the safety literature, 1941 to 1996. Clin Ther 1997; 19:383–404; Discussion 367–368.

63. Chesnut CH, 3rd, Ivey JL, Gruber HE et al. Stanozolol in postmenopausal osteoporosis: therapeutic efficacy and possible mechanisms of action. Metabolism 1983; 32:571–580.

64. Westaby D, Ogle SJ, Paradinas FJ et al. Liver damage from long-term methyltestosterone. Lancet 1977; 2:262–263.

65. Ettinger B, Fireman B. Estrogen-androgen hepatotoxicity? Am J Obstet Gynecol 1998; 178:627–628.

66. Sarrel P, Dobay B, Wiita B. Estrogen and estrogen-androgen replacement in postmenopausal women dissatisfied with estrogen-only therapy. Sexual behavior and neuroendocrine responses. J Reprod Med 1998; 43:847–856.

67. Gitlin N, Korner P, Yang HM. Liver function in postmenopausal women on estrogen-androgen hormone replacement therapy: a meta-analysis of eight clinical trials. Menopause 1999; 6:216–224.

68. Slayden SM. Risks of menopausal androgen supplementation. Semin Reprod Endocrinol 1998; 16:145–152.

69. Futterweit W, Deligdisch L. Histopathological effects of exogenously administered testosterone in 19 female to male transsexuals. J Clin Endocrinol Metab 1986; 62:16–21.

70. Cardozo L, Gibb DM, Tuck SM et al. The effects of subcutaneous hormone implants during climacteric. Maturitas 1984; 5:177–184.

71. Zhou J, Ng S, Adesanya-Famuiya O et al. Testosterone inhibits estrogen-induced mammary epithelial proliferation and suppresses estrogen receptor expression. Faseb J 2000; 14:1725–1730.

72. Hall RE, Aspinall JO, Horsfall DJ et al. Expression of the androgen receptor and an androgen-responsive

protein, apolipoprotein D, in human breast cancer. Br J Cancer 1996; 74:1175–1180.

73. Park JJ, Irvine RA, Buchanan G et al. Breast cancer susceptibility gene 1 (BRCAI) is a coactivator of the androgen receptor. Cancer Res 2000; 60:5946–5949.

74. Lobaccaro JM, Lumbroso S, Belon C et al. Male breast cancer and the androgen receptor gene. Nat Genet 1993; 5:109–110.

75. Labrie F, Luu-The V, Labrie C et al. Endocrine and intracrine sources of androgens in women: inhibition of breast cancer and other roles of androgens and their precursor dehydroepiandrosterone. Endocr Rev 2003; 24:152–182.

76. Somboonporn W, Davis SR. Testosterone effects on the breast: implications for testosterone therapy for women. Endocr Rev 2004; 25:374–388.

77. Ando S, De Amicis F, Rago V et al. Breast cancer: from estrogen to androgen receptor. Mol Cell Endocrinol 2002; 193:121–128.

78. Birrell SN, Roder DM, Horsfall DJ et al. Medroxy-progesterone acetate therapy in advanced breast cancer: the predictive value of androgen receptor expression. J Clin Oncol 1995; 13:1572–1577.

79. Birrell SN, Bentel JM, Hickey TE et al. Androgens induce divergent proliferative responses in human breast cancer cell lines. J Steroid Biochem Mol Biol 1995; 52:459–467.

80. Ortmann J, Prifti S, Bohlmann MK et al. Testos-terone and 5 alpha-dihydrotestosterone inhibit in vitro growth of human breast cancer cell lines. Gynecol Endocrinol 2002; 16:113–120.

81. Xie B, Tsao SW, Wong YC. Sex hormone-induced mammary carcinogenesis in the female Noble rats: expression of bcl-2 and bax in hormonal mammary carcinogenesis. Breast Cancer Res Treat 2000; 61:45–57.

82. Yu H, Giai M, Diamandis EP et al. Prostate-specific antigen is a new favorable prognostic indicator for women with breast cancer. Cancer Res 1995; 55:2104–2110.

83. Magklara A, Grass L, Diamandis EP. Differential steroid hormone regulation of human glandular kallikrein (hK2) and prostate-specific antigen (PSA) in breast cancer cell lines. Breast Cancer Res Treat 2000; 59:263–270.

84. Secreto G, Toniolo P, Berrino F et al. Serum and urinary androgens and risk of breast cancer in postmenopausal women. Cancer Res 1991; 51:2572–2576.

85. Wysowski DK, Comstock GW, Helsing KJ, Lau HL. Sex hormone levels in serum in relation to the development of breast cancer. Am J Epidemiol 1987; 125:791–799.

86. Dorgan JF, Longcope C, Stephenson HE, Jr et al. Relation of prediagnostic serum estrogen and andro-gen levels to breast cancer risk. Cancer Epidemiol Biomarkers Prev 1996; 5:533–539.

87. Berrino F, Muti P, Micheli A et al. Serum sex hormone levels after menopause and subsequent breast cancer. J Natl Cancer Inst 1996; 88:291–296.

88. Secreto G, Toniolo P, Berrino F et al. Increased androgenic activity and breast cancer risk in pre-menopausal women. Cancer Res 1984; 44(12 Pt 1):5902–5905.

89. Lee SH, Kim SO, Kwon SW, Chung BC. Androgen imbalance in premenopausal women with benign breast disease and breast cancer. Clin Biochem 1999; 32:375–380.

90. Thomas BS, Bulbrook RD, Hayward JL, Millis RR. Urinary androgen metabolites and recurrence rates in early breast cancer. Eur J Cancer Clin Oncol 1982; 18:447–451.

91. Thomas DB, Jimenez LM, McTiernan A et al. Breast cancer in men: risk factors with hormonal implications. Am J Epidemiol 1992; 135:734–748.

92. Lipworth L, Adami HO, Trichopoulos D et al. Serum steroid hormone levels, sex hormone-binding globulin, and body mass index in the etiology of postmenopausal breast cancer. Epidemiology 1996; 7:96–100.

93. Helzlsouer KJ, Alberg AJ, Bush TL et al. A prospective study of endogenous hormones and breast cancer. Cancer Detect Prev 1994; 18:79–85.

94. Garland CF, Friedlander NJ, Barrett-Connor E, Khaw KT. Sex hormones and postmenopausal breast cancer: a prospective study in an adult community. Am J Epidemiol 1992; 135:1220–1230.

95. Dimitrakakis C, Zhou J, Bondy CA. Androgens and mammary growth and neoplasia. Fertil Steril 2002; 77(Suppl 4):S26–S33.

96. Cauley JA, Lucas FL, Kuller LH et al. Elevated serum estradiol and testosterone concentrations are associated with a high risk for breast cancer. Study of Osteoporotic Fractures Research Group. Ann Intern Med 1999; 130(4 Pt 1):270–277.

97. Zeleniuch-Jacquotte A, Bruning PF, Bonfrer JM et al. Relation of serum levels of testosterone and dehy-droepiandrosterone sulfate to risk of breast cancer in postmenopausal women. Am J Epidemiol 1997; 145:1030–1038.

98. Hill P, Garbaczewski L, Kasumi F. Plasma testos-terone and breast cancer. Eur J Cancer Clin Oncol 1985; 21:1265–1266.

99. Ballerini P, Oriana S, Duca P et al. Urinary testos-terone as a marker of risk of recurrence in opera-ble breast cancer. Breast Cancer Res Treat 1993; 26:1–6.

100. Secreto G, Toniolo P, Pisani P et al. Androgens and breast cancer in premenopausal women. Cancer Res 1989; 49:471–476.

101. Recchione C, Venturelli E, Manzari A et al. Testosterone, dihydrotestosterone and oestradiol levels in postmenopausal breast cancer tissues. J Steroid Biochem Mol Biol 1995; 52:541–546.

102. Bryan RM, Mercer RJ, Bennett RC et al. Androgen receptors in breast cancer. Cancer 1984; 54: 2436–2440.

103. Yu H, Shu XO, Shi R et al. Plasma sex steroid hormones and breast cancer risk in Chinese women. Int J Cancer 2003; 105:92–97.

104. Thomas HV, Key TJ, Allen DS et al. A prospective study of endogenous serum hormone concentrations and breast cancer risk in premenopausal women on the island of Guernsey. Br J Cancer 1997; 75:1075–1079.

105. Coulam CB, Annegers JF, Kranz JS. Chronic anovulation syndrome and associated neoplasia. Obstet Gynecol 1983; 61:403–407.

106. Anderson KE, Sellers TA, Chen PL et al. Association of Stein-Leventhal syndrome with the incidence of postmenopausal breast carcinoma in a large prospective study of women in Iowa. Cancer 1997; 79:494–499.

107. Gammon MD, Thompson WD. Polycystic ovaries and the risk of breast cancer. Am J Epidemiol 1991; 134:818–824.

108. Dimitrakakis C, Jones R, Liu A, Bondy C. Breast cancer incidence in Australian women using testosterone in addition to estrogen replacement. In: Program of 85th Annual Meeting of the Endocrine Society, Philadelphia, 2003: 574(Abstract P3–424).

109. Puy L, MacLusky NJ, Becker L et al. Immunocytochemical detection of androgen receptor in human temporal cortex characterization and application of polyclonal androgen receptor antibodies in frozen and paraffin-embedded tissues. J Steroid Biochem Mol Biol 1995; 55:197–209.

110. Hammond J, Le Q, Goodyer C, Gelfand M et al. Testosterone-mediated neuroprotection through the androgen receptor in human primary neurons. J Neurochem 2001; 77:1319–1326.

111. Bagatell CJ, Heiman JR, Matsumoto AM et al. Metabolic and behavioral effects of high-dose, exogenous testosterone in healthy men. J Clin Endocrinol Metab 1994; 79:561–567.

112. Sherwin BB, Gelfand MM. Sex steroids and affect in the surgical menopause: a double-blind, crossover study. Psychoneuroendocrinology 1985; 10: 325–335.

113. Cutolo M, Wilder RL. Different roles for androgens and estrogens in the susceptibility to autoimmune rheumatic diseases. Rheum Dis Clin North Am 2000; 26:825–839.

114. Cutolo M, Balleari E, Giusti M et al. Androgen replacement therapy in male patients with rheumatoid arthritis. Arthritis Rheum 1991; 34:1–5.

115. Olsen NJ, Kovacs WJ. Case report: testosterone treatment of systemic lupus erythematosus in a patient with Klinefelter's syndrome. Am J Med Sci 1995; 310:158–160.

116. D'Agostino P, Milano S, Barbera C et al. Sex hormones modulate inflammatory mediators produced by macrophages. Ann N Y Acad Sci 1999; 876:426–429.

117. Li ZG, Danis VA, Brooks PM. Effect of gonadal steroids on the production of IL-1 and IL-6 by blood mononuclear cells in vitro. Clin Exp Rheumatol 1993; 11:157–162.

118. Hofbauer LC, Ten RM, Khosla S. The anti-androgen hydroxyflutamide and androgens inhibit interleukin-6 production by an androgen-responsive human osteoblastic cell line. J Bone Miner Res 1999; 14: 1330–1337.

119. Hatakeyama H, Nishizawa M, Nakagawa A et al. Testosterone inhibits tumor necrosis factor-alpha-induced vascular cell adhesion molecule-1 expression in human aortic endothelial cells. FEBS Lett 2002; 530:129–132.

120. Malkin CJ, Pugh PJ, Jones RD et al. The effect of testosterone replacement on endogenous inflammatory cytokines and lipid profiles in hypogonadal men. J Clin Endocrinol Metab 2004; 89:3313–3318.

121. Rhoden EL, Morgentaler A. Risks of testosterone-replacement therapy and recommendations for monitoring. N Engl J Med 2004; 350:482–492.

122. Goumenou AG, Chow C, Taylor A, Magos A. Endometriosis arising during estrogen and testosterone treatment 17 years after abdominal hysterectomy: a case report. Maturitas 2003; 46:239–241.

123. Schneider BK, Pickett CK, Zwillich CW et al. Influence of testosterone on breathing during sleep. J Appl Physiol 1986; 61:618–623.

124. Matsumoto AM, Sandblom RE, Schoene RB et al. Testosterone replacement in hypogonadal men: effects on obstructive sleep apnoea, respiratory drives, and sleep. Clin Endocrinol (Oxford) 1985; 22:713–721.

125. Dobs AS, Nguyen T, Pace C, Roberts CP. Differential effects of oral estrogen versus oral estrogen-androgen replacement therapy on body composition in postmenopausal women. J Clin Endocrinol Metab 2002; 87:1509–1516.

126. Davis SR, Burger HG. The role of androgen therapy. Best Pract Res Clin Endocrinol Metab 2003; 17:165–175.

127. Ferriman D, Gallwey JD. Clinical assessment of body hair growth in women. J Clin Endocrinol Metab 1961; 21:1440–1447.

128. Braunstein GD. Androgen insufficiency in women: summary of critical issues. Fertil Steril 2002; 77 (Suppl 4):S94–S99.

129. Hulley S, Grady D, Bush T et al. Randomized trial of estrogen plus progestin for secondary prevention of coronary heart disease in postmenopausal women. Heart and Estrogen/progestin Replacement Study (HERS) Research Group. JAMA 1998; 280:605–613.

130. Rossouw JE, Anderson GL, Prentice RL et al. Risks and benefits of estrogen plus progestin in healthy postmenopausal women: principal results from

the Women's Health Initiative randomized controlled trial. JAMA 2002; 288:321–333.

131. Anderson GL, Limacher M, Assaf AR et al. Effects of conjugated equine estrogen in postmenopausal women with hysterectomy: the Women's Health Initiative randomized controlled trial. JAMA 2004; 291:1701–1712.

132. Espeland MA, Rapp SR, Shumaker SA et al. Conjugated equine estrogens and global cognitive function in postmenopausal women: Women's Health Initiative Memory Study. JAMA 2004; 291:2959–2968.

133. Shumaker SA, Legault C, Kuller L et al. Conjugated equine estrogens and incidence of probable dementia and mild cognitive impairment in postmenopausal women: Women's Health Initiative Memory Study. JAMA 2004; 291:2947–2958.

134. Slater CC, Souter I, Zhang C et al. Pharmacokinetics of testosterone after percutaneous gel or buccal administration. Fertil Steril 2001; 76:32–37.

Chapter 14

An introduction to androgen decline in aging males

Maurita H Carrejo, John W Culberson, and Robert S Tan

Summary

Loss of libido, erectile dysfunction, fatigue, and depression are not uncommon among male patients above 50 years of age. These symptoms may be the first clinical manifestations of an age-related decline in androgen levels, which may have begun as much as 10 years earlier. This state of lowered androgen levels is currently referred to as androgen decline in aging males (ADAM). This chapter will discuss the history of the concept of ADAM as well as the term 'andropause'; review the role of androgens in normal male physiology; examine the diagnostic difficulties of the physiologic phenomenon of ADAM; analyze the details of laboratory evaluation; explore the effects of androgen deficiency in various systems within the aging male; and consider the management of ADAM.

ADAM and Andropause

The aging process in males leads to the physiological lowering of androgens, including testosterone. This biochemical and physiological state is currently referred to as androgen decline in aging males (ADAM). It has also been referred to as androgen deficiency in aging males, partial androgen deficiency in aging males (PADAM) and andropause. In some ways it does parallel the changes in the aging female during menopause and the postmenopause period. The main distinctions lie in the fact that ADAM does not imply infertility, the process in males is usually more gradual and it does not lead to a complete deficit of hormone. ADAM may best be defined as follows:

- The decline in androgens is gradual and does not result in an absolute absence of hormone. The word *deficiency* implies a lack of sufficiency, whereas *decline* connotes a change in value, but without any judgment as to how much is 'necessary' or normal. As such, the terms ADAM or PADAM may be most appropriate at this point in our understanding of androgens in the aging male.[1]

- Because of age-related variation in other biochemicals that bind androgens, the amount of androgen physiologically available in the older male declines more rapidly than total androgen.[2] In addition to the decline in androgens and biologically available androgens, there may also be insensitivity to androgens in target organs.[3] As a result, reliance on total serum testosterone levels to define ADAM is problematic.

- This biochemical state of androgen deficiency can be symptomatic or asymptomatic.[4] Symptoms may include decreased feeling of well-being, reduced energy levels, and diminished sexual function.

- Potential long-term effects of hypogonadism include osteoporosis, muscle atrophy, and cognitive changes.

- Other illness and normal aging may obscure the effect of declining androgen levels on the patent's overall health.

An early example of research in androgen deficiency

In 1889, at the age of 72, a distinguished French physician named Charles Édouard Brown-Séquard reported in *The Lancet* that he had experienced significant improvement in several aspects of his wellbeing following self-injection of extracts from the testes of dog and guinea pig. His observations were as follows:

> *The day after the first subcutaneous injection, and still more after the two succeeding ones, a radical change took place in me... I had regained at least all the strength I possessed a good many years ago... My limbs, tested with a dynamometer, for a week before my trial and during the month following the first injection, showed a decided gain of strength... I have had a greater improvement with regard to the expulsion of fecal matters than in any other function... With regard to the facility of intellectual labour, which had diminished within the last few years, a return to my previous ordinary condition became quite manifest.*[5]

These observations spurred a movement on several continents, which came to be known as organotherapy. However, the work was refuted in a 2002 paper which reported that the amount of testosterone that would have been extracted from dog testes by the aqueous technique reported in *The Lancet* would likely have been four orders of magnitude less than what would be appropriate for testosterone replacement therapy in hypogonadal men. The authors therefore attribute the claims of Brown-Séquard to the placebo effect, and assert that this remains a challenge in testosterone therapy today.[6]

Androgens

Androgens are a group of hormones, which include testosterone, dehydroepiandrosterone (DHEA), and androstenedione, among others. Although the androgens are sometimes referred to as the 'male hormones', this is a bit of a misnomer, as these hormones are present in females as well, though at lower levels.

In a healthy man, approximately 95% of the androgens present are accounted for by testosterone produced in the testes (Figure 14.1). Luteinizing hormone (LH) is secreted by the pituitary gland, which regulates the conversion of cholesterol to testosterone in the Leydig cells. Testosterone, in turn, is metabolized to dihydrotestosterone (DHT) by 5α-reductase and undergoes aromatization to estradiol by aromatase. Dihydrotestosterone has been linked to prostate hypertrophy and male alopecia.[7] The balance of the androgen is mainly in the form of DHEA produced by the adrenal glands.

Ninety-eight percent of circulating testosterone is bound to plasma proteins, with only 2% defined as free testosterone. About 40% of the bound testosterone is bound to sex hormone binding globulin (SHBG). The remainder is weakly bound to albumin and is readily available to tissue when needed. *Bioavailable testosterone* includes free testosterone and testosterone that is loosely bound to albumin.[8]

Total testosterone levels decline in men between the ages of 40 and 70 years, falling at the rate of about 1–2% per year. Simultaneously, the level of SHBG increases by 1–2% per year. The net result is that the amount of testosterone that is physiologically available decreases by about 3% per year.[9] On the basis of total testosterone measurements alone, 20% of men older would be defined as hypogonadal.[10,11] However, when the level of testosterone physiologically available is considered, the figure rises to 50%.[2]

Spermatogenesis is primarily regulated by the effect of LH on the Leydig cells in the testes. Testosterone has only a minor effect on sperm production. As such, ADAM may not affect male fertility, although the number of sperm with normal motility and morphology may be altered.[12] In contrast, the ultimate result of menopause is total termination of function of the ovaries and complete loss of reproductive capability. This difference aside, the long-term deprivation of sex hormones in men and women can have similar results, including effects on muscle, bone, and cognition.

Diagnostic challenges in ADAM

In our study involving 302 men (most older than 60 years),[4] the dominant symptoms of ADAM

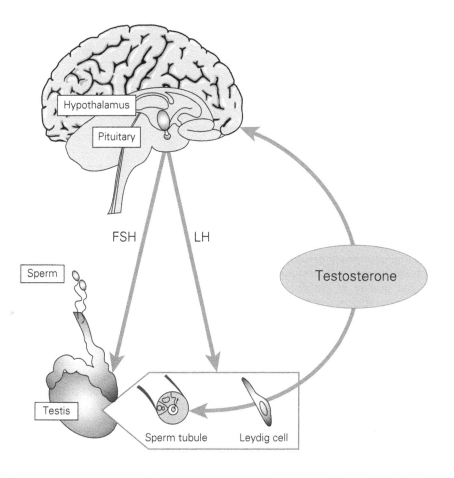

Figure 14.1

The pituitary gland secretes luteinizing hormone (LH) and follicle stimulating hormone (FSH). The LH stimulates the Leydig cells to produce testosterone. Testosterone has minimal effect on sperm production.

were loss of libido and erectile dysfunction (46%), fatigue (41%), and memory loss (36%). The correlation of symptoms to levels of testosterone is highly variable and is the subject of our ongoing investigation on relative hypogonadism.[13] At this time, the following will provide a guideline for diagnosing ADAM in routine practice:

- History and physical examination are the most important diagnostic tools. Some specific domains to be measured upon physical examination are listed in Table 14.1.
- Laboratory testing can sometimes be misleading due to numerous potential confounding factors including age, levels of albumin and SHBG and the pulsatile and diurnal nature of androgen production.
- Concomitant illnesses such as clinical depression, personality disorders, mild cognitive impairment, hypothyroidism or fibromyalgia can confound the diagnosis.
- Other confounders can include obesity, poor nutrition, stress, alcohol use, smoking, circadian rhythm, and medications.

The Androgen Deficiency in Aging Males (ADAM) questionnaire is probably the most widely used instrument to screen for hypogonadism. The ADAM questionnaire has been found to be quite sensitive, however, it is relatively nonspecific,

Table 14.1 Examination for androgen decline in aging males

Anthropometry	Exam	History
• Weight • Body mass index (BMI) • Waist/hip ratio • Body fat[14]	• Spider telangiectasia on the skin • Hair loss on the face, axilla or groin • Testicle size • Spine (for evidence of osteoporosis) • Prostate examination • Peripheral pulse • Breast development	• ADAM questionnaire for androgen deficiency • Aging Males' Symptoms (AMS) Scale • Geriatric Depression Scale • Mini-Mental State Examination • Medication History • Smoking history[4,13]

sometimes detecting clinical depression or hypothyroidism rather than androgen deficiency.[15]

The Aging Males' Symptom (AMS) scale has become commonly employed in many countries. This instrument was designed to measure health-related quality of life changes before and after androgen replacement therapy. It has been shown to have a high predictive value for the results of other scales, which only screen for androgen deficiency, while at the same time offering the ability to assess symptoms of aging more broadly.[16,17]

It is extremely important to exclude any reversible pathology that may be causing the symptoms of androgen deficiency. The number and nature of confounders may make it difficult to distinguish androgen decline from other changes of aging. If ADAM is suspected or confirmed, education is an important component of management. An understanding by patients of the process, and the perception that it is not being dismissed, along with patient-motivated lifestyle changes, may be of more value than medical treatment, especially in patients who are not significantly bothered by the symptoms.

Laboratory measurements

Most laboratories measure three categories of testosterone: total testosterone (T), free testosterone (FT), and bioavailable testosterone (BT).

- *Total testosterone* refers to all measurable testosterone, including both bound and unbound portions. Testosterone circulates in plasma and binds to SHBG and albumin. Testosterone bound to transcortin and orosomucoid is negligible. Changes in protein concentrations can alter total testosterone levels.

- *Free testosterone* represents only a small percentage of total testosterone, and may be misleading in that loosely-bound testosterone can also be biologically active.

- Testosterone is strongly bound to SHBG and loosely bound to albumin. Hence *bioavailable testosterone* is the sum of free testosterone plus that bound to albumin. Conversely, it can be viewed as total testosterone minus that bound to SHBG. In older men, the binding of testosterone to SHBG is increased, making it less likely for it to be released to become FT. In older patients, one often finds normal levels of total testosterone, with BT significantly depressed. As such, total testosterone in older men is much less reliable, and BT is the assay of choice.[18] BT is calculated as the fraction of serum testosterone not precipitated by 50% ammonium sulfate (BT). Unfortunately, most laboratories charge more for this test because it is more difficult to perform.

Free testosterone may be an appropriate middle ground between cost and utility. It has been generally agreed that FT gives a better measure of androgenicity than total testosterone.[19] The clinician should be aware of the different methods of obtaining an FT level to interpret the results correctly.

- AFTC – apparent FT; measured by equilibrium dialysis
- FT – calculated FT; total testosterone minus immunoassayed SHBG
- FAI – free androgen index; 100T/immunoassayed SHBG
- aFT – analog-free testosterone; immunoassay of free testosterone with a labeled testosterone analog.

AFTC, that is testosterone determined by equilibrium dialysis, is arguably the method of choice for measuring FT in vitro. Vermeulen et al.[18] determined the correlation of AFTC with other accepted clinical measures of testosterone. They found the correlation coefficient was 0.987 with calculated FT, 0.937 with immunoassayed free testosterone (aFT), and 0.848 with FAI. Calculated FT, therefore, approaches the accuracy of measuring testosterone by dialysis. Conditions that alter SHBG may alter the results of not only total testosterone but also FT. Conditions such as obesity, hypothyroidism and acromegaly can lead to lowered levels of SHBG, and as such confound the results of FT. Otherwise, calculated FT may be a practical means for the clinician to measure FT, as it is less time-consuming and expensive than measuring testosterone by equilibrium dialysis (AFTC).

Laboratory assessment of testosterone is also complicated by the pulsatile release and the diurnal cycle of androgens. The burst-like release of testosterone throughout the day is mediated by LH; decreases in LH levels have been shown to attenuate secretion of testosterone more in older men than in younger men.[20] Furthermore, in healthy young men, secretion of testosterone is at its maximum in the early hours of the morning, with several smaller peaks and troughs throughout the day. In older men, the circadian nature of testosterone levels is attenuated, such that late day levels may be similar to those of younger men, but early morning levels and 24-h levels are generally lower in elderly men.[21] In addition to quantification of androgens, laboratory assessment for ADAM should include at least the following to help rule out reversible causes of observed symptoms and abnormal androgen levels: serum chemistry, fasting cholesterol, and thyroid function. It cannot be reiterated too often that laboratory measures should be only one component of diagnosis and management decisions for androgen deficiency.

Consequences of androgen deficiency in aging males

Testosterone affects multiple systems in the body. As a first step toward determining when treatment may be appropriate, we review here the effects of androgen deficiency, with emphasis on the aging male.

Cognition

It is now thought that testosterone effects the brain both directly and indirectly through its aromatization to estradiol. The following findings support a direct role of androgens in cognition:

- Researchers have found many different types of androgen receptor in the brain.[22]
- Testosterone has been shown to increase intercellular communication between neurons.[23]
- Testosterone can have nongenomic effects on serotonin, dopamine, acetylcholine, and calcium signaling.[24]
- It has been demonstrated in rat models that testosterone decreases tau protein by preventing its hyperphosphorylation.[25,26] Tau protein is the precursor of amyloid tissue, the pathologic lesion often seen in brains of patients with Alzheimer disease.

The effect of testosterone on brain function appears to be domain specific, with improved performance seen in visual spatial tests as demonstrated by Janowsky et al.[27] The authors examined whether testosterone plays a maintenance role in behavior in addition to its established function in brain development. Verbal and visual memory, spatial cognition, motor speed, cognitive flexibility, and mood were assessed using a double blind design in a group of healthy older men who were given supplements with testosterone for 3 months. The increase in testosterone levels to 150% of baseline levels resulted in a significant enhancement of spatial cognition, but no change in any other cognitive domain. Testosterone supplementation influenced the endogenous production of estradiol, and estradiol was found to have an inverse relation to spatial cognitive performance. These results suggest that testosterone supplementation can modify spatial cognition in older men; however, it is possible that this occurs through testosterone's influence on estrogen.

Several clinical trials have demonstrated a positive effect of testosterone supplementation on cognition, although other studies have failed to demonstrate a significant cognitive change.[2,28–30] This could be due to different sample sizes and the use of less than optimal neuropsychological tests. In a placebo controlled pilot trial, we studied the effect of testosterone on cognitive function in ten hypogonadal patients with Alzheimer disease. Altogether 36 male patients with Alzheimer disease were screened; 10 were deemed hypogonadal as defined by a laboratory value of ≤250 ng/dl. Five subjects received testosterone enanthate (intramuscular (IM); 200 mg every 2 weeks), and five subjects received a placebo. The study subjects had monthly assessments of their testosterone, blood counts, prostate specific antigen (PSA) as well as cognitive measurements including the ADASCog and the Mini-Mental State Examination. Follow-up at 9 months failed to show a significant improvement in cognition.[28]

Sexuality

Male sexuality may be broken down into three areas: libido, erectile function, and fertility. Each of these domains depends on androgens but none does so exclusively. Any one of these areas may be impaired without the others being affected.[31] Libido is generally a central event, dependent on brain function. In contrast, erectile function is primarily a local event, relying largely on vascular function in the penis. Erectile dysfunction can sometimes result from psychologic issues including stress, and thus may have a central component.

The effect of testosterone on libido can be a result of its action on receptors in the brain as well as receptors in the penis. Studies have revealed that many, but not all, men experience improvement in libido with testosterone replacement. In a study by Hajjar et al. self-assessment of libido was dramatically improved in the testosterone-treated group ($P < 0.0001$); however, approximately a third of the subjects discontinued therapy.[32]

Testosterone may help with erectile dysfunction through its vasodilator effects. In animal models, testosterone has been shown to regulate nitrous oxide in penile cavernosal smooth muscle.[33] The clinical significance of this work is unclear. In a human study by Carani et al. nocturnal penile tumescence (NPT) and erectile response to visual erotic stimuli (VES) were measured by means of a Rigiscan device in nine hypogonadal men. This was repeated after 3 months of androgen replacement. The same assessments were carried out once in 12 eugonadal controls. The number of satisfactory NPT responses, in terms of both circumference increase and rigidity, was less in the hypogonadal men than the controls and was significantly increased by androgen replacement, confirming the results of earlier studies. In terms of circumference increase, erectile response to VES did not differ between the hypogonadal men and the controls, and did not increase with androgen replacement. In terms of rigidity, the erectile response to VES did not differ between hypogonadal men and controls. However, in terms of both duration and maximum level of rigidity, there was a significant increase following androgen replacement in the hypogonadal men.[34] A meta-analysis of testosterone supplementation for erectile dysfunction considered 16 studies that had investigated this question and which had clear measures of erectile response. The meta-analysis found an improvement in erectile function compared to placebo, with even greater effect in those with primary testicular failure and in those using transdermal delivery systems.[35]

Heart disease

Supraphysiologic doses of testosterone have been found to decrease high-density lipoprotein (HDL) levels in young body-builders.[36] Studies in older males have found no such correlation and show only modest or no change in HDL.[30,37–39] Epidemiological studies reveal a proportional relation between serum testosterone and HDL, with high levels of testosterone correlated to high levels of HDL.[40] Potential confounding factors include the relationship between exercise, diet, and HDL.

In a study on older men, Kenny et al. demonstrated that transdermal testosterone decreased HDL, but not vascular reactivity.[41] Sixty-seven men (mean age 76 ± 4 years, range 65–87) with BT levels below 4.44 nmol/L (lower limit for adult normal range) were randomized to receive transdermal testosterone (2–2.5 mg patches/day) or placebo patches for 1 year. Twenty-three men (34%) withdrew from the study. In this study, while total cholesterol, triglyceride, and low-density lipoprotein (LDL) cholesterol levels did not significantly change during the year of therapy, HDL levels ($P = 0.004$) and, specifically, HDL(2) subfraction ($P = 0.02$) decreased in men receiving testosterone supplementation. Vascular tone was measured by brachial artery reactivity in 36 men. Endothelium-dependent brachial artery reactivity did not change from baseline measurements in men receiving transdermal testosterone (0.3 ± 6.7–$1.6\pm4.6\%$; $P=0.58$) or in the placebo group (3.2 ± 5.5–$0.7\pm5.5\%$; $P=0.23$).

Contrary to previous beliefs, several studies have also demonstrated improvement in coronary blood flow after testosterone administration.[42–45] Webb et al. studied 13 men (age 61 ± 11 years) with coronary artery disease. They underwent measurement of coronary artery diameter and blood flow after a 3-min intracoronary infusion of vehicle control (ethanol) followed by 2-min intracoronary infusions of acetylcholine (10^{-7} to 10^{-5} mol/L) until peak velocity response. A dose–response curve to 3-min infusions of testosterone (10^{-7} to 10^{-5} mol/L) was then determined, and the acetylcholine infusions were repeated. Finally, an intracoronary bolus of isosorbide dinitrate ($1000\,\mu g$) was given. Coronary blood flow was calculated from measurements of blood flow velocity using intracoronary Doppler and coronary artery diameter using quantitative coronary angiography. Testosterone significantly increased coronary artery diameter compared with baseline (2.78 ± 0.74 vs. 2.86 ± 0.72 mm ($P=0.05$), 2.8 ± 0.71 mm ($P=0.038$), and 2.90 ± 0.75 mm ($P=0.005$) for baseline vs. testosterone 10^{-9} to 10^{-7} mol/L, respectively). As such, short-term intracoronary administration of testosterone, at physiological concentrations, induces coronary artery dilatation and increases coronary blood flow in men with established coronary artery disease.[44]

In conclusion, it is widely held at this time that testosterone supplementation may not be harmful to the cardiovascular system in aging males. Although there are data suggesting vasodilatory properties of testosterone, there are no trials so far to demonstrate that testosterone can indeed reduce myocardial infarction rates.

Obesity

Obesity has been increasing for all age groups and in most parts of the world. In the USA, the prevalence of obesity in older males (age 65–74) increased from 13.2 to 31.9 between 1980 and 2002.[46] Obesity is associated with hypogonadism as well as diabetes, insulin resistance and increased leptin levels. Adipose tissue can compound the hypogonadal state as it contains an abundance of the aromatase enzyme. It is believed that aromatase converts testosterone to estradiol.[47] Severe obesity also adversely influences the hypothalamic–pituitary–testicular axis.

Association does not prove causality, and as such, intervention studies may help in understanding the relationship between obesity and hypogonadism. Several investigators have reported improvement in lean body mass and decrease in fat with testosterone therapy.[2,38,39,48] For example, Snyder et al.[38] randomized 108 men over 65 years of age to wearing either a testosterone patch or a placebo patch in a double blind study for 36 months. They measured body composition by dual energy X-ray absorptiometry (DEXA) and muscle strength by dynamometer before and during treatment. Ninety-six men completed the entire 36-month protocol. Fat mass decreased (-3.0 ± 0.5 kg) in the testosterone-treated men during the 36 months of treatment, which was significantly different ($P=0.001$) from the decrease (-0.7 ± 0.5 kg) in the placebo-treated men. Lean mass increased (1.9 ± 0.3 kg) in the testosterone treated men, which was significantly different ($P<0.001$) from that (0.2 ± 0.2 kg) in the placebo-treated men. The decrease in fat mass in the testosterone-treated men was principally in the arms (-0.7 ± 0.1 kg; $P<0.001$ compared with the placebo group) and legs (-1.1 ± 0.2 kg; $P<0.001$), and the increase in lean mass was principally in the trunk (1.9 ± 0.3 kg; $P<0.001$). The change in strength of knee extension and flexion at 60 and 180°, however, was not significantly different between the two groups. They concluded that increasing the serum testosterone concentrations of normal men over 65 years of age to the midnormal range for young men decreased fat mass, principally in the arms and legs, and increased lean mass, principally in the trunk, but did not increase the strength of knee extension and flexion.[38]

Muscle mass and strength

A decrease in muscle mass would be expected to lead to loss of muscle strength.[49,50] Muscle fiber loss and selective atrophy of type II fibers results in a substantial decrease in muscle strength in men above 70 years. Muscle loss can lead to functionality loss, especially with elderly men. Most blinded and well controlled studies of testosterone replacement in older men have demonstrated an increase in body mass using computed tomography (CT) and DEXA scans.[2,37,38,51,52] Changes in measurable muscle strength have been more variable. There may be several explanations for the lack of consistency in clinical trials reporting measurable gains in muscle strength. Some studies have used relatively insensitive methods (e.g. stair walking) and significant variation in methods used to quantify strength. Different dosages and duration of treatments also created additional variability.

Of course, the actual outcome of interest is improved functionality. Bakshi et al. demonstrated that lean mass improved with a combination of testosterone and rehabilitation versus placebo and rehabilitation, and that the instrument of functional measure improved from 70.7 to 93.6 as compared with the placebo group which went from 73.7 to 78.0. This study also demonstrated that grip strength improved with testosterone from 25.08 kg to 31.16 kg ($P = 0.03$).[53]

Falls in geriatric patients are a major event, and have significant impact in the patient and the healthcare system. The most common cause of preventable falls in the elderly is muscle wasting.[54] As such, it would also be interesting to investigate whether testosterone replacement may indeed decrease falls in older males.

Interestingly, testosterone replacement has also been shown to benefit the wasting syndrome in AIDS patients.[55] This work may have implications in treating the frailty syndrome associated with the very elderly. In AIDS, endocrine hypofunction is secondary to the well known effects of severe illness. HIV-infected patients are in a catabolic state and adaptive mechanisms, which normally decrease energy expenditure and preserve lean body mass are either overridden or not operative. Strategies to reverse the catabolic state have been successfully demonstrated with anabolic hormones such as testosterone.

Bone

There is clear evidence for bone loss in both females and males with aging. Fracture rates in men lag behind women, but become comparable when men reach their eighties. Epidemiological studies have found that bone mineral density (BMD) is positively correlated to BT and estradiol.[56,57] Although bioavailable estradiol appears to be a better overall predictor of bone density, it cannot be disputed that there are androgen receptors found in osteoblasts and mesenchymal cells.[58] The effect of testosterone on bone is both a direct effect as well as through aromatization to estradiol. Most short-term studies have found that androgens reduce bone resorption rather than affecting the formation of new bone. In a study by Kenny et al.[52] 76 men (mean age 76 ± 4 years, range 65–87) with BT levels below 4.44 nmol/L (lower limit for adult normal range) were randomized to receive transdermal testosterone or placebo patches for 1 year. Outcome measures included sex hormones (testosterone, BT, SHBG, estradiol, and estrone), BMD (femoral neck, Ward triangle, trochanter, lumbar spine, and total body), bone turnover markers, lower extremity muscle strength, percent body fat, lean body mass, hemoglobin, hematocrit, prostate symptoms, and prostrate-specific antigen (PSA) levels.

Forty-four men completed the trial. In these men, BT levels increased from 3.2 ± 1.2 (SD) to 5.6 ± 3.5 nmol/L ($P < 0.002$) at 12 months in the testosterone group, whereas no change occurred in the control group. Although there was no change in estradiol levels in either group, estrone levels increased in the testosterone group (103 ± 26 to 117 ± 33 pmol/L; $P < 0.017$). The testosterone group had a 0.3% gain in femoral neck BMD, whereas the control group lost 1.6% over 12 months ($P = 0.015$). No significant changes were seen in markers of bone turnover in either group. No significant differences between the groups were seen in hemoglobin, hematocrit, symptoms or signs of benign prostate hyperplasia, or PSA levels. The investigators concluded that transdermal testosterone (5 mg/day) prevented bone loss at the femoral neck, in a group of healthy men over age 65 with low BT levels.[52] It is, therefore, possible that testosterone therapy can prevent fractures by increasing both bone and muscle strength, which in turn can prevent falls.

Other investigators have failed to find such improvements, and the effect of testosterone on bone remains somewhat controversial. An interesting concept was developed by Christmas et al.[59] in a study of the combined administration of testosterone and growth hormone. In andropausal men, testosterone administration to achieve physiologic levels did not result in significant effects on bone metabolism or BMD, whereas growth hormone plus testosterone (GH+T) increased one marker of bone formation and decreased one marker of bone resorption. Given the known biphasic actions of GH on bone and the apparent favorable biochemical effects of GH+T in men, the longer-term effects of GH+T on BMD in aged men remain to be clarified.[59]

In summary, there is evidence that testosterone may have biologic benefits on bone, but there are no long-term studies yet on whether testosterone replacement may actually decrease fracture rates in men.

Prostate

There is general agreement that testosterone administration does not cause prostate cancer.[60] This statement is based on clinical trials demonstrating insignificant rises in PSA over 3–5-year periods.[3738] It also appears that prostate cancer tends to develop in older men when endogenous testosterone is lowest.

There are several studies on effects of testosterone on other aspects of prostate health. For example, in a preliminary study, Kenny et al. they observed that after 9 weeks of treatment, there were no ill effects on prostate size, symptoms or PSA.[61] The objective of the study was to determine whether short-term testosterone administration to older men with low BT would have any immediate adverse effects, especially on the symptoms of benign prostate hyperplasia, preliminary to embarking on a long-term study of testosterone treatment. The non-randomized trial consisted of a 9-week intervention with either intramuscular testosterone, transdermal testosterone or neither, followed by a 9-week observation period. Twenty-seven men over age 70 with no medical conditions known to affect bone turnover, and total testosterone below 350 ng/dL or BT below 128 ng/dL received either testosterone via transdermal patch (TP; two 2.5 mg patches/day), intramuscular testosterone enanthate (IM; 200 mg every 3 weeks) or no testosterone for 9 weeks of treatment, followed by a 9-week observation period. Nine men were enrolled in each group. The mean age of the men was 74±3 years (range 70–83 years). While all men receiving testosterone treatment increased levels above their own baseline, only six of nine men receiving transdermal testosterone achieved BT

levels in the normal range for young men. Neither treatment group demonstrated changes in estradiol levels. No side effects were reported using the intramuscular testosterone while 5/9 men using transdermal testosterone developed a rash. There were no ill effects on prostate size, symptoms or PSA level. The results of this study were similar to others in that most studies have been over a short term and have found no correlation to prostate changes.[3738,62] Long-term data beyond 5 years are not yet available.

PSA may not be sensitive enough to pick up microscopic prostate cancer. Prostate cancer incidence increases as a function of age. At age 70, at least 50% of males may have microscopic cancer, but only 5–10% will actually develop clinical cancer, and the role of prostate biopsy remains controversial in some parts of the world. Some men with normal PSA and rectal examinations may have prostate cancer that would be detectable by biopsy.[63] It is important to discuss these points with patients before contemplating testosterone replacement therapy. There are doubtless benefits of testosterone replacement therapy for older males, but truly informed consent is mandatory. The following is the recommended prostate screening program for men on testosterone replacement therapy:[64]

- PSA and digital examination on initial visit and every 3 months
- If PSA is above 4.0 ng/dL, prostate biopsy prior to testosterone replacement
- Testosterone replacement is contraindicated if there is a history of prostate cancer
- If PSA rises more than 1.5 ng/dL over 3–6 months, repeat PSA, followed by prostate biopsy

Other domains of androgen activity

Erythrocytosis, sleep apnea, breast, fertility and health-related quality of life

Although prostate cancer is the most feared complication of testosterone replacement therapy, the most common side effect is a clinically insignificant increase in hematocrit.[3748] For this reason, testosterone replacement therapy is contraindicated in individuals with hematocrit of 52% and above. A rise of 3–5% may be expected with testosterone replacement. The effect is less with a transdermal system.[65]

It has been reported that testosterone administration can cause sleep apnea in younger males.[66,67] This is likely due to a direct effect on the laryngeal muscles. It is very infrequent in older males. Sleep apnea is a relative contraindication for testosterone replacement therapy.

Testosterone can rarely cause breast enlargement. Gynecomastia is due to estradiol, which is converted from testosterone. This can be minimized with aromatase inhibitors such as flavones and zinc. There have been rare reports of breast cancer with testosterone. This is more frequent in patients with the Klinefelter syndrome.

Testosterone administration can suppress the hypothalamic–pituitary axis, and as such inhibit LH and FSH. The possibility of sterility must be discussed with older patients prior to instituting treatment. The concept of using hormonal suppression of spermatogenesis as a method of reversible male contraception was investigated by Anderson and colleagues; they reported that the administration of testosterone to healthy adult men, aged 21–41, caused complete suppression of spermatogenesis to azoospermia in only 55% of their population. This was an undesirable finding in terms of a contraception study, but certainly a fact that should be thoroughly discussed with any patient considering testosterone therapy for androgen deficiency, who might wish to retain the option of fatherhood.[68]

Reddy et al. assessed the effect of short-term testosterone supplementation on health-related quality of life (HRQOL) in elderly males in a small study. As part of a double blind, placebo controlled study, healthy males <65 years were randomized to receive a total of four doses of 200 mg testosterone enanthanate (n = 14) or placebo (n = 8) intramuscularly every 2 weeks. HRQOL was assessed using the Short Form 36-item (SF-36) and Psychological General Well-Being (PGWB) scales, at baseline, week 8, and during therapy withdrawal at 6 weeks after the last dose. The pilot study suggests that intramuscular testosterone, administered at a dose of 200 mg every 2 weeks, does not affect the HRQOL in elderly males.[69]

Management of ADAM

Armed with the above information regarding the effects of testosterone and testosterone deficiency on the aging male, the clinician and patient may begin to consider testosterone replacement therapy, as well as other options, for the management of ADAM. We leave the thorough discussion of that topic for elsewhere in this book, but we do offer the following thoughts.

Most information related to the benefits of testosterone therapy has been garnered from studies in younger hypogonadal patients and animal models; however, there is increasing information from small trials in older men.[61] There is agreement among investigators that testosterone therapy in hypogonadal males, which brings testosterone levels into what would be considered the normal range, improves body composition and certain domains of brain function. Potential risks include erythrocytosis, edema, gynecomastia, prostate stimulation, and suppression of sperm production. The possibility of increased risk of clinically significant prostate cancer and cardiovascular disease with testosterone replacement therapy has been thoroughly investigated.[66]

It is estimated that approximately 5000–10 000 men need be randomized and treated for 5–7 years to assess for long-term safety and develop general recommendations on the use of testosterone therapy.[62] Currently, the following guidelines seem prudent:

- Testosterone therapy should be individualized.
- There should be a detailed discussion of the benefits and risks, and informed consent should be obtained.
- Patients should be monitored with PSA and hematocrit measurements.
- Lifestyle modifications, including exercise, weight loss and smoking cessation should be stressed.

Concern over the growing pressure to overuse testosterone has led to the development of interim best-practice guidelines for prescribing issued by the American Association of Clinical Endocrinologists.[64]

Noting the absence of convincing evidence of efficacy, a recent report of the Institute of Medicine has recommended that further research should focus on older men (>65 years) who are most likely to benefit from androgen therapy, specifically those with characteristic symptoms and low blood testosterone.[71] The report suggests that priority should be given to short-term efficacy studies involving physiologic blood testosterone concentrations to establish definite evidence of

Table 14.2 Potential benefits and risks of testosterone replacement therapy in older males

Potential benefits	Potential risks
• Decreased cardiovascular disease	• Increased cardiovascular disease
• Decreased irritability and depression	• Stimulates growth of preexisting prostate cancer
• Improved muscle mass and strength, decreased fat	• Stimulates benign growth of the prostate
• Increased bone mineral density, decreased falls	• Causes or worsens urinary symptoms
• Improved libido	• Erythrocytosis
• Improved erectile function	• Causes or aggravates sleep apnea
• Increased energy level	• Gynecomastia
• Improved cognitive function	• Oligospermia

efficacy before longer-term efficacy and safety studies are warranted.[72]

In conclusion, decisions regarding testosterone replacement therapy in older men with androgen decline should be made on a case-by-case basis, considering the androgen levels of the patient, ADAM symptoms, overall health, goals from treatment, as well as the benefits and risks delineated in Table 14.2.

Contraindications for testosterone replacement therapy

• History of prostate cancer
• History of breast cancer
• PSA of ≥4 ng/mL at baseline
• Palpable prostate abnormality (until evaluated for cancer)
• Benign prostatic hypertrophy with severe symptoms
• Baseline hematocrit >52%
• Severe sleep apnea

Conclusion: present and future implications

Given the fact that estrogens are the most prescribed drugs in the USA for the past several years, and the graying of our society, the possible economic implications of testosterone replacement are great. Since 1993, testosterone prescriptions have increased at an annual rate of 25–30%. In 2000, following the release of a topical testosterone in the USA, there was a 67% increase. Overall, there has been a 500% increase since 1993.[70] In spite of this trend, most men with ADAM have not been treated. Another consideration is that if indicated, treatment can be for life. This expense, however, may translate into long-term gains from lower or delayed incidence of osteoporosis and falls that lead to fractures. Other 'downstream' benefits may include lower incidence of cardiac, cognitive, and chronic health problems, which could have a tremendous impact on long-term healthcare expenditures.

Prevention may be at the very core of solving health issues in the modern world. Obesity is linked to many conditions including heart problems and diabetes. Hypogonadism and quality of life may be affected by obesity. As such, weight loss would seem to be an important preventative strategy. Less body fat may mean better cardiovascular health as well as less loss of bioavailable testosterone due to aromatization to estradiol.[73]

Paradoxically, investigators have found that an extremely high protein diet without fat may actually reduce blood levels of testosterone.[74] It is postulated that fat is needed along with protein to synthesize natural testosterone in the body through conversion of the cholesterol ring structure. Good fats such as those from monosaturated fats and polyunsaturated fats may be useful. Such fats are found in nuts and fish.

The response of the body to intense anaerobic exercise such as weight lifting has been studied.[75] Researchers have found that weight lifting, rather than aerobic exercise, may increase blood testosterone. Testosterone levels peak 20 minutes after exercise and return to baseline in another 10 minutes. Several mechanisms of elevated testosterone have been postulated including hemoconcentration, decreased metabolic clearance and increased synthesis. Researchers have found that the rise in testosterone is LH independent, which suggests that the elevation in testosterone could be local at the Leydig cell level. Testosterone response to exercise has also been observed in older men.[76]

The search continues for the ideal androgen for replacement therapy. It should target bone, muscle, and the brain specifically, without undesired effects on the prostate or heart. The major goal of androgen therapy is to replace testosterone at levels as close to physiologic levels as possible. Testosterone enanthate and testosterone cipionate (150–200 mg), administered intramuscularly every 2–3 weeks have been the mainstay of testosterone therapy. A major disadvantage is the strongly fluctuating levels of plasma testosterone, which are not in the physiological range at least 50% of the time. Lower doses given more frequently (50–100 mg), administered intramuscularly every 7–10 days produce more sustained levels, but may be less practical for long-term therapy.[77] These prohormones are converted peripherally to dihydrotestosterone (DHT) and 17β-estradiol (E_2), generating supraphysiologic levels. The significance of this is unclear, however, it has been suggested that continuous or repeated supraphysiologic levels may increase the risk of prostate cancer.[78] Orally administered testosterone is almost completely inactivated by its first pass through the liver, although testosterone undecanoate, by virtue of a lipophilic sidechain, is absorbed through gastric lymphatics and has been an acceptable oral alternative in Europe for some time. Transdermal delivery systems allow for absorption directly into the systemic circulation at a controlled rate (4–6 mg testosterone/day), thus alleviating the fluctuations in levels. Transdermal scrotal patches were developed to take advantage of the highly permeable scrotal skin; however, high concentrations of 5α-reductase present in the scrotal skin leads to higher levels of DHT, a testosterone metabolite of concern regarding prostatic hyperplasia and cancer. Nonscrotal patches have been developed. However, because enhancers are needed to increase absorption, local skin irritation has been reported. Second-generation patches have reduced skin side effects. Gel preparations applied directly to nongenital skin have been shown to provide some of the same beneficial effects as injectables and patches.[79] A transbuccal (gum surface) delivery system has also recently received FDA approval.[80]

One synthetic androgen, 7α-methyl-19-nortestosterone (MENT), has been investigated for male contraception and found to not be affected by α-reductase; it may have some benefits for aging males.[81] DHT has been studied as an alternative to testosterone, as it does not undergo aromatization and may not show adverse prostate effects.[82]

A new class of compounds may eventually provide viable options for the management of ADAM. Selective estrogen receptor modulators, (SERMs), have been used for some time to treat female osteoporosis and in breast cancer therapy. Now, the search is underway for a selective androgen receptor modulators (SARM) that will act as an antagonist or weak agonists in the prostate, but act as full agonist in muscle and pituitary. The concept is that tissue-selective activation of the androgen receptor by a SARM could reduce the side effects of the antiandrogens that are currently used to treat prostate disease, as well as be used in male contraception and in the treatment of ADAM, without adverse effect on the prostate. Animal studies to date have been promising.[83,84]

In conclusion, it is anticipated that the demand for androgen replacement will continue to grow as new and safer products are available for patients and as more clinical trials document efficacy. Although many studies support the biological effects of testosterone in many organ systems, evidence-based long-term clinical effects are not yet available.

Conclusion

The physiologic decline in androgen levels with aging, particularly bioavailable testosterone, is undeniable. The extent and individual impact of the decline vary considerably. Returning testosterone levels to the normal range for young men may have beneficial effects on a number of domains, including sense of wellbeing, cognition, bone mineral density, libido and erectile function, among others. However, these benefits have generally been seen in small trials; larger and longer trials are needed to study the long-term safety and efficacy of testosterone therapy in ADAM. It is important to address other factors that may contribute to clinical manifestations, including obesity, poor nutrition, smoking, medications, and other medical conditions.

References

1. Morales A, Heaton JP, Carson CC, III. Andropause: a misnomer for a true clinical entity. J Urol 2000; 163:705–712.
2. Sih R, Morley JE, Kaiser FE et al. Testosterone replacement in older hypogonadal men: a 12-month randomized controlled trial. J Clin Endocrinol Metab 1997; 82:1661–1667.
3. Chatterjee B, Roy AK. Changes in hepatic androgen sensitivity and gene expression during aging. J Steroid Biochem Mol Biol 1990; 37:437–445.
4. Tan RS, Philip PS. Perceptions of and risk factors for andropause. Arch Androl 1999; 43:97–103.
5. Brown-Séquard CE. Note on the effects produced on man by subcutaneous injections of a liquid obtained from the testicles of animals. Lancet 1889; 2:105–107.
6. Cussons AJ, Bhagat CI, Fletcher SJ, Walsh JP. Brown-Sequard revisited: a lesson from history on the placebo effect of androgen treatment. Med J Aust 2002; 177:678–679.
7. E Nieschlag, HM Behre (Eds.). Testosterone: Action, Deficiency, Substitution, 2nd ed. 1998:58–66. Berlin: Springer-Verlag.
8. Basaria S, Dobs AS. Hypogonadism and androgen replacement therapy in elderly men. Am J Med 2001; 110:563–572.
9. Feldman HA, Longcope C, Derby CA et al. Age trends in the level of serum testosterone and other hormones in middle-aged men: longitudinal results from the Massachusetts male aging study. J Clin Endocrinol Metab 2002; 87:589–598.
10. Smith KW, Feldman HA, McKinlay JB. Construction and field validation of a self-administered screener for testosterone deficiency (hypogonadism) in ageing men. Clin Endocrinol (Oxford) 2000; 53:703–711.
11. Tenover JS. Androgen administration to aging men. Endocrinol Metab Clin North Am 1994; 23:877–892.
12. Gallardo E, Simon C, Levy M et al. Effect of age on sperm fertility potential: oocyte donation as a model. Fertil Steril 1996; 66:260–264.
13. Tan RS. Andropause: introducing the concept of 'relative hypogonadism' in aging males [Letter]. Int J Impot Res 2002; 14:319.
14. Ukkola O, Gagnon J, Rankinen T et al. Age, body mass index, race and other determinants of steroid hormone variability: the HERITAGE Family Study. Eur J Endocrinol 2001; 145:1–9.
15. Morley JE, Charlton E, Patrick E et al. Validation of a screening questionnaire for androgen deficiency in aging males. Metabolism 2000; 49:1239–1242.
16. Heinemann LA, Saad F, Heinemann K et al. Can results of the Aging Males' Symptoms (AMS) scale predict those of screening scales for androgen deficiency? Aging Male 2004; 7:211–218.
17. Heinemann LAJ, Zimmermann T, Vermeulen A et al. A New 'Aging Male's Symptoms' (AMS) Rating Scale. Aging Male 1999; 2:105–114.
18. Vermeulen A, Verdonck L, Kaufmann JM. A critical evaluation of simple methods for the estimation of free testosterone in serum. J Clin Endocrinol Metab 2001; 86:2903.
19. Nahoul K, Roger M. Age-related decline of plasma bioavailable testosterone in adult men. J Steroid Biochem 1990; 35:293–299.
20. Liu PY, Takahashi PY, Roebuck PD et al. Age-Specific changes in the regulation of LH-dependent testosterone secretion: assessing responsiveness to varying endogenous gonadotropin output in normal men. Am J Physiol Regul Integr Comp Physiol 2005; May 12; [Epub ahead of print].
21. Bremner WJ, Vitiello MV, Prinz PN. Loss of circadian rhythmicity in blood testosterone levels with aging in normal men. J Clin Endocrinol Metab 1983; 56:1278–1281.
22. Simerly RB, Chang C, Muramatsu M, Swanson LW. Distribution of androgen and estrogen receptor mRNA-containing cells in the brain: an in situ hybridization study. J Comp Neurol 1990; 294:76–95.
23. Herve J, Pluciennik F, Verrecchia F et al. Influence of molecular structure of steroids on their ability to interrupt gap junctional communication. J Membr Biol 1996; 149:179–187.
24. Tobin VA, Millar RP, Canny BJ. Testosterone acts directly at the pituitary to regulate gonadotropin-releasing hormone-induced calcium signals in male rat gonadotropes. Endocrinology 1997; 138:3314–3319.
25. Gandy S, Almeida OP, Fonte J et al. Chemical andropause and amyloid-beta peptide. JAMA 2001; 285:2195–2196.
26. Papasozomenos SC. Heat shock induces rapid dephosphorylation of tau in both female and male rats followed by hyperphosphorylation only in female rats: implications for Alzheimer's disease. J Neurochem 1996; 66:1140–1149.
27. Janowsky JS, Oviatt SK, Orwoll ES. Testosterone influences spatial cognition in older men. Behav Neurosci 1994; 108:325–332.
28. Tan RS & Pu SJ. The andropause and memory loss: is there a link between androgen decline and dementia in the aging male. Asian J Androl 2001; 3:169–174.
29. Cherrier MM, Asthana S, Plymate S et al. Testosterone supplementation improves spatial and verbal memory in healthy older men. Neurology 2001; 57:80–88.
30. Van Goozen SH, Cohen-Kettenis PT, Gooren LJ et al. Gender differences in behaviour: activating effects of cross-sex hormones. Psychoneuroendocrinology 1995; 20:343–363.

31. Kaiser FE, Viosca SP, Morley JE et al. Impotence and aging: clinical and hormonal factors. J Am Geriatr Soc 1988; 36:511–519.

32. Hajjar RR, Kaiser FE, Morley JE. Outcomes of long-term testosterone replacement in older hypogonadal males: a retrospective analysis. J Clin Endocrinol Metab 1997; 82:3793–3796.

33. Lugg JA, Rajfer J, Gonzalez-Cadavid NF. Dihydro-testosterone is the active androgen in the mainte-nance of nitric oxide-mediated penile erection in the rat. Endocrinology 1995; 136:1495–1501.

34. Carani C, Granata AR, Bancroft J, Marrama P. The effects of testosterone replacement on noctur-nal penile tumescence and rigidity and erectile response to visual erotic stimuli in hypogonadal men. Psychoendocrinology 1995; 20:743–753.

35. Jain P, Rademaker AW, McVary KT. Testosterone supplementation for erectile dysfunction: results of a meta-analysis. J Urol 2000; 164:371–375.

36. Hurley BF, Seals DR, Hagberg JM et al. High-density lipoprotein cholesterol in bodybuilders vs. power-lifters. Negative effects of androgen use. JAMA 1984; 242:507–513.

37. Tenover JS. Effects of testosterone supplementa-tion in the aging male. J Clin Endocrinol Metab 1992; 75:1092–1098.

38. Snyder PJ, Peachey H, Hannoush P et al. Effect of testosterone treatment on body composition and muscle strength in men over 65 years of age. J Clin Endocrinol Metab 1999; 84:2647–2653.

39. Morley JE, Perry HM, III, Kaiser FE et al. Effects of testosterone replacement therapy in old hypogo-nadal males: a preliminary study. J Am Geriatr Soc 1993; 41:149–152.

40. Khaw KT, Barrett-Connor E. Endogenous sex hormones, high-density lipoprotein cholesterol, and other lipoprotein fractions in men. Arterioscler Thromb 1991; 11:489–494.

41. Kenny AM, Prestwood KM, Gruman CA et al. Effects of transdermal testosterone on lipids and vascular reactivity in older men with low bioavail-able testosterone levels. J Gerontol A Biol Sci Med Sci 2002; 57:460–465.

42. Jaffe MD. Effect of testosterone cypionate on post-exercise ST segment depression. Br Heart J 1977; 39:1217–1222.

43. Rosano GM, Leonardo F, Pagnotta P et al. Acute anti-ischemic effect of testosterone in men with coro-nary artery disease. Circulation 1999; 99:1666–1670.

44. Webb CM, McNeill JG, Hayward CS et al. Effects of testosterone on coronary vasomotor regulation in men with coronary heart disease. Circulation 1999; 100:1690–1696.

45. Ong PJ, Patrizi G, Chong WC et al. Testosterone enhances flow-mediated brachial artery reactivity in men with coronary artery disease. Am J Cardiol 2000; 85:269–272.

46. Centers for Disease Control and Prevention, National Center for Health Statistics, National Health and Nutrition Examination Survey. http://www.agingstats.gov/chartbook2004/tableshealthrisks.html#Indicator%2025

47. Cohen PG. Aromatase, adiposity, aging and disease. The hypogonadal-metabolic-atherogenic-disease and aging connection. Med Hypotheses 2001; 56:702–708.

48. Wang C, Swedloff RS, Iranmanesh A et al. Trans-dermal testosterone gel improves sexual function, mood, muscle strength, and body composition parameters in hypogonadal men. Testosterone Gel Study Group. J Clin Endocrinol Metab 2000; 85:2839–2853.

49. Frontera WR, Hughes VA, Lutz KJ, Evans WJ. A cross-sectional study of muscle strength and mass in 45- to 78-year old men and women. J Appl Physiol 1991; 71:644–650.

50. Harris T. Muscle mass and strength: relation to function in population studies. J Nutr 1997; 127 (5 Suppl):1004S–1006S.

51. Marin P. Androgen treatment of abdominally obese men. Obes Res 1993; 1:245–251.

52. Kenny AM, Prestwood KM, Gruman CA et al. Effects of transdermal testosterone on bone and muscle in older men with low bioavailable testos-terone levels. J Gerontol A Biol Sci Med Sci 2001; 56:M266–M272.

53. Bakhshi V, Elliot M, Gentili A et al. Testosterone improves rehabilitation outcomes in older men. J Am Geriatr Soc 2000; 45:550–553.

54. Tan RS & Pu SJ. Testosterone replacement in andropause as restorative therapy for older home-bound males. Home Health Care Consul 2002; 9:9–13.

55. Grinspoon SK, Donovan DS, Jr, Bilezikian JP. Aetiology and pathogenesis of hormonal and metabolic disorders in HIV infection. Bailliéres Clin Endocrinol Metab 1994; 8:35–55.

56. Greendale GA, Kritz-Silverstein D, Seeman T, Barrett-Conner E. Higher basal cortisol predicts verbal memory loss in postmenopausal women. The Rancho Bernardo study. J Am Geriatr Soc 2000; 48:1655–1658.

57. Khosla S, Melton LJ, Jr, Atkinson EJ et al. Relationship of serum sex steroid levels and bone turnover markers with bone mineral density in men and women: a key role for bioavailable estrogen. J Clin Endocrinol Metab 1998; 83:2266–2274.

58. Colvard DS, Eriksen EF, Keeting PE et al. Identi-fication of androgen receptors in normal human osteoblast-like cells. Proc Natl Acad Sci USA 1989; 86:854–857.

59. Christmas C, O'Connor KG, Harman SM et al. Growth hormone and sex steroid effects on bone metabolism and bone mineral density in healthy aged women and men. J Gerontol A Biol Sci Med Sci 2002; 57:12–18.

60. Bhasin S, Woodhouse L, Casaburi R et al. Testosterone dose-response relationships in healthy young men. Am J Physiol Endocrinol Metab 2001; 281:E1172–E1181.

61. Kenny AM, Prestwood KM, Raisz LG. Short term effects of intramuscular and transdermal testosterone on bone turnover, prostate symptoms, cholesterol and hematocrit over age 70 with low testosterone levels. Endocr Res 2000; 26:153–168.

62. Bhasin S, Buckwalter JG. Testosterone supplementation in older men: a rational idea whose time has not yet come. J Androl 2001; 22:718–731.

63. Morgentaler A, Bruning CO, III, DeWolf WC. Occult prostate cancer in men with low serum testosterone levels. JAMA 1996; 276:1904–1906.

64. American Association of Clinical Endocrinologists. American Association of Clinical Endocrinologists Medical Guidelines for clinical practice for the evaluation and treatment of hypogonadism in adult male patients. Endocr Pract 2002; 8:440–456.

65. Dobs AS, Meikle AW, Arver S et al. Pharmacokinetics, efficacy, and safety of a permeation-enhanced testosterone transdermal system in comparison with bi-weekly injections of testosterone enanthate for the treatment of hypogonadal men. J Clin Endocrinol Metab 1999; 84:3469–3478.

66. Matsumoto AM. Andropause: clinical implications of the decline in serum testosterone levels with aging in men. J Gerontol A Biol Sci Med Sci 2002; 57:M76–M99.

67. Schneider BK, Pickett CK, Zwillich CW et al. Influence of testosterone on breathing during sleep. J Appl Physiol 1986; 61:618–623.

68. Anderson RA, Wu FC. Comparison between testosterone enanthate-induced azoospermia and oligozoospermia in a male contraceptive study. II. Pharmacokinetics and pharmacodynamics of once weekly administration of testosterone enanthate. J Clin Endocrinol Metab 1996; 81:896–901.

69. Reddy P, White CM, Dunn AB et al. The effect of testosterone on health-related quality of life in elderly males – a pilot study. J Clin Pharm Ther 2000; 25:421–426.

70. IMS Sales Data, IMS Health, Inc., Westport, CN, 2001.

71. CT Liverman, DG Blazer (Eds.). Testosterone and Aging: Clinical Research Directions. Institute of Medicine 2004. Washington DC: National Academies Press.

72. Handelson DJ, Liu PY. Andropause: invention, prevention, rejuvenation. Trends Endocrinol Metab 2005; 16:39–45.

73. Cohen PG. Aromatase, adiposity, aging and disease. The hypogonadal-metabolic-atherogenic disease and aging connection. Med Hypotheses 2001; 56:70–78.

74. Volek JS, Kraemer WJ, Bush JA et al. Testosterone and cortisol in relationship to dietary nutrients and resistance exercise. J Appl Physiol 1997; 82:49–54.

75. Stepto NK, Carey AL, Staudacher HM et al. Effect of short-term fat adaptation on high-intensity training. Med Sci Sports Exerc 2002; 34:449–455.

76. Kraemer WJ, Hakkinen K, Newton RU et al. Effects of heavy-resistance training on hormonal response patterns in younger vs. older men. J Appl Physiol 1999; 87:982–992.

77. Gooren LJ, Bunck MC. Androgen Replacement Therapy: present and future. Drugs 2004; 64:1861–1891.

78. Shaneyfelt T, Husein R, Bubley G, Mantzoros CS. Hormonal predictors of prostate cancer: a meta-analysis. J Clin Oncol 2000; 18:847–853.

79. Wang C, Cunningham G, Dobs A et al. Long-term testosterone gel (AndroGel) treatment maintains beneficial effects on sexual function and mood, lean and fat mass, and bone mineral density in hypogonadal men. J Clin Endocrinol Metab 2004; 89:2085–2098.

80. Korbonits M, Kipnes M, Grossman AB. Striant SR: a novel, effective and convenient testosterone therapy for male hypogonadism. Int J Clin Pract 2004; 58:1073–1080.

81. Sundaram K, Kumar N. 7alpha-methyl-19-nortestosterone (MENT): the optimal androgen for male contraception and replacement therapy. Int J Androl 2000; 23(Suppl 2):13–15.

82. Kunelius P, Lukkarinen O, Hannuksela ML et al. The effects of transdermal dihydrotestosterone in the aging male: a prospective, randomized, double blind study. J Clin Endocrinol Metab 2002; 87:1467–1472.

83. Gao W, Kearbey JD, Nair VA et al. Comparison of the pharmacological effects of a novel selective androgen receptor modulator (SARM), the 5α-reductase inhibitor finasteride, and the antiandrogen hydroxyflutamide in intact rats: new approach for benign prostate hyperplasia (BPH). Endocrinology 2004; 145:5420–5428.

84. Chen J, Hwang DJ, Bohl CE et al. A selective androgen receptor modulator for hormonal male contraception. J Pharmacol Exp Ther 2005; 312:546–553.

Index

Printed and bound by CPI Group (UK) Ltd, Croydon, CR0 4YY

23/10/2024

01777691-0003